Methods in Neurosciences

Volume 26

PCR in Neuroscience

Methods in Neurosciences

Editor-in-Chief

P. Michael Conn

Methods in Neurosciences

Volume 26
PCR in Neuroscience

Edited by
Gobinda Sarkar

Department of Orthopedic Research
Mayo Clinic
Rochester, Minnesota

ACADEMIC PRESS

San Diego   New York   Boston   London   Sydney   Tokyo   Toronto

Front cover photograph: Photograph illustrates amplification of a segment (red) of genomic DNA (green) by means of bacterial cloning (upper panel) and segments by PCR (lower panel). In the former method, the genomic DNA is converted to small segments by digestion with a restriction enzyme. The digested DNA is then ligated into a suitable vector (yellow) and inserted into bacteria followed by screening and identification of the desired bacterial clone. The desired clone can then be amplified by growing in appropriate conditions. In PCR, the genomic DNA is mixed with oligonucleotide primers (small gray bars). Then denaturation, annealing, and primer extension reactions are carried out in the presence of a heat-stable DNA polymerase by changing temperature with a thermal cycler. One cycle consists of one round of denaturation, annealing, and extension reactions. Template copies are doubled after each round, which usually takes between 3 to 10 minutes. Specific DNA synthesis after three cycles is shown in red (courtesy of Drs. Tamas Vidovszky and Gobinda Sarkar, Mayo Clinic and Foundation, Rochester, MN).

Copyright © 1995 by ACADEMIC PRESS, INC.

All Rights Reserved.
No part of this publication may be reproduced or transmitted in any form or by any means, electronic or mechanical, including photocopy, recording, or any information storage and retrieval system, without permission in writing from the publisher.

Academic Press, Inc.
A Division of Harcourt Brace & Company
525 B Street, Suite 1900, San Diego, California 92101-4495

United Kingdom Edition published by
Academic Press Limited
24-28 Oval Road, London NW1 7DX

International Standard Serial Number: 1043-9471

International Standard Book Number: 0-12-185296-2 (Hardcover)

International Standard Book Number: 0-12-619255-3 (Paperback)

PRINTED IN THE UNITED STATES OF AMERICA
95 96 97 98 99 00 EB 9 8 7 6 5 4 3 2 1

Table of Contents

Section V Application of PCR in Mutation Detection

Section VI Generation of Probes by PCR

Section VII PCR in the Context of Cloning and Constructing Libraries

Contributors to Volume 26

Article numbers are in parentheses following the names of contributors. Affiliations listed are current.

NORMAN ARNHEIM (8), Molecular Biology Section, University of Southern California, Los Angeles, California 90089

BENTLEY A. ATCHISON (26), Victorian Institute of Forensic Pathology and Department of Forensic Medicine, Monash University, Melbourne, Victoria 3205, Australia

OMAR BAGASRA (23), Division of Infectious Disease, Department of Medicine, Jefferson Medical College, Thomas Jefferson University, Philadelphia, Pennsylvania 19107

NABEEL BARDEESY (11), Department of Biochemistry, McGill University, Montreal, Québec, Canada H3G 1Y6

SAILEN BARIK (21), Department of Biochemistry and Molecular Biology, College of Medicine, University of South Alabama, Mobile, Alabama 36688

F. BARRE-SINOUSSI (24), Unité de Biologie des Retrovirus, Paris, France

MICHAEL BECKER-ANDRÉ (9), Glaxo Institute for Molecular Biology, Plan-les-Ouates, CH-1228 Geneva, Switzerland

B. S. BLUMBERG (24), Fox Chase Institute, Philadelphia, Pennsylvania 19111

MARK E. BOLANDER (3, 10), Department of Orthopedics, Mayo Clinic, Rochester, Minnesota 55905

NANCY D. BORSON (4), Department of Biochemistry and Molecular Biology, School of Medicine, University of Minnesota, Duluth Campus, Duluth, Minnesota 55812

MARK BRUDNAK (19), Faculty of Biological Science, University of Tulsa, Tulsa, Oklahoma 74104

V. BRYZ-GORNIA (25), Department of Medicine, State University of New York-Health Science Center at Syracuse, Syracuse, New York 13210

TAPAN K. CHATTERJEE (3), Department of Pharmacology, University of Iowa, Iowa City, Iowa 52242

THERESA M. CHENG (14), Department of Neurosurgery, Mayo Clinic, Rochester, Minnesota 55905

ANNETTE CHRISTOPH (27), Institute for Genetics, University of Cologne, D-50674 Cologne, Germany

ANDRÉ DARVEAU (6), Department of Biochemistry, Laval University, Ste-Foy, Québec, Canada G1V 7P4

MICHAEL DEAN (13), Laboratory of Viral Carcinogenesis, Frederick Cancer Research and Development Center, National Cancer Institute, Frederick, Maryland 21702

ANDREA M. DOUGLAS (26), Bone Marrow Research Laboratories, Royal Melbourne Hospital, Melbourne, 3050 Victoria, Australia

LESTER R. DREWES (4), Department of Biochemistry and Molecular Biology, School of Medicine, University of Minnesota, Duluth Campus, Duluth, Minnesota 55812

D. K. DUBE (24, 25), Department of Medicine, and Anatomy and Cell Biology State University of New York-Health Science Center at Syracuse, Syracuse, New York 13210

S. DUBE (24, 25), Department of Medicine, State University of New York-Health Science Center at Syracuse, Syracuse, New York 13210

L. DYSTER (24), Cellular Products, Buffalo, New York 14202

M. RAAFAT EL-GEWELY (2), Department of Biotechnology, Institute of Medical Biology, University of Troms, N-9037 Troms, Norway

S. ERENSOY (25), Department of Medicine, State University of New York-Health Science Center at Syracuse, Syracuse, New York 13210

J. F. FERRER (24), Comparative Leukemia and Retroviruses Unit, University of Pennsylvania, New Bolton Center, Pennsylvania 19348

RORY A. FISHER (3), Department of Pharmacology, University of Iowa, Iowa City, Iowa 52242

THEODOR M. FLIEDNER (5), Department of Clinical Physiology, Occupational, and Social Medicine, University of Ulm, 89070 Ulm, Germany

MICHELLE FRENCH (1), Burnet Clinical Research Unit, Walter and Elisa Hall Institute, Melbourne, Victoria 3000, Australia

Y. FURUICHI (18), Agene Research Institute, Kamakura, Kanagawa 247, Japan

VINOD GANJU (14), Department of Hematology-Oncology, Mayo Clinic, Rochester, Minnesota 55905

G. S. GETZ (12), Department of Medicine, Pathology, Biochemistry, and Molecular Biology, The University of Chicago, Chicago, Illinois 60637

J. B. GLASER (24), Staten Island University Hospital, Staten Island, New York 10305

DAMJAN GLAVAČ (13), National Institute of Chemistry, Llubljana, Slovenia

GERALD J. GLEICH (10), Department of Immunology, Mayo Clinic, Rochester, Minnesota 55905

E. HARA (18), Department of Biological Science and Technology, Science University of Tokyo, Noda, Chiba 278, Japan

W. J. HARRINGTON, JR. (24), Division of Hematology/Oncology Center for Blood Diseases, Silvester Cancer Center, Miami, Florida 33136

MICHAEL J. HELLER (28), Nanogen, San Diego, California 92121

V. M. A. HERVE (24), Institut Pasteur, Bangui, Central African Republic, Africa

GUNNAR HUSBY (2), Oslo Sanitetsforening Rheumatism Hospital, N-0172 Oslo, Norway

KRISHNA JAYARAMAN (7), Biotex Resources, Inc., The Woodlands, Texas 77380

ROBERT B. JENKINS (14), Department of Laboratory Medicine and Pathology, Mayo Clinic, Rochester, Minnesota 55905

RAJENDRA P. KANDPAL (20), Fels Institute for Cancer Research and Molecular Biology, Temple University School of Medicine, Philadelphia, Pennsylvania 19140

DAVID KOVALIC (17), Pharmacology Department, University of Wisconsin Medical School, Madison, Wisconsin 53706

M. VIJAY KUMAR (22), Department of Urology Research, Mayo Clinic, Rochester, Minnesota 55905

CHRISTA P. LAMPING (5), Department of Clinical Physiology, Occupational, and Social Medicine, University of Ulm, 89070 Ulm, Germany

SHERRY LEONARD (16), Department of Pharmacology, University of Colorado Health Sciences Center, Denver, Colorado 80262

ANDREW LEW (1), Burnet Clinical Research Unit, Walter and Elisa Hall Institute, Melbourne, Victoria 3000, Australia

J. LOVE (24), Department of Medicine, State University of New York-Health Science Center at Syracuse, Syracuse, New York 13210

PETER W. MELERA (15), Department of Biological Chemistry, School of Medicine, University of Maryland at Baltimore, Baltimore, Maryland 21201

KENTON S. MILLER (19), Faculty of Biological Science, University of Tulsa, Tulsa, Oklahoma 74104

INGE NILSEN (2), Department of Biotechnology, Institute of Medical Biology, University of Troms, N-9037 Troms, Norway

BJØRN-YNGVAR NORDVÅG (2), Department of Rheumatology, Institute of Clinical Medicine, University of Troms, N-9037 Troms, Norway

K. ODA (18), Department of Biological Science and Technology, Science University of Tokyo, Noda, Chiba 278, Japan

MICHAEL PANACCIO (1), Department of Molecular Biology, Victorian Institute of Animal Science, Attwood, Victoria 3049, Australia

L. PAPSIDERO (24), Cellular Products, Buffalo, New York 14202

B. PAUL (25), Department of Medicine, State University of New York-Health Science Center at Syracuse, Syracuse, New York 13210

ALEX PELLETIER (6), Bio-Mega and Boehringer Ingelheim Recherche, Inc., Laval, Québec, Canada H7S 2G5

JERRY PELLETIER (11), Department of Biochemistry, McGill University, Montreal, Québec, Canada H3G 1Y6

JOSÉE PERREAULT (6), Department of Biochemistry, Laval University, Québec, Canada G1V 7P4

B. J. POIESZ (24, 25), Department of Medicine, State University of New York-Health Science Center at Syracuse, Syracuse, New York 13210

ROGER J. POMERANTZ (23), Division of Infectious Disease, Department of Medicine, Jefferson Medical College, Thomas Jefferson University, Philadelphia, Pennsylvania 19107

HILDE MONICA F. RIISE (2), Department of Clinical Chemistry, Institute of Medical Biology, University of Troms, N-9037 Troms, Norway

STEVE R. RITLAND (14), Department of Medical Genetics, Mayo Clinic, Rochester, Minnesota 55905

ROBERT A. ROBINSON (28), Department of Pathology, University of Iowa, Iowa City, Iowa 52242

N. K. SAKSENA (24), Department of Medicine, State University of New York-Health Science Center at Syracuse, Syracuse, New York 13210

WILMAR L. SALO (4), Department of Biochemistry and Molecular Biology, School of Medicine, University of Minnesota, Duluth Campus, Duluth, Minnesota 55812

A. SANYAL (12), Department of Medicine, The University of Chicago, Chicago, Illinois 60637

GOBINDA SARKAR (3, 10, 14), Department of Orthopedic Research, Mayo Clinic, Rochester, Minnesota 55905

M. P. SHERMAN (24), Department of Medicine, State University of New York-Health Science Center at Syracuse, Syracuse, New York 13210

NAY WEI SOONG (8), Department of Gene Therapy, Norris Cancer Hospital, University of Southern California, Los Angeles, California 90033

C. STEPHENS (25), Department of Medicine, State University of New York-Health Science Center at Syracuse, Syracuse, New York 13210

SANJIV SUR (10), Section of Allergy and Immunology, Department of Medicine, East Carolina University School of Medicine, Greenville, North Carolina 27858

HANS-JÜRGEN THIESEN (27), Basel Institute for Immunology, CH-4005 Basel, Switzerland

STEFAN J. THOMA (5), Department of Clinical Physiology, Occupational, and Social Medicine, University of Ulm, 89070 Ulm, Germany

CHRISTIAN A. THOMAS (5), Department of Physiology and Cellular Biophysics, College of Physicians and Surgeons, Columbia University, New York, New York 10032

DONALD J. TINDALL (22), Departments of Urology Research and Biochemistry/Molecular Biology, Mayo Clinic, Rochester, Minnesota 55905

BERNARD WEISBLUM (17), Pharmacology Department, University of Wisconsin Medical School, Madison, Wisconsin 53706

SHERMAN M. WEISSMAN (20), Department of Genetics, Yale University School of Medicine, New Haven, Connecticut 06510

A. E. WILLIAMS (24), National Red Cross, Rockville, Maryland 20855

R. YANAGIHARA (24), Frederick Cancer Research Facility, Frederick, Maryland 21702

HONGHAO YANG (15), Department of Biological Chemistry, School of Medicine, University of Maryland at Baltimore, Baltimore, Maryland 21201

BENEDIKT L. ZIEGLER (5), Department of Clinical Physiology, Occupational, and Social Medicine, University of Ulm, 89070 Ulm, Germany

Preface

The polymerase chain reaction (PCR) allows amplification of a segment in a nucleic acid sequence. This amazingly simple process has changed virtually every field of biological research. For his efforts, Dr. Kary Mullis, the inventor of PCR, was awarded a Nobel prize in 1993. This reaction has transformed fiction into reality and has opened doors where none ever existed before! This "technique of the decade" is being embraced by researchers at an exponential rate, suggesting its general utility and value. So many novel methods and applications have resulted from PCR that no single book can describe and do justice to all of them.

The utility of PCR extends broadly in biological research. Therefore the title of this volume "PCR in Neuroscience" may surprise some readers. This is not to imply that neuroscientists are unaware of the general utility of PCR. It is, however, an effort to create an easily recognizable source for presenting some cardinal aspects of PCR that may help devise simpler routes to solving problems pertinent to neuroscience. Although some topics in this volume are described elsewhere, they are dealt with in this book in greater detail, with additional novel information applicable to the neurosciences. There is also information in this volume not found elsewhere that has been presented in a manner to be of value to students and teachers alike. Thus the volume will be an invaluable reference source for all PCR users.

I express my appreciation to Dr. Mark E. Bolander whose encouragement and support have been invaluable. I am also grateful to Ms. Kristy Toogood for her patient assistance in all stages of this undertaking. I am indebted to the series editor Dr. P. Michael Conn and Shirley Light of Academic Press for their help and encouragement. I thank my wife Sukla who put up with me while I was busy working on this volume when I should have been concentrating on *bona fide* domestic activities. Finally, I extend my appreciation to all the contributors for presenting their fine work, which is the essence of a volume such as this one.

GOBINDA SARKAR

Methods in Neurosciences

Section I

Direct PCR on Clinical Specimens

[1] Formamide Low-Temperature PCR: Applications for Direct PCR from Clinical Material

Michael Panaccio, Michelle French, and Andrew Lew

Introduction

Since the advent of thermostable DNA polymerases (1) the PCR technique has become one of the most important tools in the biological sciences. One of the few limitations of the PCR technique is that it can easily be inhibited by many substances (2). This is of minor consequence in a research setting where purified DNA is the starting material for most PCR reactions. However, this is a major limitation when the PCR technique is applied to diagnostic applications. As a consequence, target preparation methods are necessary when PCR is applied to clinical material. Thus, often DNA preparation methods become the rate-limiting step in applying PCR to biological specimens. A further disadvantage is that DNA preparation methods increase the cost for diagnosis as well as increasing the risk of both sample and operator contamination.

The most important source of biological material for diagnostic purposes is blood. The inhibition of PCR by blood has been reported to be due to porphyrin compounds derived from heme (2). Heparin, a commonly used anticoagulant, has also been reported to inhibit PCR amplication (3–5). Most protocols for amplifying DNA from whole blood involve lysing blood cells and removing heme products from the nuclear pellet through extensive washing of the DNA pellet (6). A potential problem with these approaches is that even small levels of contamination can lead to inhibition. In general, even samples that have enough hemoglobin to produce a slight red tinge are inhibitory. Because the amount of contamination is variable from sample to sample this makes the diagnostic use of PCR on blood samples somewhat unreliable. To overcome these problems and to enable the handling of large numbers of samples we were interested in developing a PCR protocol that was robust enough to be used directly on whole blood. This was achieved through the use of formamide low-temperature PCR.

FoLT PCR is a rapid PCR protocol that allows direct amplification of DNA from whole blood and tissues without any preparative steps, i.e., the raw material can be put directly into the tube containing the PCR mixture.

Methods in Neurosciences, Volume 26

It entails the use of 18% formamide, reduced incubation temperatures (80, 40, and 60°C) and *Thermus thermophilus* (*Tth*) DNA polymerase. We have applied this technique to amplify histocompatibility genes and enzyme genes in several species including mouse and human. Blood and solid tissues have been used successfully. In this chapter we also demonstrate its use in screening transgenic mice.

Principle of Formamide Low-Temperature PCR

Formamide low-temperature PCR was developed based on the observation that the apparent inhibition of PCR amplification was in the main not due to the presence of a classic DNA polymerase inhibitor but due to the inability of the enzyme to interact with the target DNA (6). This is presumably because the target DNA is trapped within the coagulated organic material that occurs during the first heating step of the PCR protocol. The answer was simple. PCR could be applied directly to whole blood as long as the coagulation of blood proteins could be inhibited. This could be achieved by either lowering the highest temperature of the PCR protocol (the 95°C denaturation of the double-stranded DNA) or by increasing the solubility of the blood proteins. In fact, FoLT PCR does both. It is based on the use of formamide as well as reduced incubation temperatures to reduce the amount of target entrapment that occurs by blood proteins. Formamide low-temperature PCR uses an alternative thermostable DNA polymerase, *Tth* DNA polymerase (derived from *T. thermophilus* HB8). Two intrinsic properties of *Tth* DNA polymerase make the FoLT PCR protocol possible. First, unlike *Taq* DNA polymerase, *Tth* DNA polymerase is not inhibited by the presence of porphyrin compounds or heparin. Second, *Tth* DNA polymerase can tolerate high concentrations (up to 25%, v/v) of formamide. In contrast *Taq* DNA polymerase can only tolerate 10% (v/v) formamide. Thus FoLT PCR is based on the use of a low-temperature PCR protocol that is possible by the use of 18% formamide together with *Tth* DNA polymerase.

Formamide low-temperature PCR allows direct amplification of DNA from whole blood and solid tissues without the need for any preparative steps (7, 8). As such it saves considerable time and is economical when compared with competing methodologies. Another important characteristic of the FoLT PCR protocol is that even though it is a rapid direct method it does not compromise sensitivity as compared to protocols that involve DNA purification (7).

Materials and Methods

Formamide Low-Temperature PCR

For 100 μl Reaction

1. Mix 1 μl of whole blood with 18 μl of deionized formamide and heat the sample to 95°C for 5 min to solubilize all the blood (this step increases the sensitivity of FoLT PCR by at least 10-fold).

2. Make up the reaction mix as follows (for x samples multiply all volumes by x):

10 μl 10 × PCR buffer	(100 m*M* Tris, pH 9.0 (at 25°C), 500 m*M* KCl, 15 m*M* MgCl$_2$, 0.1% gelatin, 1% Triton X-100)
10 μl dNTP stock	[2 m*M* of dATP, dCTP, dTTP, and dGTP (Pharmacia, Sweden)]
1 μl forward primer	(2 μ*M*)
1 μl reverse primer	(2 μ*M*)
57 μl H$_2$O	
1 μl *Tth* polymerase	(0.5–2.5 units, Toyobo, Japan)

3. Using a pipette add 81 μl of the reaction mix with the blood formamide mixture. Do not spin the tubes. Overlay with liquid paraffin if appropriate. Amplify for 30–40 cycles. The optimal temperatures and incubation times vary between models of PCR machines.

Technical Tips

1. As a guide, conditions for two different machines are given below.
   (a) A robotic arm Gene Machine (Innovonics, Australia) with three water baths: 80°C, 30 sec; 40°C, 30 sec; and 70°C, 30 sec.
   (b) For the Perkin–Elmer (Norwalk, CT) 9600: 80°C, 10 sec; 40°C, 10 sec; and 60°C, 10 sec.

2. Formamide low-temperature PCR reactions can be carried out in as little as 20 μl. Adjust all volumes accordingly. However, when using small volumes accurate pipetting is essential since the final percentage of formamide in the reaction mixture is critical.

3. Up to 10% (v/v) whole blood can be used in a FoLT PCR reaction. However, we have found that using more blood did not result in greater sensitivity probably because the increase in target number may be negated by the increase in organic matter.

4. After step 1, the samples can be left indefinitely at room temperature before going onto step 2. This is a good way to store samples for later analysis or for transportation.

5. For hot start PCR, a pastille of paraffin wax (BDH, Kilsyth, Vic) can be added to step 1. The wax solidifies at room temperature. After the pretreatment the other ingredients can be added on top in a separate compartment. During PCR cycling the wax melts, ascends to the top of the tube allowing the PCR reagents to be mixed.

Solid Tissues

For solid tissue samples follow the standard FoLT PCR procedure except that 1 mm^3 slices of tissue are placed in 18 μl of 100% formamide and cycled between 95°C, 10 sec and 72°C, 10 sec for 30 cycles prior to the rest of the reagents being added. Once the tissue sample has been cycled in formamide they can be left at room temperature for at least 3 months.

Primers

HLA-DO primers which corresponded to the 5′ untranslated region of the human major histocompatibility complex class II gene are 5′ TGCAGG-CAAACAATGGTTGAG 3′ and 5′ GGACCCACCCAGAACCCAT 3′. The PCR product using the HLA-DO primers is 320 bp. Primers MinstF (5′ CCTGCCTATCTTTCAGGTC 3′) MinstR (5′ TAGTTGCAGTAGTTCTC-CAG 3′) are directed against the mouse insulin gene. Primers B2MF (5′ ATACTCACGCCACCCACCGG 3′) and B2MR (5′ TTATACTACGACA-TATTAT 3′) are directed against the mouse β_2-microglobulin gene. The cathepsin primers are as follows: ICEF, 5′ ACAGCTGAGGATCCGGCTG-TACCCGACA 3′; MP1, 5′ GAATTGGTTCAATCCCA 3′; MP2, 5′ ATACT-GTCCCTCCATAG 3′; MP4, CACGAAGCGGTGAACAA 3′. The transgene used to inject mouse oocytes is a chimera of the promoter of the mouse class II gene, IE (5′ ATAGGACCTGGTTGCAAGGAACCC 3′), and the cDNA of mouse glutamate decarboxylase (5′ ATGGGCTACGCCACACCAAG-TATC 3′).

Anticoagulants

The following anticoagulants are used to collect blood from a single individual: Lithium heparin (60 USP units/10 ml, Becton–Dickinson, NJ), sodium heparin (60 USP units/10 ml, Becton–Dickinson), fluoride heparin, ammonium oxalate (6 mg/5 ml), fluoride oxalate, potassium oxalate (4 mg/5 ml), K$_3$EDTA (7.2 mg/5 ml), disodium EDTA (10.5 mg/7 ml), sodium citrate

(0.105 *M*), sodium citrate (0.129 *M*), Alsever's solution, acid–citrate–phos-phate–dextrose (ACPD), acid–citrate–dextrose (ACD) solution A, and ACD solution B.

PCR products are resolved by electrophoresis in 2% agarose.

Results

Use of Different PCR Machines

The FoLT PCR procedure was initially developed on a Innovonics PCR machine that consists of a robotic arm that carries the samples over three water baths. When the same FoLT PCR conditions were applied to the Perkin–Elmer 9600 no DNA amplification was observed. To optimize FoLT PCR conditions, FoLT PCR was performed on both the Innovonics and Perkin–Elmer 9600 PCR machines using a range of different incubation temperatures (Fig. 1). Surprisingly the amount of PCR product observed when using the Innovonics PCR machine was enhanced by dropping the first incubation temperature to 80°C and raising the synthesis temperature to 70°C. No PCR product was observed when 85, 40, and 60°C were used on the

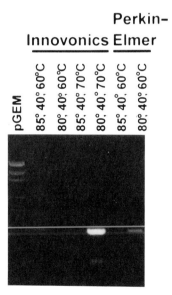

FIG. 1 Different PCR incubation temperatures for FoLT PCR for different PCR machines. The two PCR machines used were the Perkin–Elmer 9600 and the Gene Machine (Innovonics, Australia). The incubation temperatures are indicated.

Perkin–Elmer 9600 even though these conditions give consistent results when using the Innovonics PCR machine. In contrast, DNA amplification was observed by dropping the first incubation temperature by 5°C. Since different types of PCR machines differ greatly in the type of system employed for heating and cooling, it is not then surprising that the actual temperatures reached during the incubation steps vary from those set. For PCR machines that have a very accurate temperature control mechanism, like the Per-kin–Elmer 9600, 80°C is the optimal denaturation temperature. Our results suggest 85°C in 18% formamide must be at or very close to the temperature at which *Tth* DNA polymerase is denatured/inactivated.

Anticoagulants

The types of anticoagulant used in blood collections have an important effect on the quality of the DNA that is recovered from blood samples stored at room temperature, as determined by Southern analysis (9). Previously we had determined the suitability of a range of anticoagulants in FoLT PCR (10). An extension of that study is shown in Fig. 2. Human blood was collected using a range of anticoagulants and stored at room temperature for 1 year before being subjected to FoLT PCR. Ten of the fourteen anticoagulants tested gave a strong signal. The signal strength for sodium heparin, lithium heparin, and ACD solution B was markedly reduced after storage for 1 year. This is in contrast to the finding that ACD solution B is the anticoagulant of choice for Southern analysis (9). Given its low cost and availability, EDTA is the recommended anticoagulant for collecting blood to be used in FoLT PCR.

Screening Transgenic Mice

Detection of transgenic mice has traditionally involved Southern blot analysis of tail DNA. This procedure is time-consuming and requires considerable sample handling. Techniques have been developed to screen for transgenic mice using PCR of samples of DNA from blood or tails. Although these techniques are much simpler and faster compared to Southern blot analysis, they still require some degree of sample preparation (11–13). Formamide low-temperature PCR is theoretically sensitive enough to detect transgenes in blood based on the following calculations. It was previously estimated that 10 targets would be required per microliter of blood to allow for detection using FoLT PCR (7). If we assume that 1 μl of blood contains 10^4 leukocytes and that the transgene is integrated only once in 10% of the cells, then there

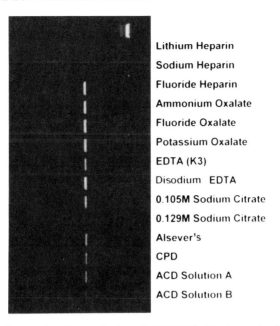

Lithium Heparin

Sodium Heparin

Fluoride Heparin

Ammonium Oxalate

Fluoride Oxalate

Potassium Oxalate

EDTA (K3)

Disodium EDTA

0.105M Sodium Citrate

0.129M Sodium Citrate

Alsever's

CPD

ACD Solution A

ACD Solution B

FIG. 2 Effect of type of anticoagulant on FoLT PCR. Photograph of a 2% agarose gel stained with ethidium bromide. Each track contains 20 μl of a 100-μl FoLT PCR reaction using the HLA-DO primers. The whole blood used (1 μl/reaction) was collected in vacutainer tubes (Becton–Dickinson) containing the anticoagulants as indicated. After being left at room temperature for 12 months, the samples were subjected to 30 cycles of 30 sec for each of the following temperatures: 85, 40, and 60°C.

would still be 100 times the number of targets required for detection of the transgene by FoLT PCR. To generate transgenic mice, NOD/Lt embryos were microinjected with DNA for glutamate decarboxylase with a heterologous promoter (an MHC class II promoter) and transferred to foster mothers. When the litters of mice were obtained, we were able to test whether FoLT PCR could indeed detect transgenic animals. Figure 3 shows the FoLT PCR screening of offspring from one of these transfers. Primers were chosen on either side of the junction between the genes for the MHC class II promoter and glutamate decarboxylase so that a PCR product of 300 bases could be amplified if the mice were carrying the transgene. Our results suggest that FoLT PCR is a rapid and simple procedure for screening transgenic mice. Although the blood samples were obtained from these mice at 21 days of age, it is conceivable, given the small amount of blood required (1 μl), that mice could be screened at a much earlier age.

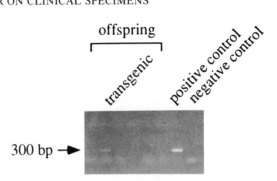

FIG. 3   Use of FoLT PCR to screen transgenic mice. Photograph of a 3% (w/v) agarose gel stained with ethidium bromide. Each tract contains 25 μl from a 100-μl FoLT PCR reaction perfomed as described under Materials and Methods. The six offspring are from NOD/Lt embryos microinjected with the transgene. Each PCR reaction contains 1 μl of blood obtained via a retroorbital bleed. The positive control contained 1 μl of blood from a normal mouse and 2 pg of the transgene used in the microinjection. No DNA was used in the negative control. Samples were subjected to 30 cycles of 60 sec for each of the following temperatures: 85, 45, and 60°C.

Solid Tissues

A variation of the standard FoLT PCR procedure can be used to amplify DNA directly from solid tissues (8). It utilizes prior cycling of 1-mm^3 slices of tissue in 100% formamide instead of heating at 95°C for 5 min. Using two different primer sets target DNA was directly amplified from a range of tissues (Figs. 4 and 5). Inconsistent results were obtained when spleen and

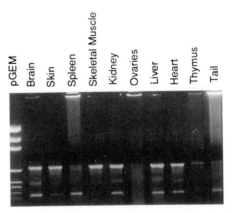

FIG. 4   Direct FoLT PCR from mouse tissue. Photograph of a 1% (w/v) agarose gel stained with ethidium bromide. The primers used are B2MF and B2MR2. The tissue used in each reaction is indicated.

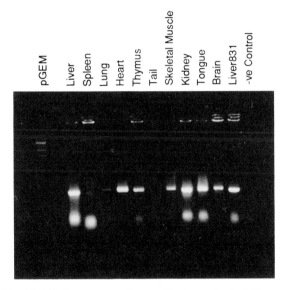

FIG. 5   Direct FoLT PCR from mouse tissue. Photograph of a 2% agarose gel stained with ethidium bromide. The primers (MinstF and MinstR) directed against the insulin gene. The tissue used in each reaction is indicated. The negative control contains no tissue.

tail were used as the source of tissue. In the case of spleen the failure to amplify the desired DNA fragment can be overcome by either adding less tissue to the reaction or by removing the tissue slice from the formamide after the precycling but before the FoLT PCR reaction is set up. It appears that too much spleen tissue in the reaction inhibits FoLT PCR. In contrast the failure to amplify sufficient PCR product from tails probably relates to the fibrous nature of this tissue.

Mapping Intron/Exon Boundaries Directly from Parasite Tissue

To illustrate the usefulness of FoLT PCR to amplify DNA directly from solid tissues, we mapped the intron–exon structure of a cathepsin gene from the trematode parasite *Fasciola hepatica* (Fig. 6). A single forward primer corresponding to the 5' terminus of the gene was used. This was used in combination with three reverse primers predicted from the cDNA sequence of a cathepsin sequence (14). The expected size fragments from each primer combination were as follows: 220, 440, and 790 bp. The PCR fragments generated using the tissue FoLT PCR protocol were the same size as predicted from a *F. hepatica* cathepsin cDNA clone indicating that the cathepsin

Reverse Primer	Expected Products
MP1	220
MP2	440
MP4	790

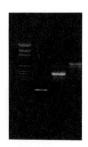

FIG. 6   Intron–exon arrangement of a cathepsin gene. Direct FoLT PCR from parasite tissue. Formamide low-temperature amplification of 1-mm³ slices of *Fasciola hepatica* tissue using the conditions described in Fig. 1. The primers (ICEF 5' ACAGCTGAGGATCCGGCTGTACCCGACA 3', MP1 5' GAATTGGTTCAATC-CCA 3', MP2 5' ATACTGTCCCTCCATAG 3', MP4 CACGAAGCGGTGAACAA 3') are designed against the cathepsin cDNA Fhcat-1 (14). The standards are the pGEM DNA markers from Promega (Madison, WI).

gene does not have any introns. The finding of no introns in trematode genes is not unusual. This experiment clearly demonstrates the generic nature of the tissue FoLT PCR protocol and its usefulness when the availability of tissue is limited.

Discussion

Formamide low-temperature PCR is a rapid PCR protocol that was designed to allow direct PCR amplification from whole blood. A slight modification of the precycling procedure allows FoLT PCR to be reproducibly applied to solid tissue samples. When using solid tissue as the source of target it is important to limit the amount of tissue that is added to the PCR tubes. In cases where inhibition is encountered, it can be overcome by removing the tissue sample after the precycling in formamide but before setting up the rest of the FoLT PCR relation. It seems that enough DNA is released from the tissue sample during precycling to allow for efficient amplification.

Formamide low-temperature PCR is not recommended for use in samples that may contain mucus. We have found mucus to be a potent inhibitor of both standard PCR and FoLT PCR. In such cases, DNA purification is recommended for consistent results.

One of the advantages of FoLT PCR is that it is suitable for use with most widely used anticoagulants. The only anticoagulants that are not recommended for routine use are lithium heparin, fluoride heparin, and sodium citrate. All three anticoagulants can be successfully used in FoLT PCR but the results obtained are somewhat variable. For example, when using fluroide heparin it is extremely important to add the correct volume of blood. Having a slightly higher concentration of fluoride heparin than that recommended will lead to inhibition presumably by binding Mg^{2+}.

Another advantage of the FoLT PCR procedure is that it is well suited for studies involving the transportation of samples. Blood samples can be collected in a large selection of anticoagulants and transported at room temperature without fear that the samples will deteriorate. We have demonstrated that blood samples stored for 1 year at room temperature are still suitable for FoLT PCR. In countries where high temperatures for a prolonged period are likely to be encountered, blood and formamide can be mixed in the appropriate ratio (1 : 18, v/v) and heated to 95°C for 10 min. The samples are then likely to be stable indefinitely. Thus the FoLT PCR procedure provides a simple method for collection, transportation, and storage of blood samples for latter analysis by PCR.

Formamide low-temperature PCR is a generic PCR platform that allows direct PCR from a variety of clinical material. As such it provides a major advantage over PCR protocols that involve DNA purification steps. We have demonstrated the use of FoLT PCR in genetic screening directly from blood samples, screening transgenic mice, and mapping intron–exon boundaries directly from solid tissues. Formamide low-temperature PCR has applications in both a research and a diagnostic setting. Any existing PCR test can be simply and rapidly converted to FoLT PCR by the addition of formamide, the use of *Tth* DNA polymerase instead of *Taq* polymerase, and the use of FoLT PCR incubation temperatures. In general the annealing temperature of any existing PCR test can be converted to the FoLT PCR format by reducing it by 10°C.

Acknowledgment

The authors acknowledge the excellent technical abilities of Michael Georgesz without whom much of this work could not have been achieved.

References

1. R. K. Saiki, D. H. Gelfand, S. Stoffel, S. J. Scharf, R. Higuchi, G. T. Horn, K. B. Mullis, and H. A. Erlich, *Science* **239,** 487 (1988).
2. R. Higuchi, *Amplifications* **2,** 1 (1989).
3. E. Beutler, T. Gelbart, and W. Kuhl, *BioTechniques* **9,** 166 (1990).

4. M. Holodniy, S. Kim, D. Katzenstein, M. Konrad, E. Groves, and T. Merigan, *J. Clin. Microbiol.* **29,** 676 (1991).
5. J.-T. Wang, T.-H. Wang, J.-C. Sheu, S.-M. Lin, J.-T. Lin, and D.-S. Chen, *J. Clin. Microbiol.* **30,** 750 (1992).
6. E. S. Kawasaki, *in* "PCR Protocols: A Guide to Methods and Applications" (M. A. Innis, D. H. Gelfand, J. J. Sninsky, and T. H. White, eds.), p. 146. Academic Press, San Diego, 1990.
7. M. Panaccio and A. Lew, *BioTechniques* **14**(2), 238 (1993).
8. M. Panaccio, M. Georgesz, C. Hollywell, and A. Lew, *Nucleic Acids Res.* **21,** 4656 (1993).
9. S. Gustafson, J. A. Proper, E. J. W. Bowie, and S. S. Sommer, *Analy. Biochem.* **175,** 294 (1987).
10. M. Panaccio and A. Lew, *in* "PCR Technology: Current Innovations" (H. G. Griffin and A. M. Griffin, eds.), CRC Press, Boca Raton, FL, 1994.
11. J. Singer-Sam, R. Tanguay, and A. D. Riggs, *Amplifications* **3,** 11 (1989).
12. D. G. Skalnik and S. Orkin. *BioTechniques* **8,** 34 (1990).
13. G. Winberg, *PCR Methods Appl.* **1,** 72 (1991).
14. G. L. Wijffels, M. Panaccio, L. Salvatore, L. Wilson, I. D. Walker, and T. W. Spithill, *Biochem. J.* **299,** 781–790 (1994).

[2] Direct Use of Blood in PCR

Bjørn-Yngvar Nordvåg, Hilde Monica F. Riise,
Gunnar Husby, Inge Nilsen, and M. Raafat El-Gewely

Introduction

The polymerase chain reaction (PCR) is a powerful technique for amplification of specific gene sequences. It has become an indispensable method in molecular biology and has dramatically facilitated diagnosis of genetic diseases and detection of genetic factors described to be involved in an increasing number of human disorders (1). Also, PCR has become an important and a most sensitive tool in the detection of infectious, pathogenic agents like human immunodeficiency virus (HIV) (2), hepatitis C virus (HCV) (3), and human cytomegalovirus (HCMV) (4), causing serious human diseases.

Blood is readily available and has always been extensively used in medical diagnostic analyses. The nuclei of white blood cells contain all the genetic information of the individual. Consequently blood is used as the main DNA source for genetic or molecular studies. Blood can also be used for early detection of foreign DNA or RNA of bacterial or viral infectious agents, frequently present in the bloodstream. Routinely DNA or RNA has been purified from blood using laborious and time-consuming methods, including the use of hazardous chemicals like phenol and chloroform (5). The numerous steps of sample treatment involved implies risks of DNA contamination, intermixing of test tubes, and risk of exposition to the analyzer of potentially infectious agents.

Different techniques have been introduced to simplify DNA isolation from blood or to facilitate target amplification by omitting DNA isolation. Such techniques include DNA extraction using denaturing and cationic detergents for lysis of the blood and precipitation of DNA (6), amplification of DNA directly from proteinase K-treated blood cell lysates and use of nonionic detergents in the PCR buffer (7), addition of protease to a small blood sample directly in the PCR buffer (8), or addition of a specific DNA binding protein (32 protein of T4 gene) and use of an alternative DNA polymerase [*Thermus thermophilus* (*Tth*) polymerase] in the PCR (9) to overcome the inhibiting effect of blood itself for the PCR reaction. Despite such methodological improvements a lot of sample handling and the use of various chemicals and/or enzyme treatments are still required.

The technique described in this chapter aims at using blood directly in PCR and minimizing sample size and manipulation, as well as the risk of contamination and exposition to health hazards. It is particularly suitable for screening of large numbers of blood samples for detection of specific DNA sequence alterations.

Amplification of DNA Directly from Blood Cells

Simple amplification of genomic and bacterial DNA using crude cell lysates (2, 10) or intact bacterial cells (11) directly in the PCR mixture have been reported. Also, using microvolumes of serum, the detection of virus RNA in a single tube reaction by reverse transcription PCR has been reported (12). Previously we have shown that DNA can easily be amplified directly from blood cells with a minimum of sample manipulation (13). Washing of the blood sample and boiling of washed cells are the only treatment steps needed prior to PCR. All this is done in a single tube, allowing rapid initiation of the reactions. As little as 2 μl blood is sufficient for successful amplifications. The results are comparable to using purified DNA in the amplifications (13). The technique speeds DNA studies and permits analyses, such as restriction enzyme digestions, Southern blotting, or sequencing of the PCR product, to be done within few hours. It provides a method for qualitative DNA studies, and has been used successfully for DNA analysis of both human and animal genome in our laboratory. A description of the technique, including possible applications and limitations, is given below. The protocol is also summarized in Table I.

The described technique was used in a molecular diagnostic study using blood samples from 100 individuals in a Danish family afflicted with lethal familial amyloid cardiomyopathy (FAC). FAC is an autosomal dominantly inherited disease releated to a specific point mutation (Met for Leu-111) in the transthyretin (TTR) protein (14). We have verified the heterozygote adenine for cytosine mutation in the first position of codon 111 in exon 4 of the TTR gene as the cause of this amino acid substitution (15). Several point muations have been detected in this protein and the majority of them have been found to be associated with different forms of inherited amyloidosis (16). Carriers of the TTR Met-111 mutation among the Danish family members were easily detected by restriction enzyme analysis of an amplified 292-bp DNA fragment, using only a few microliters of blood from the individuals (17). Also, a 299-bp DNA fragment representing exon 2 with flanking introns of the TTR gene was later amplified from the stored blood samples of the family members using this technique.

TABLE I   Protocol for Direct Use of Blood Cells in PCR Amplification of
           Genomic DNA[a]

1. Aliquot 2 μl[b] fresh or thawed, anticoagulated blood[c] into 0.5-ml sterile PCR microtubes.
2. Add 400 μl washing solution (10 mM EDTA/10 mM NaCl). Mix the tube contents and
   centrifuge at 13,000 rpm for 3 min at room temperature. Remove the supernatant by
   pipetting and repeat the washing once.[d]
3. Centrifuge 1 min (13,000 rpm at room temperature) to collect the remaining liquid and
   remove it by careful pipetting.
4. Add 50 mM Tris–HCl (pH 8.0)[e] to the washed cell pellet and place the tube in boiling
   water for 4–5 min. Centrifuge briefly.
5. Add the premade PCR cocktail mix[f] and bring the final reaction volume to 50–100 μl.
6. Perform 30–35 cycles of amplification.[g]

[a] See text for details.
[b] Larger volumes (≤100 μl) can be used if required, but samples >10 μl should be frozen before PCR manipulations.
[c] EDTA, sodium heparin or sodium citrate can be used for anticoagulation.
[d] Sample washing should be repeated twice if more than 10 μl blood is used.
[e] Use the appropriate volume for a final 50–100 μl reaction.
[f] 10× reaction buffer, dNTP's, primers, $MgCl_2$, and *Taq* DNA polymerase. See text for discussion of concentrations.
[g] Oil on the top of the reaction mixture is not required.

The blood samples are collected into EDTA-containing vacutainer tubes.
Aliquots of 1–2 ml are frozen in small plastic tubes and shipped on dry ice
for DNA analysis in our laboratory. The samples are thawed and 2 or 5 μl
blood is transferred to 0.5-ml sterile Eppendorf tubes. The subsequent washing and boiling steps are performed as described below. For DNA amplifications two sets of 25-bp primers are used. The PCR primers are

P1: 5′ GTGTGTCATCTGTCACGTTTTTCGG 3′,
P2: 5′ TCTCTGCCTGGACTTCTAACATAGC 3′,
P3: 5′ TTCGCTCCAGATTTCTAATACCACA 3′
P4: 5′ ATGTGAGCCTCTCTCTACCAAGTGA 3′

P1/P2 defines a 299-bp fragment from TTR exon 2 with flanking introns
whereas P3/P4 defines a 292-bp DNA fragment from exon 4 and flanking
region of intron 3 of the TTR gene.

   The reactions contain 1 μg of each primer, 1.5 or 2.0 mM $MgCl_2$, 200
μM of each dNTP, 1.25 or 2.5 U *Taq* DNA polymerase and reaction buffer
[final concentrations: 50 mM KCl, 10 mM Tris–HCl, pH 8.3, and 0.01%
(w/v) gelatin]. The PCR reactions are initiated by 3 min denaturation to
ensure total separation of the DNA template strands, followed by 30–35
cycles of amplification in the Perkin–Elmer Cetus (Norwalk, CT) DNA thermal cycler, using 30 sec denaturation at 94°C, 30 sec annealing at 54°C, and

1 min elongation at 72°C, expanded to 5 min elongation in the final cycle. The amplified DNA is visualized by agarose gel electrophoresis (Fig. 1) and subjected to restriction enzyme analysis (Fig. 2).

Discussion and Comments

Blood Anticoagulant

Heparin has been reported to be an inhibitor for PCR in amplifications using purified genomic or viral DNA/RNA (18, 19). We tested amplification of DNA from several blood samples anticoagulated with sodium-heparin or sodium-citrate in addition to the EDTA samples described. The inhibiting effect of heparin could not be detected. DNA was amplified in comparable

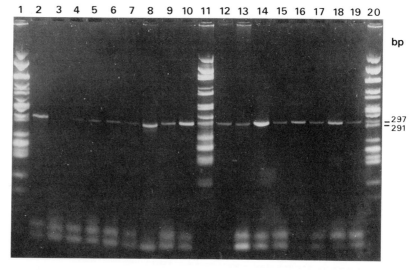

FIG. 1 Visualization of 299 and 291 bp (lane 8) TTR exon 2 and 4 DNA fragments amplified by PCR directly from DNA of washed blood cells, subsequent to electrophoresis in a 2% (w/v) low-melt agarose gel and ethidium bromide staining. A total of 10 μl was loaded in the wells. Blood sample anticoagulants and conditions for sample storage (temperature and time) for individual reactions were as presented in Table II. The reactions in lanes 16–19 contained 1.25 U/100 μl *Taq* DNA polymerase whereas 2.5 U/100 μl was used in the other samples. Final reaction volumes were 50 μl in samples represented in lanes 18 and 19. Lanes 1, 11, and 20 are 800 ng of *Hinc*II digested φX 174 DNA fragments, used as molecular weight standard.

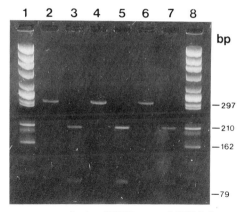

FIG. 2   Restriction enzyme analysis of TTR exon 2 DNA fragments amplified from washed blood cells. Anticoagulants used for blood sampling were EDTA (lanes 2, 3), sodium heparin (lanes 4, 5), and sodium citrate (lane 6, 7). The digestion fragments (206 and 93 bp) were visualized by 2% (w/v) low-melt agarose gel electrophoresis and ethidium bromide staining. A total of 15 μl amplified reaction mixtures was digested by 5 U *Msp*I at 37°C for 2 hr and loaded on the gel, whereas 10 μl undigested reaction mixtures were used as controls (lanes 2, 4, and 6). *Hinc*II digested ϕX 174 DNA fragments (1.2 μg) were used as molecular weight standard in lanes 1 and 8.

amounts from the blood cells irrespective of the anticoagulant chosen for sampling (Fig. 1, Table II).

Storing Conditions

Blood samples can be used in the direct PCR technique whether or not they have been previously frozen. Unfrozen blood can be stored at room temperature for several hours before aliquoting, but it is advisable to keep the samples on ice to minimize possible degradation. PCR product was obtained by amplifying DNA from blood stored at room temperature for 7 hr, but with reduced efficiency (Fig. 1, Table II). DNA could also be amplified from buffy coat samples stored at room temperature for more than 24 hr (results not shown).

Blood stored at 4°C can be used for PCR after several days (Fig. 1, Table II). Moreover, we could amplify DNA from a few SAGMAN (sodium–adenine–glucose–mannitol) erythrocyte samples stored at 4°C for 35 days in a blood bank, however, with low efficiency (results not shown).

TABLE II   Effect of Anticoagulant Used for Blood Sample Collection and Storage
Temperature and Time on PCR Amplifications[a]

Anticoagulant	Storage temperature (°C)	Storage time	PCR product	Lane number
EDTA-K	22	1 hr	+	2
EDTA-K	22	7 hr	(+)	3
EDTA-K	4	6 days	+	4
EDTA-K	−20	7 hr	+	5
EDTA-K	−20	6 days	+	6
EDTA-K	−20	3 weeks	+	7
EDTA-K	−20	4 months	+	8
EDTA-K	−20	11 months	+	9
EDTA-K	−20	15 months	+	10
EDTA-K	−20	16 months	+	16, 18
Sodium heparin	4	1 hr	+	12
Sodium heparin	−20	2 weeks	+	13
Sodium citrate	4	24 hr	+	14
Sodium citrate	−20	6 day	+	15, 17, 19

[a] Using washed blood cells. The data present results given in Fig. 1. Corresponding lane numbers in Fig. 1 are given.

We have not observed amplification problems that could be related to how long samples had been stored frozen. DNA from blood stored at −20°C for more than 1 year could be amplified without any significant loss of the product yield after thawing (Fig. 1, Table II). To ensure the highest DNA amplification yield, we recommend that blood samples not be used immediately for DNA analysis should be stored at −20 or −70°C (storage for years). The samples should first be split into smaller, sterile plastic tubes to allow quick thawing.

Use of Frozen Samples

Frozen blood samples are thawed at room temperature and placed on ice. High temperatures should be avoided to reduce possible sample degradation. Having aliquoted the desired volume for use in PCR, the thawed sample can be refrozen for possible later use.

Thawed blood samples seems to be better suited for the direct DNA amplification technique, probably because the red blood cells are completely lysed by the freezing and thawing. This improves the efficiency of the washing step (see below) and also allows DNA amplification using larger amounts of blood (10–100 μl) for the reaction (13).

Blood Volumes

Aliquots of 2 μl blood are sufficient for most PCR reactions. In healthy humans 1 μl of blood will contain about 5000 white blood cells, each containing a copy of the genome and a template for amplification. Due to potential loss of cells in the washing step (see below), a volume less than 2 μl is not recommended (Table I, step 1).

The technique might also work for detection of foreign DNA in white blood cells (like virus DNA or RNA). In such analyses larger amounts of blood may be required since the infection rate in the white cells is usually low (10^{-3}–10^{-4}) (2). A total of 100 μl of thawed blood (probably even more) can be used if extensive washing is performed (see below).

The blood is aliquoted into sterile 0.5-ml PCR tubes that are pretreated in a microwave oven at 800–1000 W for 5 min to secure sterility as well as destruction of any PCR-susceptible contamination.

Washing Step

Washing solution is added to the aliquoted blood volume which is thereby dissolved (Table I, step 2). Complete dissolution is secured by shaking the tubes using a standard rotator mixer at highest speed for a few seconds. The washing solution lyses the red cells, whereas the white cells are collected by centrifugation and kept in the tube by carefully removing the supernatant by pipetting. The small pellet will be reddish if unfrozen blood is washed, or grayish when thawed blood is used. The washing should be repeated twice if larger samples are analyzed (>10 μl) to ensure removal of all possible inhibiting factors. Subsequently, the samples should be centrifuged briefly to collect the remaining liquid from the tube walls. This is carefully removed by pipetting. Final pellet volume is approximately 1 μl.

Boiling of Washed Blood Cells

The boiling step (Table I, step 3) is essential for successful DNA amplification. Tris–HCl (50 mM) is added to the washed cells and the tubes are placed in boiling water. Approximately 75 μl Tris–HCl will be required for each sample in 100-μl reactions, depending on the concentrations of individual

PCR reactants mixed in the cocktail. The boiled samples are used directly in the PCR reaction subsequent to addition of the PCR reactants and a brief centrifugation.

Washed samples may be frozen at $-20°C$ and stored in the buffer for months before they are boiled and used for DNA amplification. In our studies, more than 90 washed samples were stored for 6–7 months before they were boiled and subjected to PCR. The efficiency observed was not significantly reduced compared to amplifications performed directly after the washing step. However, occasionally one additional DNA band was observed after electrophoresis of amplified PCR reaction mixtures when prewashed and stored cells had been used (results not shown).

PCR

The PCR cocktail mixture is prepared using amounts of reactants adjusted to give an optimal amplification yield. In addition to the specific conditions discussed above, several other variables like nucleotide and magnesium concentrations influence the PCR efficiency (Table I, step 4). In our reactions 200 μM of dNTP and 1.5 or 2.0 mM MgCl$_2$ were found to be suitable amounts (see above), but the concentrations should be optimized for different DNA amplifications. Also, the reaction parameters, particularly the annealing temperature, should be adjusted for the primer set to be used.

The primer amount can be significantly reduced compared to the amount used in our studies. In other reactions, 0.5 μg (60 pmol) of primers was successfully used (results not shown). Furthermore, 1.25 and 2.5 U Taq DNA polymerase were found equally sufficient for DNA amplifications (Fig. 1). Successful amplifications were also done using 50 μl final reaction volumes (Fig. 1), whereas no PCR product was observed in smaller volume (25 μl) (result not shown).

In our experiments, the cycling parameters were identical with those used for amplification of purified DNA in previous studies. Sufficient DNA for further analysis was amplified by 30–35 cycles in all samples. A few reactions were cycled only 25 times, still displaying visible DNA bands in the agarose gel. There is no need to overlay the reaction samples with mineral oil before the thermal cycling is started. However, if small reaction volumes are used, this may increase the PCR yield.

Generally, the PCR yield was equally good in most of the samples amplified. However, thawed blood samples tended to give higher yields than unfrozen samples (Fig. 1). In exceptional cases of no amplification, good results were obtained from another frozen aliquot.

Analysis of PCR Product

PCR products are usually visualized by ethidium bromide staining after agarose gel electrophoresis. The amplified DNA can be analyzed by restriction enzyme digestion without purification, or the product may be purified by various techniques for cloning, sequencing studies, or probing blots.

For detection of mutations in the TTR gene, we have digested the PCR products with various restriction enzymes. Irrespective of the choice of blood anticoagulant, the amplified DNA fragments were equally digestible (Fig. 2). When using 100-μl reactions, the amount of amplified DNA is sufficient for multiple digestions, sequencing reactions, or other studies.

An outline of the protocol is summarized in Table I.

Other Published Methods for Use of Blood in PCR

Reports have suggested other methods for direct use of blood in PCR. Mercier *et al.* (20) reported successful use of small aliquots of blood (1 or 2 μl) directly in 100-μl PCR reactions with no treatment other than a two-step heating incubation, repeated three times, before the PCR started. However, as little as 4 μl of blood totally inhibited the PCR reaction by this technique. This technique was not found to be reproducible by others (21). McCusker *et al.* (22) published a method by which up to 45 μl blood could be amplified directly in 100-μl PCR reactions. This could be done subsequent to mixing the sample with sterile water up to 50 μl and heating at 95°C for 15 min before adding the PCR cocktail. The PCR mixture they used contained 4 mM MgCl$_2$ and 100 μl of oil was used to overlay each reaction. We have tried this method with 2 and 10 μl blood used for PCR. DNA amplification was obtained in all samples, however, with a lower PCR yield when compared to using washed blood cells (results not shown). The amplified DNA was equally suitable for restriction enzyme digestion (results not shown). However, the samples were discolored and coagulated material remained in the tube, reducing the available volume for analysis of amplified DNA. For detection of a target DNA found mainly in serum (e.g., virus detection), this method may, however, have an advantage because it also includes serum in the PCR reaction mixture.

Another published method for direct DNA amplification from whole blood utilizes formamide low-temperature (FoLT) PCR (21). In this technique 1–10 μl blood was added to 18 μl 18% formamide and heated to 95°C for 5 min prior to PCR, using an alternative polymerase [*T. thermophilus* (*Tth*) polymerase] necessary for effective amplification. The temperature of individual PCR steps was reduced by approximately 10°C and the samples were overlaid by liquid paraffin. However, if more than 1 μl blood was used the sensitivity of the PCR was found to be significantly reduced. This method was not effective in our hands, using 2 or 10 μl blood and the more available *Taq* DNA polymerase, overlaying the reaction with mineral oil (Sigma, St. Louis, MO) instead of liquid paraffin. However, an amplification product was observed in one of eight reactions.

Conclusions

Direct use of washed and boiled blood cells in the PCR reaction is a simple and reliable method for DNA amplification. The technique offers a tool for qualitative DNA studies and is feasible for analysis of specific DNA sequences. Washed blood cells from 2 to 100 μl of blood can be used in 50 or 100 μl PCR reactions. The described technique eliminates time-consuming DNA purification with the use of toxic chemicals and enzymes for protein digestion. The samples are handled in a single tube, reducing the risk for contamination or intermixing of tubes. Exposure to health hazards is minimized, and the expenses can be kept low by optimizing the concentrations of individual reactants in the PCR.

Blood samples collected in tubes containing EDTA-K, sodium heparin, or sodium citrate are equally suitable for PCR. Unfrozen or thawed blood samples can be used and the amplifications may be done after repeated freezing and thawing of a sample. Generally, the PCR yield is better if thawed blood is used. Washed cell samples may be frozen in buffer and stored for later boiling and PCR.

Amplified DNA may be utilized in different analyses, like restriction enzyme digestion, sequencing cloning, and probe blotting. It is feasible for diagnosis of point mutations involved in hereditary diseases, genetic polymorphisms, and tissue HLA typing. Foreign DNA or RNA from virus or bacteria might also be amplified using this technique.

References

1. D. N. Cooper and J. Schmidtke, *Hum. Genet.* **92**, 211 (1993).
2. M. C. Poznansky, B. Walker, W. A. Hazeltine, J. Sodroski, and E. Langhoff, *J. Acquired Immune Defic. Syndr.* **4**, 368 (1991).
3. J. Bartolomé, I. Castillo, J. A. Quiroga, S. Navas, and V. Carreño, *J. Hepatol.* **17**, Suppl. 3, S90 (1993).
4. V. M. Ratnamohan, J. M. Mathÿs, A. McKenzie, and A. L. Cunningham, *J. Med. Virol.* **38**, 252 (1992).

5. J. Sambrook, E. F. Fritsch, and T. Maniatis, "Molecular Cloning: A Laboratory Manual," 2nd ed., Vol. 2, pp. 9.17–9.19. Cold Spring Harbor Lab., Cold Spring Harbor, NY, 1989.

6. S. Gustincich, G. Manfiolette, G. Del Sal, C. Schneider, and P. Carninci, *BioTechniques* **11,** 298 (1991).

7. M. E. Balnaves, S. Nasioulas, H.-H. M. Dahl, and S. Forrest, *Nucleic Acids Res.* **19,** 1155 (1991).

8. R. H. McHale, P. M. Stapleton, and P. L. Bergquist, *BioTechniques* **10,** 20 (1991).

9. M. Panaccio and A. Lew, *Nucleic Acids Res.* **19,** 1151 (1991).

10. R. K. Saiki, T. L. Bugawan, G. T. Horn, K. B. Mullis, and H. A. Erlich, *Nature* (*London*) **324,** 163 (1986).

11. A. K. Joshi, V. Baichwal, and G. F.-L. Ames, *BioTechniques* **10,** 42 (1991).

12. N. Ali and S. Jameel, *BioTechniques* **15,** 40 (1993).

13. B. Y. Nordvåg, G. Husby, and M. R. El-Gewely, *BioTechniques* **12,** 490 (1992).

14. M. Nordlie, K. Sletten, G. Husby, and P. J. Ranløv, *Scand. J. Immunol.* **27,** 119 (1988).

15. B. Y. Nordvåg, H. M. F. Riise, and G. Husby, *Hum. Genet.* **93,** 484 (1994).

16. M. D. Benson, *J. Med. Genet.* **28,** 73 (1991).

17. B. Y. Nordvåg, H. M. F. Riise, I. Ranløv, and G. Husby, *in* "Amyloid and Amyloidosis 1993" (R. Kisilevsky, M. D. Benson, B. Frangione, J. Gauldie, T. Muckle, and I. D. Young, eds.), Partenon Publishing, New York pp. 471–473 (1994).

18. E. Beutler, T. Gelbart, and W. Kuhl, *BioTechniques* **9,** 166 (1990).

19. M. Holodniy, S. Kim, D. Katzenstein, M. Konrad, E. Groves, and T. C. Merigan, *J. Clin. Microbiol.* **29,** 676 (1991).

20. B. Mercier, C. Gaucher, O. Feugeas, and C. Mazurier, *Nucleic Acids Res.* **18,** 5908 (1990).

21. M. Panaccio, M. Georgesz, and A. M. Lew, *BioTechniques* **14,** 238 (1993).

22. J. McCusker, M. T. Dawson, D. Noone, F. Gannon, and T. Smith, *Nucleic Acids Res.* **20,** 6747 (1992).

Section II

Application of Reverse Transcription-Mediated PCR

[3]   Use of PCR for Isolation of Neuropeptide Receptor Genes

Tapan K. Chatterjee, Gobinda Sarkar, Mark E. Bolander, and Rory A. Fisher

Introduction

The simplicity and ease by which specific DNA segments can be amplified enormously by polymerase chain reaction (PCR) provides a powerful approach for isolation of gene segments of interest. This method requires two oligonucleotides (PCR primers) complementary to sequences that lie on opposite strands of the target DNA molecule and a thermostable DNA polymerase to amplify the DNA segment exponentially between the two primers. Thus, if the sequence of two different regions of a gene is known, PCR primers can be designed with specificity for these known sequences to PCR amplify the DNA segment between these two regions.

Molecular cloning of various neurotransmitter receptor genes has revealed the existence of conserved sequences among receptors within a particular family. Such conserved sequences have been used as targets for priming oligonucleotides to amplify cDNA sequences in an effort to identify cDNA's encoding subtypes of a particular receptor or those encoding new members of the receptor family. Degenerate priming oligonucleotides are often used in such studies to increase the probability of an individual primer being a perfect match for the target sequence, i.e., due to potential differences in codon preferences among different receptors. Following amplification and isolation of the sequence of interest, the partial DNA sequence can be used as a probe to screen cDNA libraries in an effort to isolate the full-length cDNA encoding the receptor. However, isolation of full-length cDNAs by library screening is labor intensive and often unsuccessful. The ease of isolating a full-length cDNA by screening a cDNA library is dependent on the quality of the library and the abundance of the cDNA. Rare mRNAs can be lost during construction of the library and incomplete cDNA clones in the library can confound isolation of a full-length cDNA sequence. This is particularly problematic with large mRNA's, due to the possibility of incomplete first-strand cDNA synthesis.

A PCR-based approach to isolate full-length receptor cDNA's can overcome many of the problems inherent in the conventional procedure for cDNA cloning. Unfortunately, the application of PCR to retrieve full-length clones of a receptor cDNA is limited by the fact that nucleotide sequences at cDNA ends do not appear to be conserved within receptor families. Without sequence information from these regions, it is not possible to design primers to the cDNA ends to PCR amplify full-length receptor cDNAs.

This limitation of PCR was subsequently circumvented by adopting procedures where cDNA ends were modified by incorporating a stretch of known sequence. One such approach (1) involves modification of the 3' end of cDNA by terminal transferase reaction, generally with GTP or CTP, to produce a homopolymeric G or C tail. This tail can then be used as a target sequence for one of the PCR primers, enabling amplification of the 3' end of the cDNA. An alternate procedure (2) employs ligation of a synthetic oligonucleotide of known sequence at the 3' end of cDNA to similarly serve as a target for one of the PCR primer pairs. PCR amplification of the 5' end of cDNAs can be accomplished using the poly(T) sequence at the 5' end of oligo(dT)-primed cDNAs as a target sequence for one of the PCR primer pairs. The use of such PCR-based methods could provide a simple and highly effective procedure for molecular cloning of neurotransmitter receptor cDNAs. Furthermore, the enormous amplification of cDNA molecules by PCR provides an advantage in isolation of cDNAs of rare mRNAs, difficult to obtain by conventional approaches.

Our interest was to isolate a cDNA encoding the pituitary adenylate cyclase-activating polypeptide (PACAP) receptor, which we hypothesized to be a member of the vasoactive intestinal peptide (VIP)/secretin/parathyroid hormone (PTH)/calcitonin receptor family. Cloning of the VIP, secretin, PTH, and calcitonin receptors (3–6) suggests that these receptors represent a new family of receptors in the superfamily of seven transmembrane-spanning G-protein-coupled receptors. Sequence comparison of these receptors revealed considerable homologies in their transmembrane domains. We hypothesized that these conserved sequences are a general structural feature of the receptors in this family and that these sequences would also be conserved in the PACAP receptor. Thus, we targeted these conserved sequences to design PCR primers in an effort to amplify gene segments for the PACAP receptor and other novel receptors within this family. On the basis of sequence information obtained from sequencing cDNA clones obtained by PCR with degenerate primers, we employed PCR to isolate a full-length cDNA encoding the PACAP receptor. This communication describes detailed procedures of this novel PCR strategy for molecular cloning of new neurotransmitter receptor cDNAs.

Procedures

RNA Extraction

Total RNA from various rat tissues is prepared by a standard guanidinium hydrochloride/cesium chloride centrifugation method (7) and the quality of the preparations is checked by electrophoresis on 2% (w/v) agarose gel.

First-Strand cDNA Synthesis

First-strand cDNA is synthesized using avian myeloblastosis virus (AMV) reverse transcriptase (Promega, Madison, WI). First-strand cDNA synthesis mixture (20 μl) contains 10 μg of total RNA (prepared as described above), 10 μl of hexanucleotide mixture (Boehringer-Mannheim), 300 ng of oligo(dT)$_{15}$, 2 mM dNTPs, 10 U of RNasin (Promega), and 15 U of reverse transcriptase (RT) (Promega). The reaction mixture is incubated at 42°C for 2 hr and diluted at the end of incubation with 30 μl of sterile double-distilled water.

PCR with Degenerate Primers

The conserved amino acid sequences within the third and seventh transmembrane domains of the cloned VIP, secretin, PTH, and calcitonin receptors serve as the basis for synthesis of three degenerate oligonucleotides for use as primers in our initial PCR. The amino sequences within the third and seventh transmembrane domains (TM) of the VIP, secretin, calcitonin, and PTH receptors are shown below and the underlined regions indicate amino acid sequences selected for oligonucleotide synthesis.

	3rd TM
VIP	AAVVFFQYCVMANFFWLLVEGLYL
SECRETIN	LVMIFFQYCIMANYAWLLVEGLYL
PTH	VAVTVFLYFLTTNYYWILVEGLYL
CALCITONIN	VLHFFHQYMMSCNYFWMLCEGVYL

	7th TM
	........FQGFVVAILYCFLNGEVQA
	........FQGLVVAVLYCFLNGEVQL
	........FQGFFVAIIYCFCNGEVQA
	........FQGFFVAIIYCFCNHEVQG

The forward primer we synthesized has nucleotide sequence 5' TGGATT-CTTGTTGA(A/G)GGT(C/G)T(A/T/G/C)TA(T/C)(C/T)T 3' (primer A) and represents conserved amino acid sequence W(L/I/M)L(V/C)EG(L/V)YL found within the third transmembrane domain of these receptors. Of the two reverse primers synthesized, one has nucleotide sequence 5' TGAAC(T/C)TCACCATTA(A/C)(G/A)(A/G)AA(A/G)CA(A/G)TA 3' (primer B) representing conserved amino acid sequence YCF(C/L)N(G/H)EVQ found within the seventh transmembrane domain of these receptors; the other has nucleotide sequence 5' (A/G/C)GC(A/T)AC(A/G/C)A(A/C)(A/G/C)A(A/G)(A/T)CCCTGGAA 3' (primer C) representing conserved amino acid sequence FQG(F/L)(F/V)VA.

PCR Conditions

Our routine PCR mixture (20 μl) contains 50 mM Tris–HCl (pH 8.3), 1.5 mM MgCl$_2$, 200 μM dNTPs, 0.5 U of *Taq* DNA polymerase (Perkin–Elmer Cetus, Norwalk, CT), and 20 pmol of both reverse and forward primers. The standard PCR condition involves initial heating at 94°C for 5 min and holding at 80°C during the addition of *Taq* DNA polymerase, followed thereafter by 30 cycles of denaturation at 94°C for 1 min, primer annealing at 50°C for 2 min, and primer extension at 72°C for 3 min.

Three degenerate primers allow us to undertake two successive rounds of PCR for 30 cycles each. In the first round of PCR, we use primer combinations of A and B. At the end of 30 cycles, a 1-μl aliquot of this PCR mixture is diluted 100-fold with sterile double-distilled water and a 1-μl aliquot of this diluted sample is used as a template for a second round of seminested PCR with primer combinations of A and C. The final PCR mixture (5 μl) is subjected to 2% (w/v) agarose gel electrophoresis. A single band of ~500 bp was observed (Fig. 1). The size of the PCR product is consistent with that expected for amplification of DNA segments targeted in receptors within the VIP/secretin/calcitonin/PTH family.

Ligation of PCR Products into Plasmid Vector

PCR products are ligated to pCR™II vector DNA (Invitrogen) using T$_4$ DNA ligase. Non-template-dependent activity of *Taq* DNA polymerase adds a single deoxyadenosine residue at 3' ends of PCR-amplified duplex DNA to produce 3' A overhangs. This modification provides convenient sticky ends for incorporation and efficient ligation of PCR products with pCR™II vector which contains single-base complementary 3' T overhangs at the insertion site.

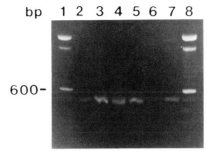

FIG. 1   Reverse transcription PCR products from different rat tissues. Degenerate oligonucleotides were designed on the basis of conserved regions found within the third and seventh transmembrane domains in VIP/secretin/calcitonin/PTH receptors and used as primers to PCR amplify corresponding DNA segments. cDNA derived from total RNA of several rat tissues served as templates in these PCRs. PCR conditions and primer combinations were as detailed under Procedures. PCR products (5-μl aliquot) were resolved on a 2% TAE agarose gel and stained with ethidium bromide. Lanes 1 and 8, 100-bp DNA ladder (Life Technologies); lanes 2 to 6 represent PCR products from heart, lung, spinal cord, vas deferens, and cerebellum. Lane 7 represents the PCR product from a rat brain cDNA library (Invitrogen).

Ligation of PCR Products with pCR™II Vector

The ligation mixture (total volume 11 μl) contains 2 μl of PCR mixture, 50 ng of pCR™II vector (obtained from Invitrogen and reconstituted in sterile double-distilled water), ligation buffer, and 1 U of T$_4$ DNA ligase. The incubation is continued for 16 hr at 12°C.

Incorporation of Ligation Products into Competent Bacteria and Isolation of Individual Colonies

An aliquot (5 μl) of the ligation mixture is used to transform competent bacteria (INVαF′). Transformed cells are plated on ampicillin-containing LB agar plates covered with X-Gal solution (5-bromo-4-chloro-3-indolyl-β-D-galactopyranoside, Boehringer-Mannheim) in dimethylformamide. Insertion of PCR products into vector DNA produces a frame shift of its *lacZ* gene to produce white colonies while self-ligated vector expresses the *lacZ* gene resulting in blue colonies in the presence of the chromogenic substrate X-Gal. Individual white colonies are picked for preparation of plasmid DNA.

Preparation of Plasmid DNA and Identification of Clones with Appropriate Insert

Up to 25 white colonies are picked and minipreparation plasmid DNA is prepared using the alkaline/sodium dodecyl sulfate (SDS) lysis method (8). Appropriate aliquots of these plasmid DNAs are subjected to PCR for 30 cycles under standard conditions in the presence of 2 pmol each of SP-6 (5′ TATTTAGGTGACACTATAG 3′) forward and T-7 (5′ TAATACGACT-CACTATAGGGAGA 3′) reverse primers. Since the site of PCR product insertion within the vector is flanked by SP-6 and T-7 promoter sequences, the inserted DNA is expected to be amplified following PCR with these primers. The examination of such amplification products on TAE 1.5% (w/v) agarose gel electrophoresis indeed showed that plasmid DNA prepared from several of these colonies had inserts of varying sizes (Fig. 2). We selected products of appropriate sizes for further processing to analyze nucleotide sequences of the individual clones.

Transcription of Selected PCR Products with T-7 and SP-6 RNA Polymerase

PCR products amplified with SP-6 and T-7 primers contain RNA polymerase recognition sequences at both ends. Therefore, selected PCR products are transcribed with either T-7 or SP-6 RNA polymerase to obtain RNA transcripts for nucleotide sequencing.

Transcription Reaction Protocol

Routine transcription reaction (20 μl) mixtures contain 2 μl of the PCR mixture; 40 mM Tris–HCl, pH 7.5; 6 mM MgCl$_2$; 2 mM spermidine; 10 mM NaCl; 10 mM dithiothreitol (DTT); 20 U RNasin; 0.5 mM each of rATP, rGTP, rCTP, and rUTP; and 10 U of either T-7 or SP-6 RNA polymerase (Promega). Reaction mixtures are incubated at 37°C for 2 hr and RNA transcripts are used subsequently for nucleotide sequencing with ^{32}P-end-labeled primer and dideoxynucleotides.

Sequencing of RNA Transcript with End-Labeled Primer

Sequencing Reaction Protocol

For dideoxy sequencing reaction, 2 μl of the RNA transcript is mixed with 10 μl of annealing buffer (250 mM KCl, 10 mM Tris–HCl, pH 8.3) and 1 μl of ^{32}P-labeled oligonucleotide (5 ng, prepared as described below). The

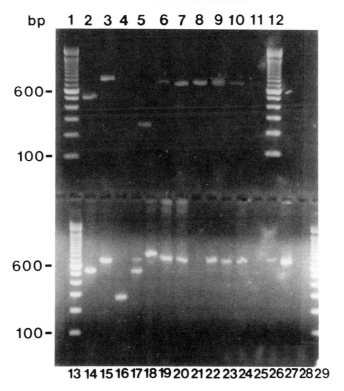

FIG. 2   Insert size of individual clones of rat spinal cord RT-PCR products. Reverse transcription PCR products of rat spinal cord cDNA were cloned and the presence of inserted DNA in individual clones was evaluated by agarose gel electrophoresis following PCR amplification of plasmid DNA from individual clones with SP-6 and T-7 primers. Lanes 1, 12, 13, and 29, 100-bp DNA ladder; lanes 2–11 and 14–28, PCR-amplified DNA inserts from individual clones of rat spinal cord RT-PCR product (some clones have no inserts).

annealing reaction mixture is heated at 80°C for 3 min and after cooling to 55°C, a 2-μl aliquot is added to reverse transcriptase reaction medium containing 24 mM Tris–HCl, pH 8.3, 16 mM MgCl$_2$, 8 mM DTT, 0.8 mM dATP, 0.4 mM dCTP, 0.8 mM dGTP, 1.2 mM dTTP, 1 U of reverse transcriptase, and 0.25 mM each of dideoxynucleotides. The reverse transcriptase reaction mixture (final volume, 6 μl) is incubated at 55°C for 45 min and stopped thereafter by the addition of 4 μl of stop solution containing 85% formamide, 25 mM EDTA, 0.1% bromphenol blue and xylene cyanol FF. The mixture is then heated at 80°C for 3 min and cooled on ice and aliquots (1–2 μl) are separated by electrophoresis through polyacrylamide/

urea gel. After being dried, the gel is exposed overnight to X-ray film (Kodak, Rochester, NY).

End Labeling Reaction Protocol

The primers used for sequencing are end-labeled using T_4 polynucleotide kinase. Routine end-labeling reaction mixture (total volume 13 μl) contains 50 mM Tris–HCl buffer, pH 7.4, 10 mM MgCl$_2$, 5 mM DTT, 0.1 mM spermidine, 100 μCi [γ-^{32}P]ATP (5000 Ci/mmol), 10 units of T_4 polynucleotide kinase, and 100 ng of appropriate primer. After incubation for 30 min at 37°C, the reaction mixture is diluted with 7 μl of double-distilled water and stored frozen for subsequent use in sequencing reaction.

Examination of Sequence Homology and Uniqueness

Nucleotide and amino acid sequences of these partial clones are analyzed by GCG software package using the PILEUP program (9). The examination of sequence homology revealed that our PCR strategy amplified several new clones having varying degrees of homology to already published sequences for receptors in the VIP/secretin/calcitonin/PTH receptor family.

Amplification of cDNA Ends

For further study, we selected a partial clone that was most homologous to the VIP receptor and we attempted to PCR amplify the full-length cDNA for complete sequence analysis. The selection of this clone is based on our assumption that the PACAP receptor is structurally similar to the VIP receptor. The amino acid sequence of this partial clone is shown in Fig. 3. Since the nucleotide sequence at the 3′ end of this cDNA was unknown, we modify this end by ligating a synthetic oligonucleotide of known sequence to serve as a target for forward PCR primer annealing.

For ligation of the synthetic oligonucleotide at the 3′ end of cDNA, we

WLLVEGLYLFTLLVETFFPERRYFYWYTIIGWGTPTVCVTVWAVLRLYFDDAGCWDMNDSTALW

WVIKGPVVGSIMVNFVLFIGIIIILVQKLQSPDMGGNESSIYLRLARSTLLLIPLFGIHYTVFAFSPEN

VSKRERLVFELGLGSFQGFVVA

FIG. 3 Predicted amino acid sequence of a cDNA clone derived from PCR amplification of rat spinal cord cDNA with degenerate primers. The underlined regions indicate sequences to which PCR primers were synthesized for additional PCR amplifications.

utilize the known ability of T_4 RNA ligase to accept, albeit less efficiently, two single-stranded DNA molecules as substrates for ligation. Since contaminating RNA molecules as well as PCR primers would compete with cDNA as more efficient substrates, cDNA purification is necessary before undertaking this ligation reaction.

Purification of cDNA for Ligation Reaction

Twenty microliters of diluted first-strand cDNA synthesis reaction mixture from rat spinal cord is mixed with 3 μl of 3 N NaOH and incubated at 65°C for 30 min to hydrolyze RNA. The mixture is then cooled and single-stranded cDNA is precipitated by the addition of 3 μl of 3 N acetic acid, 2 μl of glycogen (20 mg/ml), and 84 μl of 95% (v/v) ethanol. After overnight precipitation at −20°C, cDNA is pelleted by centrifugation, dissolved in 20 μl of double-distilled water, and purified through GlassMax spin cartridge (Life Technologies) according to the manufacturer's suggestion. After the column is washed, bound cDNA is eluted with 40 μl of sterile double-distilled water (65°C) and reprecipitated by incubation for 30 min in dry ice following addition of 4 μl of 5 M sodium acetate, pH 5.5, 2 μl of glycogen (20 mg/ml), and 140 μl of 95% (v/v) ethanol. The precipitate is washed once with 70% (v/v) ethanol and dissolved in 5 μl of sterile double-distilled water.

Ligation of Synthetic Oligonucleotide to cDNA End with T_4 RNA Ligase

To the 3' end of purified single-stranded cDNA, we ligate a 24-base-long synthetic oligonucleotide of known sequence (anchor oligo). The ligation reaction mixture contains 2.5 μl of GlassMax purified cDNA, 5 μl of 2× ligation buffer, 0.5 μl of T_4 RNA ligase (10 U), and 2 μl of anchor oligo (4 pmol, 31 ng). The composition of 2× ligation buffer is 100 mM Tris–HCl, pH 8.0, 20 mM MgCl$_2$, 20 μg/ml acetyl BSA (bovine serum albumin) (New England BioLab), 2 mM hexamminecobalt chloride (Sigma, St. Louis, MO), 40 μM dATP, and 50% polyethylene glycol (Sigma). The anchor oligonucleotide is blocked at the 3' end by amidation to prevent self-ligation and has the following nucleotide sequence: 5' P-CTATCGATTCTGGAACCTTCAGAG-NH$_2$ 3'. The ligation reaction is performed at room temperature for 24 hr.

PCR Amplification of 3' End of cDNA

One microliter of ligation reaction mixture is used as a template for PCR under standard conditions using 20 pmol each of forward and reverse primers. The forward primer is complementary to the anchor oligonucleotide (i.e., CTCTGAAGGTTCCAGAATCGATAG; primer D) and primer B is used as the reverse primer. One-microliter aliquot of this PCR mixture is diluted to 100 μl with sterile double-distilled water and 1 μl aliquot of this sample is subjected to another 30 cycles of PCR with the same forward primer D but substituting the reverse primer this time with a nested reverse primer C. This PCR mixture is diluted 1 : 100 and a 1-μl aliquot is used as a template for another 30 cycles of PCR with another nested reverse primer with nucleotide sequence 5′ GGTGTACCAGTAGAAATATCTCCT 3′ (E) designed based on a unique stretch of eight amino acids RRYFYWYT found in the partial clone we selected. The final PCR mixture (5 μl) is analyzed on TAE 1.5% (w/v) agarose gel. Several distinct bands ranging from 150 to 850 bp were observed in our experiments (Fig. 4). The PCR products are ligated to pCR™II vector (Invitrogen) and the ligated product is used to transform competent bacteria (INVαF′). After blue/white colony selection, individual white colonies are picked and plasmid DNA is prepared from each of them. Plasmid DNAs are subjected to PCR amplification with SP-6 forward and T-7 reverse primers; subsequent preparation of RNA transcripts and nucleotide sequencing is performed as described above. Sequence analysis of inserts from several different clones revealed that each of these clones represented partial sequences found in the largest of these clones (850 bp). A consensus

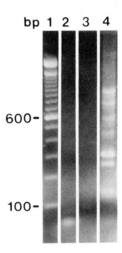

FIG. 4   PCR amplification of 3′ end of cDNA. The 3′ end of cDNA was modified by ligation with a synthetic oligonucleotide (anchor) and the modified cDNA was PCR-amplified with a primer complementary to this anchor sequence (primer D) and primer B. The product of the first PCR was diluted and was used for a second round of PCR with primers D and C. The product of the second round PCR was diluted and was used for a third round of PCR with primers D and E. PCR mixtures were resolved on an agarose gel and stained with ethidium bromide. Lane 1, 100-bp DNA ladder; lanes 2–4 represent PCR products (5 μl) from the first, second, and third round of PCR, respectively.

sequence for translation start site was present in the 850-bp clone and the amino acid sequence deduced on the basis of this initiation site exhibited varying degrees of similarity to sequences of the previously cloned VIP, secretin, PTH, and calcitonin receptors. Sequencing of multiple clones revealed that two clones had A instead of G in one place within the entire 850-bp sequence and these differences may have resulted from *Taq* polymerase errors during PCR amplification.

PCR Amplification of 5' End of cDNA

For amplification of the 5' end of cDNA, we utilize the existing poly(T) tail at the 5' end of the cDNA as a target for a reverse PCR primer. One microliter of diluted first-strand cDNA synthesis reaction mixture from rat spinal cord (see above) is subjected to PCR amplification with 2 pmol of forward primer F (representing amino acid and nucleotide sequences, respectively, of YF-WLFIE and 5' TACTTCTGGCTGTTCATTGAG 3') and 4 pmol of reverse primer G of nucleotide sequence 5' ATTAACCCTCACTAAAGGGAT$_{25}$ 3'. To increase the likelihood of successful amplification of the 5' cDNA end, we perform two additional PCRs with two different forward primers. The forward primer in one PCR is H (representing amino acid and nucleotide sequences, respectively, of RRYFYWY and 5' AGGAGATATTTCTACTG-GTAC 3') and in the other PCR is I (representing amino acid and nucleotide sequences, respectively, of GCWDMND and 5' GGATGCTGGGGATAT-GAATGAC 3'). One-microliter aliquots of a 100-fold diluted sample of these PCR mixtures are subjected to another 30 cycles of PCR using 4 pmol of the same reverse primer (G) but the forward primer F is replaced with 2 pmol of forward primer H. The forward primers H and I in the other two PCRs are replaced, respectively, with 2 pmol of primer I and primer J (representing amino acid and nucleotide sequences, respectively, of HYTV-FAF and 5' CACTACACAGTATTCGCCTTC 3'). These forward primers were designed on the basis of partial sequence information we obtained on this clone and represented stretches of amino acid sequences unique in comparison to sequences of other receptors cloned within the family. The location of the amino acid sequences corresponding to primers H, F, I, and J in the partial clone can be seen in Fig. 3. The resulting products from these PCRs were analyzed on TAE 1.5% (w/v) agarose gel and bands ranging from 1000 to 700 bp were seen (Fig. 5). These PCR products are processed further for sequencing as described above. Sequencing of multiple clones did not reveal any differences in sequences within clones. All of these clones had a stop codon and 5' untranslated sequence indicating successful amplification of the 5' cDNA end. Sequence alignment of clones corresponding to the 3' and 5' cDNA ends revealed that these clones were overlapping, yielding a

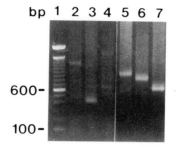

FIG. 5   PCR amplification of 5′ end of cDNA. Rat spinal cord cDNA was subjected to PCR amplification with oligo(dT) reverse primer (G) and forward primers F, H, and I. PCR mixtures were diluted 100-fold and subjected to seminested PCR with the same reverse primer (G) and new forward primers H, I, or J as described under Procedures. Lane 1, 100-bp DNA ladder; lanes 2–4, first-round PCR products with primers G and F (lane 2), G and H (lane 3), and G and I (lane 4); lane 5, nested PCR with primers G and H using lane 2 sample as template; lane 6, nested PCR with primers G and I using lane 3 sample as template; lane 7, nested PCR with primers G and J using lane 4 sample as template.

full-length cDNA with an open reading frame of 1404 bp encoding a unique protein of 468 amino acids.

Ligation of PCR Fragments to Obtain Full-Length DNA

After obtaining the complete nucleotide sequence of the full-length clone, we synthesize a new pair of primers with restriction enzyme recognition sites (not present in the cDNA) at their 5′ ends. The forward primer K (37 nucleotides long) represents nucleotides −30 to −9 upstream of the initiation codon and contain, in addition, a *Hind*III recognition sequence at its 5′ end and a stretch of 9 nonspecific nucleotides thereafter (5′ ATCCGTACC<u>AAGC-TT</u>AATAGCCAGAGATAGTGGCTTG 3′). The reverse primer L (37 nucleotides long) represents a nucleotide stretch from the translation stop codon to 22 nucleotides downstream and contains, in addition, a *Xho*I site at its 5′ end and a stretch of 9 nonspecific nucleotides following the restriction enzyme recognition sequence (5′ GGTACTGTT<u>CTCGAG</u>AGGAGGAGGGAGA-CACGCCTCA 3′). Restriction enzyme-sensitive sites (underlined sequences) are included in these PCR primers to facilitate ligation of PCR fragments to cloning sites within pcDNA3 (Invitrogen). A stretch of 9 nonspecific nucleotides is added at the 5′ end of restriction enzyme recognition sequences to enhance the sensitivity of these sites for digestion by their respective restriction enzymes. In addition, a forward primer representing nucleotides 710–731 (primer M) and a reverse primer representing nucleotides 749 to 767 (primer N) are also synthesized for use in recombinant PCR (below).

Appropriate first-round PCR templates are nested with forward primer K and reverse primer N or, alternatively, with forward primer M and reverse primer L in an attempt to create overlapping PCR products corresponding to nucleotides (−)30-767 and 710-(+)22, respectively. These two PCR fragments represent two halves of the entire sequence with an overlap in the middle of 58 nucleotides. Denaturation and renaturation of a mixture of these two PCR products will cause some of the complementary strands to anneal at the overlapping sequence. Products annealing at the overlapping sequence would provide template for PCR amplification of complete sequence with primer combination of K and L.

Both PCR products are, thus, mixed and purified through GlassMax spin column cartridge (Life Technologies) to remove contaminating primers. One microliter sample of each purified PCR product is subjected to PCR with forward primer K and reverse primer L. An aliquot (5 μl) of this PCR mixture is resolved on TAE 1% (w/v) agarose gel. An intense band of approximately 1.4 kb was observed using either *Pfu* or *Taq* DNA polymerase in our studies (Fig. 6). The intensity of the *Taq*-amplified product was considerably greater than that of the *Pfu*-amplified product.

Cloning of Full-Length cDNA in Eukaryotic Expression Vector pcDNA3

To obtain sufficient amounts of the full-length cDNA PCR product for further manipulation, we perform the ligation PCR in multiple tubes and these tubes are pooled. A 100-μl aliquot of this pool is extracted twice with phenol/chloroform followed by two extractions with chloroform/isoamyl alcohol. After final extraction, the aqueous phase is mixed with 50 μl of cold 7.5 M ammonium acetate and 450 μl of cold 95% ethanol to precipitate the PCR-amplified DNA. DNA is pelleted by centrifugation, dissolved in 100 μl of 10 mM Tris–HCl (pH 8.0) containing 5 mM EDTA and 0.5% (w/v) SDS, and incubated at 37°C for 30 min following addition of 2 μl of proteinase K (3 mg/ml). Following proteinase K digestion, DNA is extracted twice with phenol/chloroform followed by two additional extractions with chloroform/isoamyl alcohol. After the final extraction, the aqueous phase is mixed with 10 μl of 5 M sodium acetate, pH 5.5, and 220 μl of 95% ethanol to precipitate the DNA. The DNA precipitate is dissolved in 48 μl of double-distilled water and then mixed with 6 μl of Buffer B (Boehringer-Mannheim) and 2 μl each of *Hind*III and *Xho*I. DNA is digested for 20 hr at 37°C and then subjected to 1% agarose gel electrophoresis. The band of approximately 1.4 kb size is cut out of the gel and purified through a GlassMax spin cartridge column.

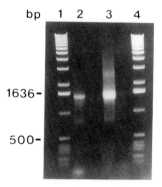

FIG. 6   PCR amplification of full-length receptor cDNA. Two PCR products encompassing the full-length cDNA and containing a 58-nucleotide overlapping sequence were used to PCR amplify the full-length cDNA. The two purified PCR products were mixed and subjected to PCR with forward primer K (3′ primer) and reverse primer L (5′ primer). Lanes 1 and 4, 1-kb DNA ladder (Life Technologies); lane 2, PCR product obtained using *Pfu* DNA polymerase; lane 3, PCR product obtained using *Taq* DNA polymerase.

This purified DNA is ligated to *Hind* III and *Xho*I cut pcDNA3 with T_4 DNA ligase. Competent INVαF cells (Invitrogen) are transformed with the ligated DNA and plated on ampicillin-containing LB agar plate. Plasmid DNA is prepared from several of these colonies and subjected to DNA sequence analysis. Sequence analysis of this PCR-amplified full-length cDNA revealed absolute identity to the two overlapping clones sequenced earlier. The predicted amino acid sequence of the clone and its alignment with the rat VIP receptor is shown in Fig. 7.

Discussion

While we were performing experiments to evaluate the functional activity of this clone, Pisegna and Wank (10) and Hosoya *et al.* (11) simultaneously reported cloning of the PACAP receptor by homology screening with a VIP receptor cDNA. Hosoya *et al.* (11) found both a short and long form of the receptor while Pisegna and Wank (10) reported cloning only the long form. Analysis of these sequences of the PACAP receptor revealed that our clone is identical to the sequence of the short form of the PACAP receptor. The long form contains a 28-amino acid insert in the third intracellular loop that arises presumably by alternative splicing of the primary transcript. Subse-

```
           1                                                          50
  PACAP    .....MARVL  QLSLTALLLP  VAI.AMHSDC  IFKKEQAMCL  ERI....QRA
  VIP      MRPPSPPHVR  WLCVLAGALA  CALRPAGSQA  ASPQHECEYL  QLIEIQRQQC

           51                                                         100
  PACAP    NDLMGLNESS  PGCPGMWDNI  TCWKPAQVGE  MVLVSCPEVF  RIFNPDQVWM
  VIP      LEEAQLENET  TGCSKMWDNL  TCWPTTPRGQ  AVVLDCPLIF  QLFAPIHGY.

           101                                                        150
  PACAP    TETIGDSGFA  DSNSLEITDM  GVVGRNCTED  GWSEPFP.HY  FDACGFDDYE
  VIP      .........   .........   .NISRSCTEE  GWSQLEPGPY  HIACGLNDRA

           151                                                        200
  PACAP    P..ESGDQDY  YYLSVKALYT  VGYSTSLATL  TTAMVILCRF  RKLHCTRNFI
  VIP      SSLDEQQQTK  FYNTVKTGYT  IGYSLSLASL  LVAMAILSLF  RKLHCTRNYI

           201                                                        250
  PACAP    HMNLFVSFML  RAISVFIKDW  ILYAEQDSSH  CFVSTVECKA  VMVFFHYCVV
  VIP      HMHLFMSFIL  RATAVFIKDM  ALFNSGEIDH  CSEASVGCKA  AVVFFQYCVM

           251                                                        300
  PACAP    SNYFWLFIEG  LYLFTLLVET  FFPERRYFYW  YTIIGWGTPT  VCVTVWAVLR
  VIP      ANFFWLLVEG  LYLYTLLAVS  FFSERKYFWG  YILIGWGVPS  VFITIWTVVR

           301                                                        350
  PACAP    LYFDDAGCWD  MNDSTALWWV  IKGPVVGSIM  VNFVLFIGII  IILVQKLQSP
  VIP      IYFEDFGCWD  TIINSSLWWI  IKAPILLSIL  VNFVLFICII  RILVQKLRPP

           351                                                        400
  PACAP    DMGGNESSIY  LRLARSTLLL  IPLFGIHYTV  FAFSPENVSK  RERLVFELGL
  VIP      DIGKNDSSPY  SRLAKSTLLL  IPLFGIHYVM  FAFFPDNFKA  QVKMVFELVV

           401                                                        450
  PACAP    GSFQGFVVAV  LYCFLNGEVQ  AEIKRKWRSW  KVNRYFTMDF  KHRHPSLASS
  VIP      GSFQGFVVAI  LYCFLNGEVQ  AELRRKWRRW  HLQGVLGWSS  KSQHPWGGSN

           451                            482
  PACAP    GVNGGTQLSI  LSK.SSSQLR  MSSLPADNLA  T
  VIP      GATCSTQVSM  LTRVSPSARR  SSSFQAEVSL  V
```

FIG. 7   Predicted amino acid sequence of PCR-derived PACAP receptor cDNA clone and its alignment with the rat VIP receptor sequence.

quently, evidence for additional splice variants of the PACAP receptor was reported by Spengler *et al.* (12). The exact match in the nucleotide sequences observed between our clone and those isolated by library screening underscores the reliability of this PCR-based strategy for cloning novel neuropeptide receptor genes.

In summary, we have described a new approach for cloning novel neuropeptide receptor genes that relies entirely on the use of PCR. We have documented the ability of this procedure to amplify a full-length cDNA sequence of the PACAP receptor from total RNA. These results document the feasibility, reliability, and applicability of this PCR strategy to isolate novel neuropeptide receptor genes. The procedures described here are likely to be useful in cloning nonreceptor cDNAs for which limited sequence information is available. In addition, this method obviates some of the difficulties associated with traditional cloning strategies and may be particularly useful in isolation of rare cDNAs due to the enormous amplification afforded by PCR.

References

1. E. Y. Loh, J. F. Elliot, S. Cwirla, L. L. Lanier, and M. M. Davis, *Science* **243,** 217 (1989).
2. J. B. Dumas, M. Edwards, J. Delort, and J. Mallet, *Nucleic Acids Res.* **19,** 5227 (1991).
3. T. Ishihara, S. Nakamura, Y. Kaziro, T. Takahashi, K. Takahashi, and S. Nagata, *EMBO J.* **10,** 1635 (1991).
4. T. Ishihara, R. Shigemoto, K. Mori, K. Takahashi, and S. Nagata, *Neuron* **8,** 811 (1992).
5. H. Y. Lin, T. L. Harris, M. R. Flannery, A. Aruffo, E. H. Kaji, A. Gorn, L. F. Kolakowski, Jr., H. Lodish, and S. R. Goldring, *Science* **254,** 1022 (1991).
6. H. Juppner, A-B. Abou-Samra, M. Freeman, X. F. Kong, E. Schipani, J. Richards, L. F. Kolakowski, Jr., J. Hock, J. T. Potts, Jr., H. M. Kronenberg, and G.V. Segré, *Science* **254,** 1024 (1991).
7. R. J. Macdonald, G. H. Swift, A. E., Przybyla, and J. M. Chirgwin, *in* "Methods in Enzymology" (S. L. Berger and A.R. Kimmel, eds.), Vol. 152, p. 219. Academic Press, San Diego, 1987.
8. H. Miller, *in* "Methods in Enzymology" (S. L. Berger and A. R. Kimmel, eds.), Vol. 152, p. 145. Academic Press, San Diego, 1987.
9. J. Devereaux, P. Haebrli, and O. Smithies, *Nucleic Acids Res.* **12,** 387 (1984).
10. J. R. Pisegna and S. A. Wank, *Proc. Natl. Acad. Sci. U.S.A.* **90,** 6345 (1993).
11. M. Hosoya, H. Onda, K. Ogi, Y. Masuda, Y. Miyamoto, T. Ohtaki, H. Okazaki, A. Arimura, and M. Fujino, *Biochem. Biophys. Res. Commun.* **194,** 133 (1993).
12. D. Spengler, C. Waeber, C. Pantaloni, F. Holsboer, J. Bockaert, P. H. Seeburg, and L. Journot, *Nature (London)* **365,** 170 (1993).

[4]　Lock-Docking Rapid Amplification of cDNA Ends PCR: Strategies and Applications

Nancy D. Borson, Wilmar L. Salo, and Lester R. Drewes

Polymerase chain reactions (PCR) are often performed in searches for genes of interest, or their mRNA transcripts. However, the direct amplification and sequencing of cDNA products that encompass 3' and 5' ends have been problematic. The oligo(dT) primer that is traditionally used in the cDNA synthesis step can anneal at any position along the length of a natural (3') or appended (5') poly(A) tail (1). Subsequently, PCR products of a single, discrete size are not obtained. To enable the acquisition of discrete, first-round PCR products, a "lock-docking" cDNA synthesis primer and accompanying PCR procedure (the "lock-docking system"), are described. These PCR products can be directly sequenced (2).

This lock-docking primer system may be applied to a novel method for searching for previously unidentified gene family members (3). While PCR targets in the internal, coding regions tend to be of similar lengths, targets in the 3' regions (including the untranslated regions) tend to be of varying lengths. Thus, internal PCR products are difficult to separate for further study, while products from 3' regions may be separated by agarose gel electrophoresis.

Isolation of PCR Products for 3' Ends

Underlying Principles

The lock-docking primer (Fig. 1) is a modification of the oligo(dT) cDNA synthesis primer used in the 5' and 3' rapid amplification of cDNA end (RACE) procedures of Frohman (4). The primer is designed to anneal to the poly(A)$^+$ RNA at the junction of gene-specific sequence and polyadenylation (Fig. 2). When the junctional sequence of a polyadenylated mRNA is considered, the nucleotide just preceding the first A will be a U, C, or G. The penultimate nucleotide preceding the first A will be an A, U, C, or G. Thus, a mixture of oligo(dT) primers including all 12 permutations at the 3' end was synthesized to enable primer annealing to all possible mRNA polyadenylation

$$5'-(mcs)\,TTTTTTTTTTTTTTTTVN-3'$$

FIG. 1   The lock-docking primer. V is A, C, G; N is A, C, G, T; mcs, multiple cloning site. The lock-docking primer was synthesized by Bio-Synthesis, Inc. (Denton, TX) at no extra charge for the degeneracy at the 3′ end. Alternatively, one can purchase bulk CPG-linked nucleotides and empty columns from various suppliers (Applied Biosystems, Foster City, CA, or Cruachem, Sterling, VA). From these components, one can mix any combination of the four CPG-linked nucleotides to start a synthesis.

junction sites. Only one primer synthesis is required to generate this primer set, which we refer to as the lock-docking primer.

An additional feature of the lock-docking primer is a multiple cloning site (mcs) attached at the 5′ end. The reason for including the mcs is that mcs primers are used in subsequent polymerase chain reactions. Higher annealing temperatures are allowed with mcs primers than are possible with oligo(dT) primers. Thus, an upper-strand, gene-specific primer with a relatively high melting temperature can be selected and used in conjunction with the mcs

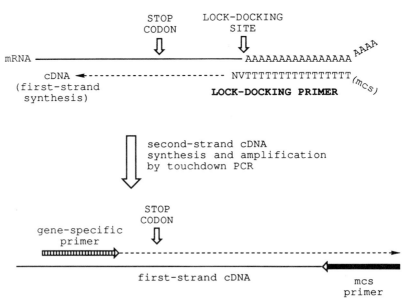

FIG. 2   Procedure for generation of 3′ end PCR products. First-strand cDNA synthesis is primed with the lock-docking primer. The first-strand cDNA serves as template in the subsequent touchdown PCR. One of the primers for the touchdown PCR is gene-specific, the other is the Tmcs primer described under Methods for Amplification of 3′ Ends.

primer. The mcs region may be made long enough to enable the synthesis and use of heminested mcs primers.

The strategy for the PCR step should include choosing primers that are (a) gene-specific primers with slightly higher melting temperatures (3–4°C higher) than mcs primers, (b) preferably, gene-specific primers that contain a G or a C at their 3' ends, and (c) mcs primers that contain an A or a T at their 3' ends. This results in a combination of primers that works effectively in a "touchdown" PCR protocol (5). In a typical touchdown protocol, annealing occurs at sequentially lower temperatures, usually dropping 1°C every two cycles. Because the gene-specific primer will be the first to bind in the early cycles of the PCR, it will enable linear amplification of the second strand of the target cDNA severalfold before the mcs primer can begin to bind. The goal is to prevent the formation of nonspecific second-strand cDNA transcripts, to which the mcs primer would also bind.

Methods for Amplification of 3' Ends

A specific example that was used to generate the 3' end PCR products for glucose transporter genes Glut3 and Glut1 from canine brain cortex is presented below. Glut3 and Glut1 are members of a family of glucose transporters that transport glucose across cell membranes via facilitative diffusion.

mRNA Isolation

Approximately 1 g of fresh canine brain cortex tissue is obtained and immediately frozen in liquid nitrogen. Poly(A)$^+$ RNA is extracted from the tissue using a commercially available kit (Micro Fast Track kit, Invitrogen, San Diego, CA).

cDNA Synthesis

First-strand cDNA synthesis is performed using 1 μg of canine brain cortex poly(A)$^+$ RNA as template and Maloney murine leukemia virus (M-MLV) reverse transcriptase (GIBCO-BRL, Grand Island, NY) as follows: To a 1.5-ml microfuge tube, additions are made, in order, of 4 μl of 5× M-MLV reaction buffer (GIBCO-BRL), 8 μl of a mixture that is 1.25 mM in each dNTP (Perkin–Elmer Cetus, Norwalk, CT), and 16 ng of the lock-docking primer dissolved in 1 μl of deionized H$_2$O. The mRNA template, diluted in deionized H$_2$O to yield a final reaction volume of 20 μl, is denatured at 75°C for 3 min and then quenched on ice before addition to the above mixture. Two hundred units of M-MLV reverse transcriptase are added to the mixture, and the reaction is incubated 40 min at 37°C and 30 min at 42°C to encourage formation of longer transcripts. The resultant cDNA–RNA hybrid is treated with 2 units of RNase H (Amersham, Arlington Heights, IL) for 20 min at 37°C, followed by enzyme inactivation at 95°C for 5 min. The cDNA is appropriately diluted for use in the PCR, without synthesis of the second strand of cDNA.

Touchdown PCR for Canine Brain Cortex Glut3

Two separate PCRs are performed on the cDNA template using two different, canine-specific Glut3 20-mer primers. Primer A (CTTCCTCATCGTCTT-CTTGG) is designed to prime synthesis at a site located 172 bases upstream of the predicted location of the termination codon of Glut3, and primer B (TTTGAGGAAATCACCCGAGC) at a site 40 bases downstream of primer A. Each of these primers is used in conjunction with a 19-mer truncated version of the mcs segment that is part of the lock-docking primer. The sequence of the 19-mer truncated mcs primer is CCGCAGATCTAGATAT-CGA (Tmcs); the entire mcs sequence is CCGCATGCGGCCGCAGATCTA-GATATCGA, which contains the restriction enzyme sites *Sph*I/*Not*I/*Bgl*II/*Eco*RV/*Cla*I. The approximate predicted sizes of the PCR products obtained with primers A/Tmcs and B/Tmcs are 2400 and 2360 base pairs, respectively (6).

The PCR conditions are based on the touchdown PCR protocol (5). The annealing temperature is decreased 1°C every second cycle from 60°C to a touchdown temperature at 50°C; this final annealing temperature is maintained for 10 cycles. Denaturation is done for 5 min at 94°C in the first cycle and 1 min in each cycle thereafter. Extension times at 72°C are gradually increased as follows: 10 cycles at 2 min each, followed by 10 cycles at 3 min each, then 10 cycles at 4 min each. The final extension time is 15 min. Increasingly longer extension times enable completion of longer transcripts (more than 2000 base pairs). Reactions are performed in final volumes of 100 μl, using AmpliWax PCR Gems (Perkin–Elmer Cetus, Norwalk, CT) to facilitate final mixing of primer and template at a temperature high enough to prevent possible undesirable primer dimerization from occurring prior to the first denaturation cycle. A lower layer consists of 2.5 μl of 10× PCR buffer (100 m*M* Tris–HCl, pH 8.3, 500 m*M* KCl), 10 μl of 25 m*M* MgCl$_2$, 16 μl of a dNTP solution that is 1.25 m*M* in each dNTP, and 20 pmol of each primer. After addition of one AmpliWax PCR Gem, heating at 80°C for 5 min, and cooling to room temperature, the upper layer is added. The upper layer consists of 60 μl of deionized H$_2$O, 10 μl of 10× PCR buffer, 2.5 units of *Taq* DNA polymerase (AmpliTaq, Perkin–Elmer Cetus), and 1 μl of a 1 : 10 dilution of the canine brain cortex cDNA (in the range of 5–10 ng) as described above. Final concentrations in the PCR reaction are 200 μ*M* in each dNTP, 62.5 mM KCl, 2.5 mM MgCl$_2$, and 12.5 mM Tris–HCl, pH 8.3. Cycling is done in a DNA thermal cycler (Perkin–Elmer Cetus).

Touchdown PCR for Canine Brain Cortex Glut1

The PCR conditions used to amplify a Glut1 3' end fragment are nearly identical to those used for Glut3. The template used is 1 μl of a 1 : 100 dilution (approximately 0.5 ng) of the canine brain cortex cDNA. An optional addition to each reaction mixture is 60 pmol of T4 gp32 protein (United States Biochemical, Cleveland, OH) (7). Two canine-specific Glut1 uptstream primers, primer C (AAGTTCCTGAGACCAAAGGC) and primer D (CGGACCTTT-GATGAGATTGC) are used in two separate PCRs, each with the Tmcs primer. Primer C is designed to prime synthesis at a site located 124 bases upstream of the predicted termination codon, and primer D at a site located 20 bases downstream from primer C. Primers C/Tmcs and D/Tmcs are predicted to amplify PCR products of 1025 and 1005 base pairs, respectively (8).

The products of all PCRs are separated by electrophoresis through 1% agarose gels (Sea Plaque GTG agarose, FMC, Rockland, ME).

Sequencing

All sequencing is done directly from PCR products as described (2).

Results of Searches for 3' Ends of Glut3 and Glut1

Primer A, when used in a PCR in conjunction with the Tmcs primer, amplified a discrete 2400-base pair product (Fig. 3, lane 2). The use of primer B amplified a 40-base smaller product (Fig. 3, lane 3). These sizes correspond to the base pair lengths predicted for canine Glut3 cDNA. Both products were isolated from agarose gels and sequenced directly. The results verified that both products were derived from canine Glut3.

Similarly, two discrete products were amplified for the 3'ends of Glut1. The first product was formed with primer C and the Tmcs primer (Fig. 4, lane 2); the second product was formed with primer D and the Tmcs primer (Fig. 4, lane 3). These products were 1025 and 1005 base pairs, respectively, as predicted for canine Glut1. The direct sequencing of these products verified that they were derived from canine Glut1.

Isolation of PCR Products for 5' Ends

Underlying Principles

The same set of lower-strand primers that is used in the lock-docking system to amplify 3' end products is used in the procedure for amplification of 5'

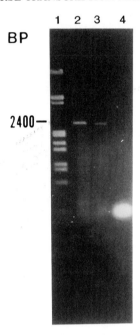

FIG. 3 Electrophoretic analysis of 3′ end PCR products of canine cortex Glut3. Primers are described under Methods for Amplification of 3′ Ends, and the products shown in lanes 2 and 3 were obtained using 1 μl of a 1 : 10 dilution of canine brain cortex cDNA as template. Lane 1: DNA standards (λDNA-*Hin*dIII + *Eco*RI; Boehringer-Mannheim, Indianapolis, IN). Sizes in base pairs are, from the bottom: 564, 831, 947, 1375, 1584, 1904, 2027, 3530, 4268, 4973, 5148, and 21226. Lane 2: The 2400-bp product obtained using the Glut3 primer A in conjunction with the Tmcs primer. Lane 3: The 2360-bp product obtained using the Glut3 primer B in conjunction with the Tmcs primer. Lane 4: Negative control (no template). Reproduced from ref. 2.

end products (Fig. 5). However, a major difference in the procedure for 5′ends is that the lock-docking primer initiates synthesis of second-strand cDNA rather than first-strand cDNA. The first-strand cDNA synthesis is primed with a gene-specific lower strand primer, following the methods of Frohman for 5′ RACE (4). The first-strand cDNA is then enzymatically poly(A) tailed, and two polymerase chain reactions are performed.

The first PCR synthesizes second-strand cDNA. Both the lock-docking primer and the gene-specific lower-strand primer are present in this reaction. This enables both second-strand synthesis and some amplification of the desired product to occur. A low annealing temperature is used in this PCR to allow for binding of the lock-docking primer.

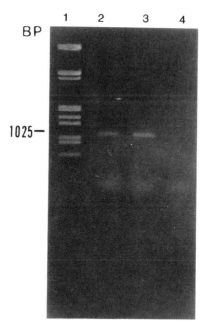

FIG. 4   Electrophoretic analysis of 3' end PCR products of canine brain cortex Glut1. Primers are described under Methods for Amplification of 3' Ends, and the products shown in lanes 2 and 3 are obtained using 1 μl of a 1 : 100 dilution of canine brain cortex cDNA. Lane 1: DNA standards (see Fig. 3). Lane 2: The 1025-bp product obtained using the Glut1 primer C in conjunction with the Tmcs primer. Lane 3: The 1005-bp product obtained using the Glut1 primer D in conjunction with the Tmcs primer. Lane 4: Negative control (no template). Reproduced from ref. 2.

In the second PCR, the Tmcs primer (now an upper-strand primer) and a second gene-specific primer are employed. This second primer is heminested to the first-strand cDNA synthesis primer and confers a level of specificity unattainable during the first-strand cDNA synthesis and the first low-stringency PCR step. A touchdown PCR protocol is again used, and the same melting point considerations apply that were given above for the 3' end PCR primers.

Methods for 5' End

Detailed below is a specific example describing amplification of the 5' end of canine brain cortex Glut3 cDNA.

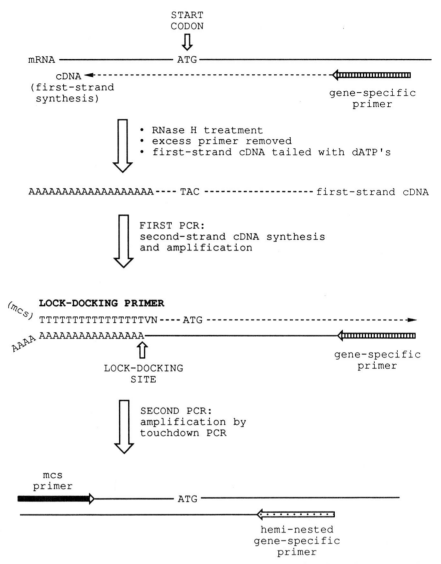

FIG. 5   Procedure for generation of 5′ ends. A gene-specific primer is used to prime synthesis of first-strand cDNA. The first-strand cDNA is synthetically polyadenylated, producing the complementary sequence for the lock-docking primer, which then primes the synthesis of second-strand cDNA. The second-strand cDNA is synthesized and both strands are amplified during the first PCR. To increase specificity, and amplify the desired product, a touchdown PCR is performed with the lock-docking primer and a heminested gene-specific primer. The template for the touchdown PCR is an aliquot of product from the first PCR.

cDNA Synthesis

The first-strand cDNA synthesis procedure used for the 5′ end is identical to that described for the 3′ end, except that the lock-docking primer is replaced with 10 pmol of canine-specific primer. This canine-specific Glut3 primer, primer E (CCAAGAAGACGATGAGGAAG), is based on the comparable sequence at base pairs 1553–1572 of the human homolog.

Spun-Column Procedure

A Sephadex G-50 (Sigma, St. Louis, MO) filtration column is prepared and preconditioned first with 100 μl of TE (pH 8), followed by 100 μl of 0.5× TE (pH 8). The cDNA synthesis reaction is brought to 100 μl by the addition of 0.5× TE (pH 8), placed on the preconditioned column, and centrifuged at 4000 g for 4 min. The collected sample is then concentrated to 20 μl with a vacuum concentrator (Speed-Vac, Savant, Farmingdale, NY). Alternatively, a commercially available spun column may be used.

Poly(A) Tailing

Poly(A) tailing is done in a 40-μl final volume consisting of the 20 μl of column-cleaned, and concentrated, cDNA synthesis product; 8 μl of 5× terminal deoxynucleotidyltransferase buffer (GIBCO-BRL, Gaithersburg, MD); 8 μl of sterile deionized H_2O, 2 μl of 10 mM dATPs (Perkin–Elmer Cetus, Norwalk, CT); and 30 units (2 μl) of terminal deoxynucleotidyltransferase (GIBCO-BRL). The mixture is incubated at 37°C for 60 min and terminated by heating for 15 min at 65°C. The tailed product is diluted 1 : 10 with sterile water for subsequent use in the first PCR.

First PCR

The first PCR is conducted using the AmpliWax PCR Gem 100 method (Perkin–Elmer Cetus). The lower layer consists of 1.25 μl of 10× PCR buffer II (Perkin–Elmer Cetus), 3 μl of $MgCl_2$ (25 mM), 8 μl of dNTPs mixture (1.25 mM in each dNTP), and 20 pmol of each primer (the lock-docking primer and primer E). An AmpliWax PCR Gem tablet is added and melted at 80°C for 5 min. After the wax is allowed to set, an upper layer is added consisting of 30 μl of deionized H_2O, 5 μl of 10× PCR buffer II (Perkin–Elmer Cetus), 0.5 μl AmpliTaq polymerase (Perkin–Elmer Cetus), and 1 μl of the poly(A) tailed product. Thermocycling conditions are as follows: one round at 94°C for 5 min, 37°C for 1 min, and 72°C for 2 min; 24 rounds at 94°C for 1 min, 37°C for 30 sec, and 72°C for 1 min. The extension time on the final cycle is increased to 10 min. In each cycle, a slow ramp time of 1 min is programmed between the annealing and extension steps to minimize detachment of the lock-docking primer. All cycling is done on a programmable DNA thermocycler (Perkin–Elmer Cetus).

Second PCR

The second PCR protocol is identical to the touchdown PCR protocol described for amplification of the 3′ end except for the primers and template. In this reaction the Tmcs primer is paired with primer F (GCTACGAAGAC-CAAGATAGC), a second canine-specific Glut3 primer homologous to human Glut3 bases 1347–1366. Note that primer F is internal to primer E. The template is 1 μl of the unprocessed PCR obtained with primer E and the lock-docking primer. The predicted size of a 5′ end product for canine Glut3 obtained with primers F/Tmcs is approximately 1400 base pairs.

Results of Search for 5′ End of Glut3

Two discrete products were generated (Fig. 6) for the 5′ end of canine brain cortex Glut3. On electrophoretic analysis, the sizes of the major and minor products were approximately 650 and 1350 base pairs, respectively. Both PCR products, on direct sequencing, were shown to originate from the 5′ end of Glut3. The 650-base pair product represents a section of sequence that originated entirely from the coding region (comparable to bases 716–1366 in human Glut3). A portion of sequence of the 1350-base pair product, showing the ATG start codon, is shown in Fig. 7.

Discussion of 3′ and 5′ End Amplifications

Messenger RNAs of eukaryotic cells normally have 3′ ends that are polyadenylated in a range from 90 to 300 bases in length (9). In PCR-based approaches to amplification of these transcripts an oligo(dT) primer is often used to prime the synthesis of cDNA. However, annealing may occur anywhere along the poly(A) tail and lead to a subsequent population of heterogeneously sized PCR products. To circumvent this problem and to generate homogeneously sized PCR transcripts a primer has been developed that selectively anneals at the junction of the poly(A) tail and gene-specific sequence. This so-called lock-docking primer leads to the formation of a discrete, homogeneously sized population of product.

The lock-docking primer system enabled the PCR amplification of discrete cDNA segments for the 3′ ends of both Glut3 and Glut1. Evidence that the lock-docking primer annealed to the poly(A)$^+$ RNA at the junction of gene-specific sequence and polyadenylation was demonstrated by the production of discrete products. Confirmation of the identity of the product was shown by independent amplifications using internal nested primers with cDNA tem-

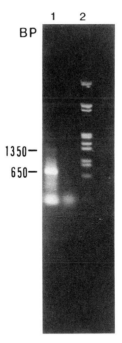

FIG. 6 Electrophoretic analysis of 5' end PCR products of canine brain cortex Glut3. Primer F and the Tmcs primer are described under Methods for Amplification of 5' Ends and Methods for Amplification of 3' Ends, respectively. The template used was 1 μl of the product from the first PCR, as described. Lane 1: The 1350 and 650 base pair products obtained with primer F in conjunction with the Tmcs primer. Lane 2: DNA standards (see Fig. 3).

plates. This lock-docking primer system has also been successfully applied with primers specific for other transcripts including glucose transporters and two other unrelated poly(A)$^+$ RNAs (data not shown).

The PCR for the 3' end of Glut3 in canine brain cortex generated a 2400-base pair product, as predicted. The use of a gene-specific, heminested primer for Glut3, when paired with the Tmcs primer, yielded the predetermined 40-base pair smaller product. Both products were sequenced directly and identified, on the basis of comparison to the known sequences of human and mouse Glut3 (6, 10), as having been amplified from the 3' ends of canine brain cortex Glut3.

Similarly, the PCR generated discrete products from the 3' end of canine brain cortex Glut1. Primer pairs C/Tmcs and D/Tmcs yielded the predicted and predetermined size products of 1025 and 1005 base pairs, respectively.

G A T C

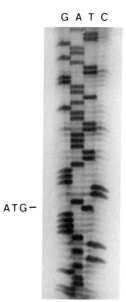

ATG—

FIG. 7   Sequence of a portion of the 5′ end of canine cortex Glut3 obtained from the 1350-base pair Glut3 PCR product. Reading from top to bottom (5′ to 3′): a portion of the 5′ untranslated region, the ATG start codon, and the first 13 bases at the 5′ end of the internal portion of canine brain cortex Glut3. A canine-specific Glut3 primer located at bases 292-312 (when compared to human) was used to obtain this sequence.

These PCR products were also directly sequenced and identified as having originated from the 3′ ends of canine brain cortex Glut1.

The 5′ end of the Glut3 transcript was amplified with the lock-docking system and yielded a predicted PCR product of approximately 1350 base pairs. The identity of this product was independently confirmed by the use of a heminested primer (data not shown). A second product of smaller size (650 base pairs) was also observed. Although both PCR products have been sequenced and shown to be overlapping 5′ end products of canine brain cortex Glut3, the reason for this is not yet known. Others have also observed this phenomenon of two products when seeking to amplify a 5′ end transcript (11).

Optimization of cDNA synthesis for the 5′ end may be required in individual circumstances. A heat-stable reverse transcriptase, such as rTth DNA polymerase (Perkin–Elmer Cetus) may be employed. The temperature at which this enzyme functions allows for denaturation of the template and high stringency annealing of the primer.

The lock-docking system has other advantages. For example, when isolating 3' end products, the lock-docking primer system will differentiate products that are the result of multiple polyadenylation sites, or the result of alternative mRNA splicing. Alternatively, when seeking to isolate products that have originated from 5' ends of poly(A)$^+$ RNA, this system has the capability of finding the full-length 5' end. Thus, the lock-docking system has the potential to detect tissue and temporal specific variance of gene transcription.

PCR Search for New Gene-Family Members

Underlying Principles

A common strategy that is used when searching for new members of a gene family is to design a pair of consensus primers based on two highly conserved regions among known family members (12, 13). Two problems arise with this approach that can be addressed by using the lock-docking system to amplify 3' ends.

First, a common feature of many gene families is that the coding regions, where high conservation of sequences is found, are often of very nearly the same base pair length. This leads to PCR products that vary little in size and are difficult to separate electrophoretically. Consequently, cloning and screening steps are required to isolate individual products. However, the noncoding 3' ends of gene-family members may vary widely in length, such as occurs with the glucose transporter family (Fig. 8). The use of lock-docked cDNA as template enables the generation of discrete-sized PCR products for each differentiable length. These PCR products are electrophoretically separable through an agarose gel and can be retrieved and directly sequenced.

A second problem that arises when using two internal consensus primers is the lowered probability that both primers will successfully find the target. In the lock-docking system only one consensus-family-specific primer must find its desired binding site, the second primer (the Tmcs primer) is complementary to a known sequence. Thus, the design of a single consensus, upper-strand primer located near the 3' end of the coding region in a highly conserved region can be used with a greater probability of desired target amplification.

Methods for Amplification of 3' Ends of Family mRNAs

The 3' ends of glucose transporter family mRNAs have been amplified as detailed below.

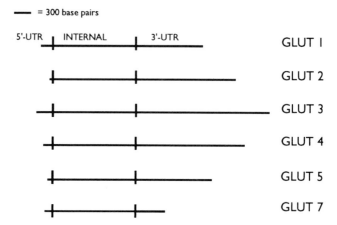

FIG. 8   Variations in mRNA lengths of human glucose transporter isoforms. Each line depicts a representative isoform mRNA, containing the 5' untranslated, coding, and 3' untranslated regions, as indicated. Sequence information was retrieved from EMBL (Glut7) and GenBank (Glut1-5). UTR, untranslated regions. Reproduced from ref. 3.

Isolation of mRNA and cDNA Synthesis

The methods for isolation of mRNA and for cDNA synthesis are as previously described above for the 3' end procedure.

Consensus Primer Design

The amino acid sequence (YF)KVPET (amino acids 448–455 in human Glut1) is highly conserved among members of the glucose transporter family as well as canine and different species (14). The canine-specific consensus primer is based entirely on nucleotide sequence in this region from Glut1 and Glut3, where W is A or T, and Y is T or C.

Consensus Primer: WCTTCAAAGTYCCTGAGACC

Amplification with this primer, in conjunction with the Tmcs primer, generates a 2350-base pair product for the 3' end of Glut3 and a 1030-base pair product for the 3' end of Glut1.

Touchdown PCR for Canine Brain Cortex Glucose Transporter Family Members

The PCR is run using the AmpliTaq Stoffel Fragment (Perkin–Elmer Cetus), and the touchdown thermocycling parameters are the same as those outlined for the isolation of 3' end products. Using an AmpliWax PCR Gem 100 protocol, a lower layer consists of 1.25 μl 10× Stoffel buffer (Perkin–Elmer Cetus), 6 μl of 25 mM MgCl$_2$, 10 μl of a dNTP solution that is 1.25 mM in each dNTP, 20 pmol of the glucose transporter family consensus primer, and 20 pmol of the Tmcs primer described above. An AmpliWax PCR Gem is added, and the tube is incubated at 80°C for 5 min and then cooled to room temperature. An upper layer is composed of 25 μl of sterile deionized H$_2$O, 5 μl of 10× Stoffel buffer, 10 units of AmpliTaq Stoffel Fragment, and 1 μl of a 1 : 10 dilution of canine brain cortex lock-docked cDNA (as described above). Final concentrations in the PCR reaction are 1.25× Stoffel buffer, 3 mM MgCl$_2$, and 250 mM in each dNTP.

Results of Glucose Transporter Family Search in Canine Brain

Five discrete products are observed after electrophoresis through an agarose gel and ethidium bromide staining (Fig. 9). These products are approximately 2350, 1425, 1375, 1030, and 830 base pairs in length. Note that the expected products for both Glut3 and Glut1, 2350 and 1030 base pairs, respectively, are observed.

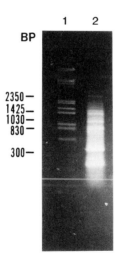

FIG. 9   Electrophoretic analysis of PCR products of a canine brain cortex glucose transporter family search. Lane 1: DNA standards (see Fig. 3). Lane 2: Products are observed at 830, 1030, 1375, 1425, and 2350 base pairs. The products at 1030 and 2350 base pairs are those expected for Glut1 and Glut3, respectively. Primers and template are described under Methods for Amplification of 3' Ends of Family mRNAs.

Discussion of Family-Member Searches

In a family search the amplified DNA will typically consist of multiple products. Each of these products needs to be identified and characterized. In our study, on electrophoretic analysis, a minimum of five potential glucose transporter 3' ends derived from canine brain cortex are observed. Based on the known transcript lengths of canine Glut1 and Glut3, the products at 1030 and 2350 base pairs are tentatively identified as Glut1 and Glut3, respectively. The remaining three products, at 830, 1375, and 1425 base pairs, require further characterization. They may be Glut2, Glut4, Glut5, Glut7, or unknown glucose transporter homologs. Or they may have resulted from alternative polyadenylation sites for any of the glucose transporters. In particular, an 830-base pair product was occasionally observed in amplification of the 3' end of canine Glut3 (data not shown). Following analysis, this product was identified as resulting from the use of an alternative polyadenylation site for canine Glut3.

A search has also been performed on canine cDNA templates produced from kidney, intestine, and brain microvessel tissues. The approximate expected lengths of 3' ends for the glucose transporters that are known to be expressed in these tissues are observed (3).

The Stoffel fragment was chosen for this 3' amplification of family members as it has optimal activity over a broader range of magnesium ion concentrations than AmpliTaq DNA polymerase. Therefore, the Stoffel fragment is more likely to amplify different-sized products simultaneously. The Stoffel fragment is also more thermostable than AmpliTaq DNA polymerase and thus higher denaturation temperatures are permitted, if desired (15, 16).

Acknowledgments

This work was supported by grants from the National Institutes of Health (NS-27229, LRD) and the American Diabetes Association, Minnesota Affiliate (WLS and LRD).

References

1. R. Jain, R. Gomer, and J. Murtagh, Jr., *BioTechniques* **12,** 58 (1992).
2. N. Borson, W. Salo, and L. Drewes, *PCR Methods Appl.* **2,** 144 (1992).
3. N. Borson, W. Salo, and L. Drewes, *in* "Frontiers in Cerebral Vascular Biology: Transport and Its Regulation" (L. R. Drewes and A. L. Betz, eds.), p. 19. Plenum, New York, 1993.
4. M. A. Frohman, *in* "PCR Protocols: A Guide to Methods and Applications"

(M. A. Innis, D. H. Gelfand, J. J. Sninsky, and T. J. White, eds.), p. 28. Academic Press, San Diego, 1990.

5. R. H. Don, P. T. Cox, B. J. Wainwright, K. Baker, and J. S. Mattick, *Nucleic Acids Res.* **19,** 4008 (1991).

6. T. Kayano, H. Fukumoto, R. L. Eddy, Y. Fan, M. G. Byers, T. B. Shows, and G. I. Bell, *J. Biol. Chem.* **263,** 15245 (1988).

7. K. Schwarz, T. Hansen-Hagge, and C. Bartram, *Nucleic Acids Res.* **18,** 1079 (1990).

8. M. Mueckler, C. Caruso, S. A. Baldwin, M. Panico, I. Blench, H. R. Morris, W. J. Allard, G. E. Lienhard, and H. F. Lodish, *Science* **299,** 941 (1985).

9. E. J. Baker, *in* "Control of Messenger RNA Stability" (J. G. Belasco, ed), p. 368. Academic Press, Boston, 1993.

10. S. Nagamatsu, J. M. Kornhauser, C. F. Burant, S. Seino, K. E. Mayo, and G. I. Bell, *J. Biol. Chem.* **267,** 467 (1992).

11. N. S. Templeton, E. Urcelay, and B. Safer, *BioTechniques* **15,** 48 (1993).

12. M. R. Al-Ubaidi, S. J. Pittler, M. S. Champagne, J. T. Triantafyllos, J. F. McGinnis, and W. Baehr, *J. Biol. Chem.* **265,** 20563 (1990).

13. T. Compton *in* "PCR Protocols: A Guide to Methods and Applications" (M. A. Innis, D. H. Gelfand, J. J. Sninsky, and T. J. White, eds.), p. 39–53. Academic Press, San Diego, 1990.

14. C. F. Burant, et al., *Recent Prog. Horm. Res.* **47,** 349 (1991).

15. F. Bárány, *PCR Methods Appl.* **1,** 5 (1991).

16. D. H. Gelfand and S. Stoffel, Roche Molecular Systems, personal communication to Perkin-Elmer, Norwalk, CT (1988).

[5] Single-Cell cDNA-PCR

Benedikt L. Ziegler, Christa P. Lamping, Stefan J. Thoma,
Christian A. Thomas, and Theodor M. Fliedner

Introduction

Conventional approaches to the analysis of gene expression at the transcriptional level involve techniques such as RNA blot analysis and nuclease protection analysis. The analysis of gene expression in small numbers of cells is extremely difficult if not impossible when using these techniques. The introduction of molecular techniques has led to a substantial increase in the sensitivity of the analysis of gene expression. The polymerase chain reaction (PCR) represents a powerful tool to amplify very small quantities of DNA or cDNA synthesized from RNA, i.e., cDNA-PCR, RNA-PCR, or RT-PCR, derived from limited numbers of cells (1–3). To determine the mRNA phenotype of cells by cDNA-PCR two oligonucleotide primers which can recognize the (+)-strand and the (−)-strand of the target gene are required. The target sequence is amplified exponentially by repeated cycles of denaturation, primer annealing, and primer extension in the presence of thermostable DNA polymerase (4). Analysis of the mRNA phenotype of a small number of cells by cDNA-PCR requires the isolation of sufficient quantities of RNA. This approach is hampered by the fact that standard protocols for the isolation of RNA cannot be applied. Therefore, techniques scaled down for the isolation of small amounts of RNA such as the micro-adapted guanidine thiocyanate (GuSCN)/CsCl gradient centrifugation (3) and protocols for the direct isolation of poly(A) RNA from cellular lysates (5) have been developed. Analysis of mRNA by cDNA-PCR often is obscured by contaminating genomic DNA. To distinguish PCR products generated from cDNA from those derived from genomic DNA, primers are selected that recognize two different exons of the same gene. Hence, in the presence of cDNA and genomic DNA, two PCR products are detectable, one smaller PCR product that corresponds to the spliced mRNA and a larger product derived from genomic DNA. However, this approach is not always possible. The cDNA sequence, but not the genomic sequence, is known for the majority of genes. In this situation, a selected pair of primers may recognize a single exon of the target gene generating one PCR product from both mRNA and genomic DNA. Furthermore, selection of primers which can distinguish between RNA and genomic DNA is not possible if the gene of interest does

Methods in Neurosciences, Volume 26

not possess any introns (e.g., bacteria or proviruses). For these reasons DNase treatment of the RNA prior to cDNA-PCR is required in order to detect unambiguously the RNA transcripts.

Here, we describe microadapted techniques to isolate mRNA or total RNA from only a single cell. The isolated mRNA is directly processed for cDNA-PCR whereas the total RNA is treated with DNase I to remove contaminating genomic DNA. The DNase I-treated total RNA is reverse-transcribed into cDNA and then used for cDNA-PCR analysis. Our techniques allow the efficient analysis of mRNA expression in single cells or small numbers of cells.

Materials and Reagents

Moloney murine leukemia virus (M-MLV) reverse transcriptase (Super-Script RNase H$^-$, 200 units/μl) (GIBCO BRL, Life Technologies, Gaithersburg, MD).

AmpliTaq DNA polymerase (5 units/μl) (Perkin–Elmer Cetus, Norwalk, CT).

DNase I immobilized on matrix G3m (25 μg DNase I corresponding to 88 Kunitz units/reaction column) (MoBiTec, Göttingen, Germany).

Recombinant RNasin ribonuclease inhibitor (40 units/μl) (Serva/Promega, Heidelberg, Germany). *Escherichia coli* rRNA (Boehringer-Mannheim, Germany).

M-MLV reverse transcriptase buffer (5×): 250 mM Tris–HCl (pH 8.3), 375 mM KCl, 15 mM MgCl$_2$, 50 mM dithiothreitol (DTT).

PCR buffer (10×): 100 mM Tris–HCl (pH 8.3), 500 mM KCl, 15 to 50 mM MgCl$_2$, 0.01% gelatin.

PCR dNTP mix: 10 mM dATP, 10 mM dCTP, 10 mM dGTP, 10 mM dTTP in distilled H$_2$O (Pharmacia, Piscataway, NJ).

DNase I reaction buffer: 20 mM Tris–HCl (pH 7.5), 5 mM MnCl$_2$.

Lysis buffer for isolation of total RNA: 4 M guanidine isothiocyanate (GuSCN), 25 mM sodium citrate (pH 5.0), 0.5% (w/v) sodium lauroyl sarcosinate, 0.14 M 2-mercaptoethanol, 0.1% (v/v) antifoam A (Sigma St. Louis, MO, A-5758).

5.7 M CsCl/25 mM sodium citrate (pH 5.0).

PolyATtract System 1000 (Serva/Promega, Heidelberg, Germany) for the isolation of poly(A) RNA provided by the manufacturer with GuSCN lysis buffer (4 M guanidine thiocyanate, 25 mM sodium citrate, pH 7.1) 2-mercaptoethanol (2%), dilution buffer [10 mM Tris–HCl, pH 7.6, 1 mM EDTA, 90 mM sodium citrate, 0.9 M NaCl, 0.25% sodium dodecyl sulfate (SDS)], biotinylated oligo(dT) (50 pmol/μl),

SSC 0.5× solution (75 mM NaCl, 7.5 mM sodium citrate), streptavidin Magne-Sphere paramagnetic particles (SA-PMP), and magnetic separation stand.

3 M potassium acetate (pH 5.2).

Oligo(dT)$_{12-18}$ (0.5 μg/ul) (Pharmacia).

Diethyl pyrocarbonate (DEPC)-treated distilled H$_2$O.

All reagents and RNA are prepared under laminar flow hoods. Pre-PCR and post-PCR areas are strictly segregated (6). Buffers and reagents are DEPC-treated with the exception of Tris–HCl and reagents provided by the manufacturers. To eliminate possible contamination, buffers and reagents used for cDNA synthesis and PCR are pretreated with 254 and 300 nm ultraviolet light (7). Screw cap tubes are used for all reactions with RNA, cDNA, and PCR products. Before opening, tubes are briefly centrifuged to prevent formation of aerosols. Disposable gloves are worn and frequently changed during all experiments.

Methods

Isolation of Total RNA from Single/Low Numbers of Cells

Single cells are obtained conveniently using a fluorescence-activated cell sorter equipped with an automatic cell deposition unit. Cultured cells are first diluted and then individual cells collected under microscopic visualization using a siliconized Pasteur pipette prefilled with a few microliters of buffer. The single cell is then transferred to 100 μl of GuSCN lysis buffer containing 20 μg *Escherichia coli* rRNA as carrier, thoroughly vortexed, and layered on top of a 100-μl 5.7 M CsCl cushion. Samples in DEPC-treated, siliconized 0.3-ml polyallomer tubes are then centrifuged for 6 hr at 45,000 rpm at 20°C in a Sorvall TST 60.4 swinging bucket rotor (DuPont, Bad Homburg, Germany) using buckets equipped with Delrin adaptors. Other ultracentrifuges (e.g., table-top centrifuges) and swinging bucket rotors may be used as well as long as they provide the required g force and can fit small-sized tubes. We do not use fixed angle rotors since these cause deposition of the RNA along the tube wall where it comes into contact with the cell lysate. Some batches of commercially available *E. coli* rRNA may contain contaminating *E. coli* DNA. Therefore, it is recommended that *E. coli* rRNA be treated with DNase followed by phenol extraction using standard procedures (8). After ultracentrifugation of the sample, the supernatant containing proteins and DNA is carefully removed to avoid mixing with the invisible RNA pellet. The tube is turned upside down for 2 min. The bottom of the tube containing the RNA pellet is then cut off with a razor blade and the RNA is dissolved in 33 μl of DEPC-treated distilled H_2O for 2 min on ice and transferred to an Eppendorf tube. This step is repeated twice. Then, 0.1 volume of 3 M potassium acetate (pH 5.2) and 2.5 volumes of 100% ethanol are added and the RNA is allowed to precipitate overnight at $-20°C$. The precipitate is pelleted at 52,000 g at 0°C for 30 min using a Biofuge 28RS table-top centrifuge (Heraeus, Hanau, Germany), washed in 70% ethanol ($-20°C$), vacuum-dried, dissolved in an appropriate buffer or distilled H_2O, and further processed for treatment with immobilized DNase I or directly used for cDNA-PCR. The overnight precipitation of the RNA and centrifugation at high speed are crucial steps to yield RNA from single or low numbers of cells. In our case, this precipitation/centrifugation procedure is superior to short precipitation times (e.g., 2–3 hr) and centrifugation at lower g forces (e.g., 12,000–20,000 g) which are achieved by commonly used bench-top centrifuges. In addition, it must be noted that extensive vacuum drying of RNA will cause difficulties in dissolving the RNA which may subsequently hinder an efficient cDNA synthesis.

Isolation of Poly(A) RNA from Single/Low Numbers of Cells by Biotinylated Oligo(dT) and Streptavidin-Conjugated Paramagnetic Particles

Several kits designed for the isolation of poly(A) RNA from small numbers of cells are commercially available but have not been tested at the level of a few cells, i.e., cell number <100. We have scaled down the PolyATtract System 1000 (Serva/Promega) to isolate mRNA from the equivalent of single cells. Similar products from other suppliers may also work at the single-cell level but have not yet been tested. The mRNA isolation was performed with slight modifications as recommended by the manufacturer. Cells are transferred to 25 μl GuSCN lysis buffer containing 2% 2-mercaptoethanol (2-ME) in a 1.5-ml polypropylene tube and immediately vortexed thoroughly for 1 min. Fifty microliters of dilution buffer preheated to 70°C, containing 1% 2-ME and 1 μl of a 1:10 dilution of 50 pmol/μl biotinylated oligo(dT) stock solution is added. After mixing, the diluted homogenate is incubated at 70°C for 5 min and then centrifuged at 12,000 g for 15 min at room temperature. This step removes cell debris and precipitated proteins. During centrifugation, 100 μl of resuspended SA-PMP (1 mg/ml) in storage solution is transferred to a 1.5-ml tube and placed into a magnetic stand. After 2 min, the storage buffer is removed and the SA-PMPs are washed three times with 0.5× SSC using magnetic separation for 2 min each and finally resuspended in 100 μl 0.5× SSC. When the centrifugation is completed, the supernatant containing poly(A) RNA hyridized to biotinylated oligo(dT) is transferred to a 1.5-ml tube containing 50 μl of SA-PMPs in 0.5× SSC, mixed, and incubated for 5 min at room temperature to allow binding of streptavidin to biotin. The tube is then placed into the magnetic separation device for 2 min and the supernatant is pipetted off which is again incubated with 50 μl SA-PMPs. The first-step SA-PMPs are immediately resuspended in 100 μl of 0.5× SSC and combined with the second-step SA-PMPs. The SA-PMPs are then washed three times each with 200 μl 0.5× SSC using magnetic separation. After complete removal of 0.5 × SSC, particles are resuspended in 50 μl of DEPC-treated distilled H_2O and placed into a magnetic stand for 2 min. The supernatant containing the dissociated mRNA is transferred to a 1.5-ml tube and placed on ice immediately. The remaining SA-PMPs are resuspended for a second time with 50 μl of DEPC-treated distilled H_2O and both supernatants combined. At this step the supernatants may be quick-spun to pellet any remaining SA-PMPs. The supernatant (100 μl) containing the mRNA is precipitated with 10 μl of 3 M potassium acetate and 250 μl of 100% ethanol (-20°C) and stored at -20°C overnight. The mRNA is then pelleted at 52,000 g for 30 min at 0°C, washed with 70% ethanol (-20°C), vacuum-dried, and further processed for cDNA-PCR. We could not detect amplification products from mRNAs hybridized to biotinylated oligo(dT) and bound to SA-PMPs which were directly processed for cDNA-PCR. This may be due to interference of biotinylated oligo(dT)-SA-PMP with the reverse transcription step and/or the polymerase chain reaction. Therefore, the mRNA elution from SA-PMPs using distilled H_2O and removal of SA-PMPs are necessary steps to allow an efficient cDNA-PCR.

Treatment of Total RNA Derived from Single Cells by Immobilized DNase I

The commercially available immobilized DNAse I reaction columns used (MoBiTec GmbH) containing 25 μg of DNase I, degrade 100 μg of DNA in 1 min. When RNA derived from a single cell is passed through these columns, cDNA-PCR products are not detectable which suggests loss of material. Therefore, the volume of G3m matrix to which the DNase I is cross-linked must be reduced. Empty reaction columns including bottom polyethylene filters (pore size 35 μm) are available from the same supplier. To decrease the matrix volume, the G3m matrix in storage buffer obtained from a ready-to-use column is gently resuspended and an aliquot of the slurry corresponding to 1 μg of DNase I is loaded onto an empty reaction column including bottom filters with a pore size of 35 μm. Depending on the amount of RNA, i.e., 1–1000 cells, loaded onto the column, the quantity of immobilized DNase I may be scaled up or down (e.g., 0.5–5 μg per column). The reaction column is briefly spun to remove the storage buffer and equilibrated with 2 ml DNase I reaction buffer (20 mM Tris–HCl, pH 7.5; 5 mM MnCl$_2$) which is gently pressed through the column using a syringe. Finally, the column is briefly centrifuged. Total RNA obtained from single cells dissolved in 10 μl DNase I reaction buffer is then loaded onto the column and allowed to incubate for 5 min at room temperature. We have tested this procedure for RNA isolated from 1–1000 cells. The RNA is then briefly centrifuged out of the column (2 sec using a bench-top centrifuge) and the eluate recycled three to eight times to achieve complete digestion. Two final washes of the column using 10 μl DNase I reaction buffer each are performed and the eluates combined. To prevent degradation of RNA, it is necessary to perform the DNase treatment as quickly as possible. After DNase I treatment, the RNA is precipitated with 0.1 volume of potassium acetate and 2.5 volumes of 100% ethanol (−20°C), washed in 70% ethanol (−20°C), dried, and processed further for cDNA-PCR. Reaction columns containing immobilized DNase I from other commercial suppliers may also work well for the described procedure but have not been tested in our laboratories. We have not detected bleeding out of the used reaction columns using ^{32}P-labeled control DNA which was incubated with DNase I reaction buffer eluted from the columns. However, the possibility of DNase I leaching off the column should always be considered if cDNA-PCR products are not obtained.

As an alternative to treatment with immobilized DNase I, we have performed standard DNase digestions of DNA-contaminated total RNA prepared from single cells. After phenol extraction and ethanol precipitation cDNA-PCR products were not detectable in single cells, which suggests that amplifiable material was lost during standard DNase treatment.

Reverse Transcription and PCR

Pellets of total RNA, poly(A) RNA, or DNase I-treated total RNA are dissolved in 10 μl reverse transcription buffer to synthesize first-strand cDNA.

1. To a 1.5-ml screw cap tube containing the RNA pellet add:
   DEPC-treated distilled H$_2$O   2.5 μl
   Oligo(dT)$_{12-18}$ (0.5 μg/μl)   1 μl
   and incubate at 70°C for 10 min to denature the RNA.
2. Briefly centrifuge, quick chill on ice, and add
   DTT (0.1 M)   1 μl

RNasin (40 units/μl) freshly 1:5 diluted with distilled H_2O	2 μl
Reverse trancriptase buffer (5×)	2 μl
dNTP mix (10 mM)	0.5 μl
M-MLV H$^-$ reverse transcriptase (200 units/μl)	1 μl
diluted 1:2 with distilled H_2O	

3. Gently mix the reaction, briefly centrifuge, and incubate at 42°C (or 45°C) for 60 min. The final concentration of the cDNA synthesis reaction in a volume of 10 μl is 50 mM Tris–HCl (pH 8.3), 75 mM KCl, 3 mM MgCl$_2$, 10 mM DTT, 500 μM of each dNTP containing 100 units M-MLV H$^-$ RTase, 16 units RNasin, and 0.5 μg oligo(dT).

If mRNA secondary structures interfere with the extension of the oligo(dT), cDNA synthesis can then be performed at higher reaction temperatures, i.e., 45°C using M-MLV H$^-$ reverse transcriptase. Other reverse transcriptases such as avian myeloblastosis virus (AMV) may work as well. In this case, sodium pyrophosphate should be added which substantially increases the yield of first-strand cDNA. Furthermore, thermostable reverse transcriptases may be used but they have not been tested in our laboratories. To avoid additional precipitation steps, use reverse transcriptases which are active in buffers which are compatible with the PCR. When several RNA samples are processed in parallel prepare two master mixes, one containing distilled H_2O and oligo(dT) and the second containing the other reagents including reverse transcriptase.

The number of precipitation steps should be minimized throughout the single-cell cDNA-PCR procedure in order to avoid loss of material.

Without precipitation the entire cDNA synthesis reaction or aliquots thereof are processed further for PCR. We usually add 2.5 μl of the cDNA synthesis product directly to the prepared 50 μl PCR. This increases slightly the molarity of the constituents in the final PCR but does not exhibit inhibitory effects on the reaction. A selective ethanol precipitation may be required when the exact molarity of individual constituents in the final PCR is of critical importance or when oligo(dT) primers and nucleotides need to be removed from the cDNA synthesis reaction (e.g., for tailing of the 3' end of the first-strand cDNA). In this case 5 μl of 7.5 M ammonium acetate and 15 μl of 100% ethanol (−20°C) are added to a 10-μl reverse transcriptase reaction. After precipitation overnight at −20°C the sample is centrifuged at 52,000 g at 0°C for 30 min, washed in 70% ethanol, and dried, and the PCR buffer is added directly to the tube. In contrast to centrifugation using Centricon 30 spin dialysis columns (Amicon, Danvers, MA) or related products which work well if larger quantities of material (e.g., cDNA or PCR products) are used, the selective precipitation allows the recovery of cDNA derived from single cells while oligonucleotides are not precipitated.

4. During cDNA synthesis the PCR buffer must be prepared (usually master mixes are used). For a 50-μl PCR add the following to a 1.5-ml screw cap tube:

PCR buffer (10×) containing 15($-$50) mM MgCl$_2$	5 μl
Upstream sequence-specific primer (0.5–10 μM)	2.5 μl
Downstream sequence-specific primer (0.5–10 μM)	2.5 μl
dNTP mix (10 mM)	1 μl
Distilled H$_2$O	36.5 μl
cDNA synthesis product	2.5 μl

Add 80 μl of light white mineral oil (Sigma, M-5904) to the tube and briefly centrifuge.

5. Place the tube into a thermal cycler and denature at 93°C for 7 min. At the end of the denaturation step, while the reaction is still at 93°C, add 2.5 μl of AmpliTaq polymerase (5 units/μl) diluted 1 : 10 with 1× PCR buffer. The *Taq* polymerase used for single-cell cDNA-PCR should always be kept at -20°C.

6. Perform at least 35–45 PCR cycles with denaturation at 91–95°C for 45–90 sec, annealing at 48–63°C for 45–120 sec, and extension at 72°C for >45 sec. Cycling conditions including the number of cycles depend largely on the type of target cDNA, the specificity of primers, and the length of the amplified sequence. The optimized cycling and reaction conditions need to be determined empirically for each target sequence and pair of primers. This specifically includes MgCl$_2$ concentrations ranging from 1.5 to 5 mM and the concentration of primers and dNTPs, as well as the pH (range 8.3–8.8) of the PCR. When a new pair of primers is tested, we use RNA isolated from 1000 cells and set up the following cycling profile for a PCR (35 cycles) containing MgCl$_2$ in the range from 1.5 to 5 mM in 0.5 increments: 90 sec, 93°C; 120 sec, 50–62°C (2°C steps); 120 sec, 72°C. After the optimal annealing temperature is determined we decrease gradually the denaturation and annealing time. Finally, the optimal extension time is determined. The cDNA derived from 1000 cells is then diluted serially and processed for PCR sensitivity testing using optimized conditions. The addition of cosolvents can be considered (9) to further enhance the cDNA-PCR sensitivity.

7. Load a 10-μl aliquot of the PCR onto a 2% (w/v) NuSieve GTG:1% (w/v) LE agarose gel (FMC, Rockland, ME) for small PCR products (e.g., < 800 bp) and stain with ethidium bromide. Transfer the PCR products onto membranes such as Genescreen Plus membranes (DuPont/NEN, Hamburg, Germany) and hybridize with ^{32}P-labeled probes and autoradiograph

on Kodak XAR X-ray films (Kodak, Rochester, NY) using standard techniques (8).

Results and Discussion

We describe a method to analyze gene expression efficiently at the transcriptional level by cDNA-PCR following isolation of total or poly(A) RNA from a single cell (Figs. 1 and 2) or small numbers of cells. When poly(A) RNA is isolated with SA-PMPs no genomic DNA can be detected as determined by subsequent cDNA-PCR by using primers spanning one intron (Fig. 2,

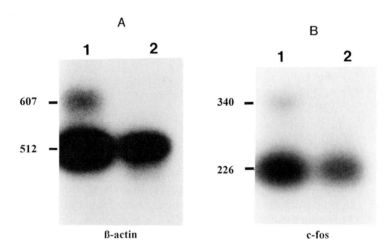

FIG. 1   Hybridization of cDNA-PCR products derived from single macrophages with ^{32}P-labeled β-actin (A) and c-*fos* (B) oligonucleotide probes. Total RNA from single cells was either not DNase-treated (A and B, lanes 1) or was DNase-treated (A and B, lanes 2), RNA was reverse-transcribed, and the cDNA product was amplified by cDNA-PCR. Ten microliters of the final PCR product was electrophoresed on an agarose gel, transferred to Genescreen Plus membranes, and hybridized with ^{32}P-labeled β-actin or c-*fos* oligonucleotide probes. Location of primers in the nucleotide sequence was β-actin, GenBank locus HUMACCYBA: positions 2096–2114; 5′ TCATGTTTGAGACCTTCAA 3′ for exon 4 and 2702–2684; 5′ GTCTTTGCGGATG-TCCACG 3′ for exon 5; and c-*fos*, GenBank locus HUMFOS: positions 2531–2550; 5′ ATGCCGCAACCGGAGGAGGG 3′ for exon 3 and 2870–2851; 5′ TGGCAGGCC-CCCAGTCAGAT 3′ for exon 4. Cycling conditions were as follows: β-actin, 90 sec, 93°C; 120 sec, 50°C; 120 sec, 72°C; and c-*fos* 60 sec 93°C; 60 sec, 60°C; 120 sec, 72°C. (Reprinted by permission of the publisher from Ziegler *et al.* (10). Copyright © 1992 by Eaton Publishing.)

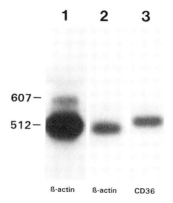

FIG. 2   Hybridization of cDNA-PCR products with ^{32}P-labeled β-actin (lanes 1 and 2) and CD36 (lane 3). Lane 1: Total RNA contaminated with genomic DNA isolated by GuSCN/CsCl centrifugation from 10 macrophages. Without DNase treatment total RNA was processed for cDNA-PCR. Ten microliters of the PCR was separated by agarose gel electrophoresis, transferred to Genescreen Plus membranes, and hybridized with ^{32}P-labeled β-actin oligonucleotide probes. Lane 2 and 3: Poly(A) RNA was isolated from the equivalent of a single cell using the PolyATract System 1000. Without DNase treatment the poly(A) RNA was reverse-transcribed and the cDNA processed for PCR in separate reactions using primer pairs for CD36 and β-actin. Ten microliters of each PCR product was run on an agarose gel, transferred to Genescreen Plus membranes, and hybridized with ^{32}P-labeled β-actin (lane 2) or CD36 (lane 3) oligonucleotide probes. Location of primers in the nucleotide sequence was CD36, GenBank locus HUMANTCD36: positions 431–450; 5' AGGAAGTGAT-GATGAACAGC 3' and 971–952; 5' AATGAGGCTGCATCTGTACC 3'; and β-actin, see legend for Fig. 1. Cycling conditions for CD36 were as follows: 90 sec, 93°C; 120 sec, 60°C; 120 sec, 72°C.

lane 2). This isolation procedure may, therefore, eliminate the need for DNase treatment prior to cDNA-PCR. However, nonspecific binding of SA-PMPs or binding of biotinylated oligo(dT) to single-stranded genomic DNA containing stretches of poly(A) may occur. In such a case, DNA will copurify with the poly(A) RNA. Therefore, a control, i.e., primers which recognize two different exons of the same gene separated by one or more introns, should be included in the cDNA-PCR to detect genomic DNA. As an alternative to poly(A) RNA isolation, total RNA can be isolated from single cells and processed for cDNA-PCR (3). We noted in some samples that genomic DNA copurifies with the total RNA (Figs. 1A and 1B, lanes 1). This requires the DNase treatment of total RNA samples prior to cDNA synthesis in order to obtain meaningful cDNA-PCR results (10) when primers which can distinguish between cDNA and genomic DNA are unavailable. The isolation procedure for total RNA has two disadvantages: First, it requires the addition of carrier (e.g., rRNA) (3) which may not be neutral in subsequent enzymatic reactions (e.g., tailing reactions, cloning of the PCR product) (11). Second, it requires a time-consuming DNase treatment during which the RNA is prone to degradation. However, after DNase treatment we did not observe a substantial decrease in the intensity of PCR signals derived from single cells (Figs. 1A and 1B, lanes 2).

The successful amplification of genes in single cells largely depends on the quality of the primers used. To reduce the chance of primer binding to partially complementary sequences, we regularly perform a computer search for similarity between the query sequence and sequences stored in a data bank (e.g., GenBank). Furthermore, to avoid formation of primer dimers, primers should be checked against each other for complementarity and sequences with significant secondary structure should also be avoided. In some cases several primer pairs must be tested to allow the detection of a certain mRNA species in single cells. A higher initial concentration of *Taq* polymerase or addition of fresh enzyme after the first 30–45 cycles can increase the yield of cDNA-PCR product but may also lead to mispriming on nontarget sequences.

To determine the optimal conditions for PCR we start with cDNA derived from 1000 cells. After the optimal $MgCl_2$ concentration, pH, and cycling conditions have been established, the cDNA is diluted serially and the PCR is then performed. Alternatively, known quantities of cDNA (e.g., vector-derived or *in vitro* transcribed target RNA) are used for cDNA-PCR optimization.

Quantitative analysis of gene expression in single cells could theoretically be achieved by competitive PCR using the described protocol in combination with cRNA which is identical to the original RNA except for a deletion (12, 13) that does not affect binding of the PCR primers. The competitive cRNA is added in varying amounts to the original RNA prior to total RNA isolation or mRNA isolation with SA-PMPs. To monitor the efficiency of the DNase treatment, an internal control consisting of a double-stranded DNA sequence with ends identical with the RNA of interest recognized by the primers, but of different length, can be included. Alternatively, primers recognizing different exons of a gene can be used to monitor the efficiency of DNase treatment.

The procedures described here may represent an important step for the construction of cDNA libraries based on single or low numbers of cells (11, 14) which has been already achieved using a few cells (11). Particularly, the SA-PMP protocol which eliminates the addition of carrier rRNA or other procedures utilizing oligo(dT)–latex particles (15) appear to be applicable. For directional cloning of cDNA derived from a single cell, a modification of the 3' end of the first-strand cDNA (e.g., G tailing) followed by sequence-independent amplification may represent a promising approach. However, attempts to construct a cDNA library from a single cell have not yet been successful.

The cDNA-PCR of single cells or small numbers of cells has many applications in the field of neurobiology, developmental cell biology, experimental hematology, embryology, and related fields where the gene expression in rare cell populations is investigated. Which genes are expressed and how the gene expression is regulated or induced are central questions. However, conventional cDNA-PCR will not resolve whether genes are translated into their protein products. To answer this question, an alternative PCR-based technique such as the immuno-PCR (16) may be applied. The cDNA-PCR may also be applied to monitor cells which contaminate small numbers of highly purified populations (e.g., cells sorted by flow cytometry) using primers which recognize marker genes (e.g., transcripts of cell membrane antigens linked to differentiation) of cells which contaminate the sorted cell population (17). This is of critical importance in order to avoid false-positive cDNA-PCR signals when the gene repertoire of a "pure" cell population is investigated. Due to the sensitivity of the cDNA-PCR several transcripts can be detected in a single cell. This would allow both the reanalysis of the phenotype identified by flow cytometry at the transcriptional level and the analysis of genes of interest which are expressed in this cell.

Acknowledgments

This research project was supported by Grant InSan I 0590-V-3892 issued by the Ministry of Defense of the Federal Republic of Germany and the European Communities. We are grateful to Professor U. Reischl for critically proofreading the manuscript.

References

1. D. A. Rappolee, C. A. Brenner, R. Schultz, D. Mark, and Z. Werb, *Science* **241,** 1823 (1988).
2. C. A. Brenner, A. W. Tam, P. A. Nelson, E. G. Engleman, N. Suzuki, K. E. Fry, and J. W. Larrick, *BioTechniques* **7,** 1096 (1989).
3. D. A. Rappolee, A. Wang, D. Mark, and Z. Werb, *J. Cell. Biochem.* **39,** 1 (1989).
4. R. K. Saiki, D. H. Gelfand, S. Stoffel, S. J. Scharf, R. Higuchi, G. T. Horn, K. B. Mullis, and H. A. Erlich, *Science* **239,** 487 (1988).
5. J. Thompson, R. Solomon, M. Pellegrino, K. Sakai, M. Lewin, M. Feild, M. Castrovinci, L. Sacramone, and D. Gillespie, *Anal. Biochem.* **181,** 371 (1989).

6. S. Kwok and R. Higuchi, *Nature (London)* **339,** 237 (1989).
7. G. Sarkar and S. S. Sommer, *Nature (London)* **343,** 27 (1990).
8. J. Sambrook, E. F. Fritsch, and T. Maniatis, "Molecular Cloning: A Laboratory Manual," 2nd ed. Cold Spring Harbor Lab., Cold Spring Harbor, NY, 1989.
9. G. Sarkar, S. Kapelner, and S. S. Sommer, *Nucleic Acids Res.* **18,** 7465 (1990).
10. B. L. Ziegler, S. Thoma, C. A. Thomas, and C. Lamping, *BioTechniques* **13,** 726 (1992).
11. A. Belyavsky, T. Vinogradova, and K. Rajewski, *Nucleic Acids Res.* **17,** 2919 (1989).
12. A. M. Wang, M. V. Doyle, and D. F. Mark, *Proc. Natl. Acad. Sci. U.S.A.* **86,** 9717 (1989).
13. J. P. Vanden Heuvel, F. L. Tyson, and D. A. Bell, *BioTechniques* **14,** 395 (1993).
14. A. W. Tam, M. M. Smith, K. E. Fry, and J. Larrick, *Nucleic Acids Res.* **17,** 1269 (1989).
15. K. Kuribayashi-Ohta K, S. Tamatsukuri, M. Hikata, C. Miyamoto, and Y. Furuichi, *Biochim. Biophys. Acta* **1156,** 204 (1993).
16. T. Sano, C. L. Smith, and C. R. Cantor, *Science* **258,** 120 (1992).
17. S. J. Thoma, C. P. Lamping, and B. L. Ziegler, *Blood* **83,** 2103 (1994).

Section III

Gene Synthesis by PCR

[6] PCR-Mediated Synthesis of Chimeric Molecules

André Darveau, Alex Pelletier, and Josée Perreault

Introduction

Introduction of the polymerase chain reaction (PCR) has revolutionized molecular biology. Not only does it allow amplification and detection of an infinitesimal amount of DNA, it also facilitates and accelerates most of the steps involved in common techniques used in every laboratory dealing with molecular biology. Furthermore, it has opened the way to the development of new technologies.

Antibodies are naturally made by joining together at a molecular level components with different functions: the variable region at the amino terminus of the molecule is involved in the recognition of a given antigen by the antibody while the constant region at the carboxy-terminal end supports the effector functions of the antibody. However, it has become more prevalent to assist nature by manipulating *in vitro* immunoglobulin genes in order to create new reagents. In our laboratory, we routinely use PCR to facilitate the creation of chimeric molecules derived from antibodies. We present three examples of increasing complexity pertaining to immunoglobulin genes. Nevertheless, the approach that is described can be used for any proteins for which DNA is available (1).

Reagents and Materials

Hybridoma cell lines are prepared and grown in our laboratory using standard procedures. Deoxynucleotide triphosphates are from Pharmacia-LKB (Baie d'Urfe, Quebec). Oligonucleotides are synthesized by Oligos etc. (Wilsonville, OR) and used directly without further purification. Moloney leukemia virus (MLV) reverse transcriptase is purchased from GIBCO/BRL (Burlington, Ontario) and *Taq* DNA polymerase from Boehringer-Mannheim (Laval, Quebec). All PCRs are performed in a Perkin–Elmer Cetus (Norwalk, CT) DNA thermal cycler.

Methods in Neurosciences, Volume 26

Methods

RNA Preparation

Total RNA is prepared from the various hybridoma cell lines by the guanidinium isothiocyanate extraction procedure (2) and purified by centrifugation through a CsCl cushion (3).

cDNA Synthesis

RNA (1–5 μg) is directly added to a reaction mixture containing 1× PCR buffer (Tris–HCl, 10 mM; MgCl$_2$, 1.5 mM; KCl, 50 mM; pH 8.3), 1 mM of each dNTP, and 10 pmol of 3' primer together with 40 units of MLV reverse transcriptase. The reaction mixture is then incubated at 42°C for 1 hr.

Polymerase Chain Reaction

Polymerase chain reactions are carried out by adding 20 μl of cDNA synthesis reaction mixture to 8 μl of 10× PCR buffer, 50 pmol of each oligonucleotide primer, and 2.5 units of *Taq* polymerase in a final volume of 100 μl. Mineral oil is overlaid on top of the reaction mixtures to prevent evaporation during PCR. Reactions are performed according to the following parameters: denaturation at 94°C for 1 min, annealing at 45 or 50°C for 2 min, and elongation at 74°C for 1 min for 30 cycles. The last cycle is followed by a 10-min incubation at 72°C.

Gel Electrophoresis

Aliquots of PCRs are analyzed by agarose gel electrophoresis in 1× TBE buffer (100 mM Tris base, 83 mM boric acid, 1 mM EDTA) containing 5 μg/ml ethidium bromide.

Applications of PCR-Mediated Ligation

Linking Two Different DNA Fragments Together

Monoclonal antibodies produced by murine B cell hybridomas (4) are now routinely used in research and diagnosis. Altering the properties of a given antibody in order to improve its efficiency was difficult before recent advances in PCR technology which have provided tools to manipulate antibodies and to create new molecules adapted to very specific needs. The ability to produce genetically engineered antibodies has been greatly facilitated by the design of degenerate oligonucleotide primers (5–7) to be used in the PCR. This technology enables the rapid cloning of specific human and mouse immunoglobulin (Ig) variable (V) regions, a primordial step in antibody engineering. Following cloning, Ig V domains can be linked to various types of Ig constant (C) regions or even to other molecules to create a variety of chimeric antibodies with different effector functions. All these products can then be transferred in various expression systems in order to produce a large amount of material to be used for diagnostic or therapeutic purposes. The following procedure describes the amplification and linking of a humanized variable region prepared from the light chain of an Ig gene to a human kappa (κ) constant region.

The strategy that has been used to link both fragments is described in Fig. 1. The humanized version of the antibody variable region is prepared as described under Multiple DNA Fragment Exchange below using oligonucleo-

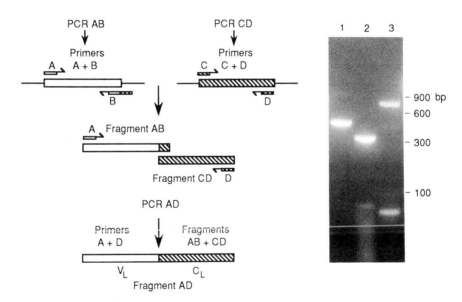

FIG. 1   Ligation of two different DNA fragments. Schema of the strategy is shown on the left-hand side. Kappa variable region is depicted by an open box and the constant region by a hatched box. The relative position of each primer is shown. Analysis of PCR fragments by gel electrophoresis is presented on the right-hand side. Lane 1, fragment AB; lane 2, fragment CD; lane 3, fragment AD.

tides A and B for the final amplification round. The human κ constant region is amplified using oligonucleotides C and D.

A: 5' GGG AAT TCA TGG ACA TG[A/G] [A/G][A/G][A/G/T]
   [C/T]CC [A/C/T][A/C/G]G [C/T][G/T]G A[C/G]C TT 3'
B: 5' CCA AGC TTC ATC AGA TGG CGG GAA GAT 3'
C: 5' ACT GTG GCT GCA CCA TCT GTC TTC 3'
D: 5' CTA ACA CTC TCC CCT GTT GAA GCT 3'

Oligonucleotide A is degenerate and is derived from a consensus sequence corresponding to a region coding for the leader peptide at the amino terminus of the κ chain. It allows the amplification of most of the human Ig κ variable regions (6). Equal volumes (1 μl) of each amplified fragment were mixed together and subjected to a second round of PCR using oligonucleotides A and D for the amplification. Both fragments overlap by 43 bp. Electrophoresis of PCR fragments shows the presence of single bands following amplification of the variable and constant regions (lanes 1 and 2, respectively). Similarly, ligation of both fragments in a single PCR reaction, using only a minor fraction of each fragment (1%) produced a single band of $\approx$800 bp (lane 3). In addition, sequencing of the resulting fragment has revealed that the ligation had been performed exactly as expected (data not shown). Cloning of the recombinant DNA into an expression vector and further expression in SP2/0, a myeloma cell line, confirmed the authenticity of the molecule, as detected by ELISA using an anti-κ chain antibody (data not shown). These data clearly demonstrate that by using the right combination of primers, it is possible to ligate together two different DNA fragments in a single PCR. However, the fragments do not have to be overlapping and can be linked through the addition of an exogenous linker as described in the example below.

Joining DNA Fragments through the Addition of a Linker

The antibody V region is sufficient by itself to recognize a given antigen. The C domain can be completely removed and replaced by unrelated peptides to introduce new properties to the antibody molecule (8, 9). In that regard, in order to simplify antibody engineering, V_L and V_H domains can be incorporated into a single-chain Fv protein (scFv) in which V_L and V_H are linked together via a specific linker (10, 11). The scFv can be further engineered into fusion proteins, combining antigen specificity of the scFv with the effector functions of the fusion partner. The addition of specific tags to the scFv can also help in the purification of recombinant molecules. The following example describes the formation of a scFv molecule and its resulting expression in *Escherichia coli.*

Figure 2 describes the strategy that has been used to join two DNA fragments through the addition of a linker. cDNAs coding for light-chain and heavy-chain V regions of an antibody molecule were amplified using oligonucleotides A and B for the κ light-chain V region and C and D for the heavy-chain V region.

A: 5′ GGG AAT TCG A[C/T]A TTG TG[A/C] T[A/G]A C[A/C]C A[A/G][G/T] [A/C]TC AA 3′

B: 5′ GGA ACC TCC GCC TCC GCT ACC ACC ACC ACC GCT ACC ACC ACC ACC TGC AGC AGC CCG 3′

C: 5′ GGA GGC GGA GGT TCC [C/G]AG GT[C/G] [A/C]A[A/G] CTG CAG 3′

D: 5′ TTA TGG GGG TGT CGT TTT GGC 3′

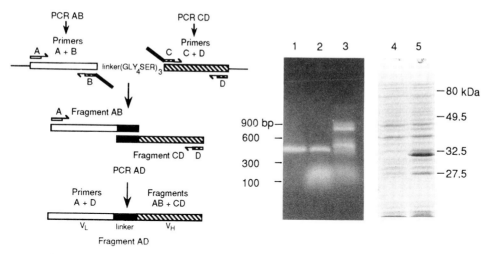

FIG. 2   Linking two DNA fragments through the addition of a linker. Schema of the strategy is shown on the left-hand side. The open box represents the variable region of the light chain and the hatched box the variable region of the heavy chain. The closed box represents the (Gly₄Ser)₃ linker. The relative position of each primer is shown. Analysis of PCR fragments by gel electrophoresis is shown in the middle. Lane 1, fragment AB; lane 2, fragment CD; lane 3, fragment AD. Sodium dodecyl sulfate–polyacrylamide gel electrophoresis of bacterial lysates not expressing (lane 4) or expressing (lane 5) fragment AD is shown on the right-hand side.

Oligonucleotides A and C are partly degenerate to allow the respective amplification of murine κ light-chain and heavy-chain V regions (12). In addition to being essential to light-chain variable region amplification, oligonucleotide B also codes for the linker $(Gly_4Ser)_3$. Oligonucleotide D is complementary to the heavy-chain cDNA and has been slightly modified to include an in-frame stop codon. Finally, oligonucleotides B and C overlap by 15 nucleotides in order to favor ligation of both DNA fragments following the first round of PCR. A second round of PCR was performed by mixing equal volumes (1 μl) of both PCRs and by using oligonucleotides A and D as primers.

Analysis of the PCR fragments on gel revealed the presence of single bands following amplification of light-chain (lane 1, Fig. 2) and heavy-chain (lane 2, Fig. 2) V regions. Simultaneous addition of both molecules in a second PCR using oligonucleotides A and D as primers produced various fragments ranging from 450 to 900 bp including a major one of the expected size at $\approx$850 bp. This fragment could be easily recovered by cloning and further analyzed to determine its sequence which was as predicted (data not shown). Insertion of the recombinant molecule into a prokaryotic expression vector allowed the expression of a protein of the expected size at $\approx$32 kDa (lane 5, Fig. 2) when bacterial lysates were analyzed by sodium dodecyl sulfate (SDS)–polyacrylamide gel electrophoresis (compare to lane 4, Fig. 2, in the absence of recombinant plasmid).

Multiple DNA Fragment Exchange

For diagnostic and therapeutic purposes, chimeric antibodies comprised of mouse variable region and human constant region have been prepared by genetic engineering (13). Yet, such antibodies are still immunogenic in humans due to a resulting immune response to the framework structure of the mouse variable region. For this reason, chimeric antibodies have been taken one step further: hypervariable regions of heavy and light chains from a human Ig gene have been replaced by specific regions from rat- or mouse-derived antibodies (14, 15). However, construction of these humanized antibodies may require a lot of work which renders this approach difficult to use in order to prepare a pool of specific antibodies directed against a given antigen. It is now possible to facilitate these manipulations through the use of PCR (16). The example below describes humanization of a murine light-chain variable region where the murine hypervariable fragments were linked to human framework regions isolated from a human antibody.

Figure 3 describes the strategy that was used for the exchange of DNA fragments. The objective was to replace complementarity-determining re-

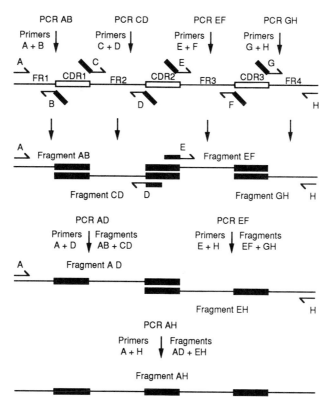

FIG. 3   Strategy for multiple DNA fragment exchanges. Open boxes represent human κ CDRs and closed boxes murine κ CDRs. The relative position of each primer is shown.

gions (CDRs) of a human κ light chain, responsible in a large part for the recognition of a given antigen, by the CDRs of a murine κ chain. Oligonucleotides were designed according to the sequences of the murine and human κ chain V regions. Joining sense and antisense oligonucleotides (B and C, D and E, F and G) overlap by 15 nucleotides.

A: 5′ GGG AAT TCA TGG ACA TG[A/G] [A/G][A/G][A/G/T] [C/T]CC [A/C/T][A/C/G]G [C/T][G/T]G A[C/G]C TT 3′
B: 5′ GCT TAA CCA AAC ATT AAT ATT CTG ACT GGC ATG GCA AGT GAT GGT GAC 3′
C: 5′ AAT GTT TGG TTA AGC TGG TAT CAG CAG AAA CC 3′
D: 5′ TGT GTG CAA GAT GGA AGC CTT ATA GAT CAG GAG TTT 3′

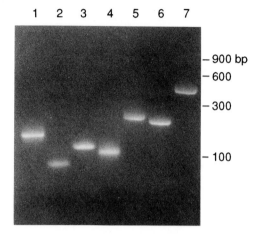

FIG. 4   Analysis of PCR fragments. Gel electrophoresis of each PCR fragment is shown. Lane 1, fragment AB; lane 2, fragment CD; lane 3, fragment EF; lane 4, fragment GH; lane 5, fragment AD; lane 6, fragment EH: lane 7, fragment AH.

E: 5′ TCC ATC TTG CAC ACA GGG GTC CCA TCA AGG 3′
F: 5′ ACT TTG ACC CTG TTG GCA GTA ATA AGT TGC 3′
G: 5′ CAA CAG GGT CAA AGT TAT CCT CTC ACG TTC GGC CAA
   GGG ACC 3′
H: 5′ CCA AGC TTC ATC AGA TGG CGG GAA GAT 3′

The κ V region was first amplified using oligonucleotides A and H. The resulting fragment was used as a template for subsequent PCR rounds using the oligonucleotide pairs A and B, C and D, E and F, G and H in four different reactions. Fragment AB was then joined to fragment CD by using an equal volume of each reaction and oligonucleotides A and D as primers. Similarly, fragment EF was juxtaposed to fragment GH using oligonucleotides E and H. Finally fragment AD and fragment EH were used in the last round of PCR using oligonucleotides A and H to produce fragment AH.

Aliquots of each reaction were analyzed by gel electrophoresis as shown on Fig. 4. In each case, single bands corresponding to the expected size of the amplified fragments could be detected. In addition, each product was sequenced and shown to contain no mutations (data not shown).

The examples that we have described demonstrate the usefulness of PCR in creating chimeric molecules. The approach that we suggest facilitates and accelerates the preparation of such molecules. It can be used not only in a variety of research applications but also in the creation of new classes of components for therapeutic and diagnostic purposes.

Acknowledgments

This work was supported, in part, by the CRCS R&D Program and by the Cutter/CRCS R&D Fund.

References

1. P. J. Dillon and C. A. Rosen, *BioTechniques* **9,** 298 (1990).
2. T. M. Chirgwin et al., *Biochemistry* **18,** 5294 (1979).
3. V. Glisin et al., *Biochemistry* **13,** 2633 (1974).
4. G. Köhler and C. Milstein, *Nature* (*London*) **256,** 495 (1975).
5. Y. L. Chiang et al., *BioTechniques* **7,** 360 (1989).
6. J. W. Larrick et al., *Bio/Technology* **7,** 934 (1989).
7. Orlandi et al., *Proc. Natl. Acad. Sci. U.S.A.* **86,** 3833 (1989).
8. M. Whitlow and D. Filpula, *Methods: Companion Methods Enzymol.* **2,** 97 (1991).
9. J. K. Batra et al., *Proc. Natl. Acad. Sci. U.S.A.* **89,** 5867 (1992).
10. R. E. Bird et al., *Science* **242,** 423 (1988).
11. J. S. Huston et al., *Proc. Natl. Acad. Sci. U.S.A.* **85,** 5879 (1988).
12. J. V. Gavilondo-Cowley et al., *Hybridoma* **9,** 407 (1990).
13. M. S. Neuberger et al., *Nature* (*London*) **314,** 268 (1985).
14. L. Riechmann et al., *Nature* (*London*) **332,** 323 (1988).
15. S. D. Gorman et al., *Proc. Natl. Acad. Sci. U.S.A.* **88,** 4181 (1991).
16. A. P. Lewis and J. S. Crowe, *Gene* **101,** 297 (1991).

[7]   PCR-Mediated Gene Synthesis

Krishna Jayaraman

Introduction

Synthesis of double-stranded DNA fragments using deoxyribooligonucleotides and polymerase chain reaction (PCR) was first described by Mullis *et al.* (1). Since then alternate and more efficient procedures have been described (2, 3). We have developed new strategies for gene synthesis using PCR that have facilitated the synthesis of genes easily and efficiently (4–6). Precise fusion of different DNA fragments can be achieved using PCR (7–9). We have developed a strategy to join DNA fragments in frame that has applications both in gene synthesis and site-directed mutagenesis (5). Details of these approaches are described in this chapter.

Strategy 1. Single-Step Ligation of All Overlapping Oligonucleotides followed by PCR Amplification

Principle of Method

The main feature of this approach is that the entire gene is synthesized and purified in a single step by using the PCR. All the oligonucleotides making up the gene are annealed and ligated and the crude ligation mixture is used as the target for PCR amplification of the product using the two extreme end oligonucleotides as primers. This procedure has been used successfully in the synthesis of several genes.

Single-Step Ligation and PCR

The synthesis of a gene for horseradish peroxidase (isozyme c) was accomplished using this strategy. Forty oligonucleotides varying in length from 32 to 60 bases long were ligated in a single step and the crude ligation reaction mixture was used as the target. The number of oligonucleotides that can be ligated in a single reaction was investigated before 40 oligonucleotides were used. The purity requirement of the oligonucleotides was also investigated. We also wanted to determine if purification of the ligation reaction mixture

Methods in Neurosciences, Volume 26

was necessary before using a target for PCR. It was found that crude oligonucleotides (desalted on NAP columns) could be used as effectively as gel or HPLC-purified oligonucleotides, but as the number of oligonucleotides increased, it was critical that the oligonucleotides be purified by gel or HPLC. From our experience, it was difficult to successfully amplify the product when more than 20 crude oligonucleotides were ligated. The presence of unligated oligonucleotides or shorter gene fragments in the ligation mixture did not seem to affect the PCR amplification of the gene. We have routinely used Centricon (Amicon, Danvers, MA) filtration to remove any contaminant that might affect the efficiency of PCR amplification. PCR amplification of a ligation mixture containing 0.25 pmol of each oligonucleotide yielded the product as efficiently as a 1 : 100 dilution of a ligation mixture containing 25 pmol of each oligonucleotide. The results are shown in Fig. 1.

Effects of Reaction Conditions on PCR Amplifications

For the amplification of ligation reaction mixtures, the optimal $MgCl_2$ and dNTP concentrations were 2.5 mM and 500 μM, respectively. Lower concentrations showed a significant difference in intensity when analyzed by agarose gel electrophoresis. The optimal $MgCl_2$ and dNTP concentrations required are in the range suggested by Eckert and Kunkel (10) for enhancing the fidelity of *Taq* polymerase enzyme. The maximum concentrations studied were 10 mM of $MgCl_2$ and 1.5 mM dNTPs. Analysis of amplification mixtures by agarose gel electrophoresis obtained using 2–10 units of *Taq* polymerase showed no difference in the intensity of the product bands. Twenty to thirty cycles were required to obtain the maximum yield. Thirty cycles were generally used.

Materials and Methods

Restriction enzymes, T4 DNA ligase, and T4 polynucleotide kinase are from BRL (Gaithersburg, MD), IBI, or New England Biolabs (Beverly, MA). *Taq* polymerase is from Perkin–Elmer/Cetus (Norwalk, CT) Agarose is obtained from Bio-Rad (Richmond, CA). Low-melting-point agarose (SeaPlaque and NuSieve) is obtained from FMC Corp (Rockland, ME). A DNA thermal cycler from Perkin–Elmer is used for the PCR. Oligonucleotides are synthesized on Applied Biosystems (Foster City, CA) Model 380 B or MilliGen (Milford, MA) Model 8750 DNA synthesizers. Purifications are done by

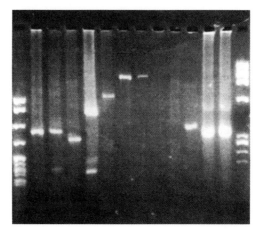

1   2   3   4   5   6   7   8   9 10 11 12 13

FIG. 1   Analysis of PCR amplification products from single-step ligation of various numbers of oligonucleotides on a 4% agarose gel (3% NuSieve/1% SeaKem). Lanes: 1, *Msp*I digest of pBR322 DNA; 2, ligation and PCR amplification of gel-purified HRP oligonucleotides 1–14; 3, ligation and PCR amplification of gel-purified HRP oligonucleotides 13–26; 4, ligation and PCR amplification of gel-purified HRP oligonucleotides 27–40; 5, ligation and PCR amplification of gel-purified HRP oligonucleotides 19–40; 6, ligation and PCR amplification of gel-purified HRP oligonucleotides 1–26; 7, ligation of oligonucleotides 1–40 and PCR amplification before Centricon-30 filtration; 8, ligation of oligonucleotides 1–40 and PCR amplification after Centricon-30 filtration; 9, ligation of 10 pmol of gel-filtered oligonucleotides 1–14 analyzed before PCR amplification; 10, ligation and PCR amplification of gel-filtered oligonucleotides 1–14; 11, ligation and PCR amplifications of 0.25 pmol of HRP oligonucleotides 13–26; 12, ligation and PCR amplifications of 0.25 pmol of HRP oligonucleotides 27–40; 13 *Hae*III digest of ϕX174 DNA. Reproduced from ref. 5.

denaturing 20% polyacryamide gel electrophoresis. The bands corresponding to the products are cut out and eluted by soaking in water or 1× TE buffer.

Synthesis of Genes Using Single-Step Ligation followed by PCR
5′ Phosphorylation

Oligonucleotides:	25 pmol each
Phosphorylation buffer:	15 μl containing 50 mM Tris–HCl (pH 7.0), 10 mM MgCl$_2$, 100 mM dithiothreitol (DTT), 100–250 pmol of ATP
Polynucleotide kinase:	2 units
Incubation:	30–45 min at 37°C

Ligations

Oligonucleotides:	Pool the entire sample of all 5′ phosphorylated oligonucleotides and the two end oligonucleotides (25 pmol each) that are not phosphorylated Heat the pooled oligonucleotide solution to 95°C, incubate for 5 min, cool to room temperature over a period of 1.5 hr
Buffer:	Add a fresh solution of 10 mM ATP and 100 mM DTT to a final concentration of 1 mM ATP and 10 mM DTT to the oligonucleotides which are in phosphorylation buffer
Enzyme:	2 to 10 units of T4 DNA ligase
Incubation:	Incubate at room temperature for 2 hr or at 12°C overnight after the addition of ATP, DTT, and ligase

Polymerase Chain Reaction

Dilute the ligation reaction mixture to 2 ml with 1× TE buffer (10 mM Tris–HCl, pH 7.6, 1 mM EDTA) or water. Remove the excess ATP, unligated oligonucleotides, or shorter ligated products using a Centricon filter of appropriate size. Usually Centricon-30 is used. Centrifuge at 2000g for 20 to 30 min at 4°C. Add another 500 μl of 1× TE and centrifuge again. Finally turn the sample reservoir upside down and centrifuge for 15 min to collect the retentate. Approximately 5 μl of the retentate is used for PCR amplification of the product.

Target:	Ligation reaction mixture as described above
Primers:	The two oligonucleotides representing the 5′ and 3′ ends of the gene, 1 μM each
dNTPs:	500 μM each
Buffer:	50 mM KCl, 10 mM Tris–HCl (pH 8.0), 2.5 mM MgCl$_2$, and gelatin (100 μg/ml)
Enzyme:	*Taq* polymerase, 2 to 5 units
Cycles:	Number 30
	Denaturation, 94°C, 1 min
	Annealing, 55°C, 30 sec
	Extension, 70°C, 45 sec

After the PCR amplification, an aliquot of the reaction mixture is run on a 4% (w/v) agarose (3% NuSieve, 1% SeaKem) gel. Since this is low melting gel, cut the band from the gel, dilute with 1× TE, and reamplify using PCR or use directly for cloning.

Charcterization of PCR Products by PCR

Preliminary evaluation of the success of PCR-mediated gene synthesis was done by agarose gel electrophoresis of the amplification reaction mixture. The presence of a band corresponding to the expected size product indicates successful synthesis of the gene of interest. Further confirmation on the arrangement of oligonucleotides can be obtained by carrying out PCR using different sets of oligonucleotides as the primers on the PCR-amplified gene product. The characterization of the horseradish peroxidase (HRP) gene by this procedure is shown in Fig. 2.

Procedure

Dissolve the PCR-amplified gene in 20 μl of 1× TE. Use 0.5 μl of this as the target for the PCR reaction. If the gene is present in a low-melting-point gel, melt the gel, dilute 5- to 10-fold with 1× TE and use 2 to 5 μl in the PCR reaction. Carry out the PCR reaction for 30 cycles as described under

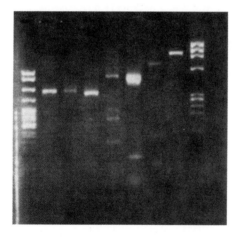

1   2   3   4   5   6   7   8   9

FIG. 2   Characterization of HRP gene by using the PCR. By using the synthetic gene as the target and several different combinations of oligonucleotide primers, the PCR as carried out and the products were analyzed on a 4% agarose gel. Lanes: 1, *Msp*I digest of pBR322 DNA; 9, *Hae*III digest of ϕX174 DNA. PCR amplifications used the following oligonucleotides as primers. Lanes: 2, oligonucleotides 1 and 14; 3, oligonucleotides 13 and 26; 4, oligonucleotides 25 and 40; 5, oligonucleotides 1 and 20; 6, oligonucleotides 19 and 40; 7, oligonucleotides 1 and 26; 8, HRP oligonucleotides 1 and 40. Reproduced from ref. 5.

PCR amplifications. Analyze the reaction on a 4% agarose gel containing 3% NuSieve and 1% SeaKem.

The single-step ligation followed by PCR offers several advantages: (i) Several sequential ligation and purification steps usually needed in the synthesis of a gene are avoided making this procedure more efficient and rapid. (ii) The entire gene can be assembled from as little as 1–5 ng of oligonucleotides thus saving material in synthesis. Although the savings in the quantity of oligonucleotides may not appear to be a crucial factor in the case of short oligonucleotides, this approach will provide significant advantages when longer oligonucleotides (ca. 100 bases long) are used. (iii) Since sufficient quantities of the gene can be generated by PCR, it can be sequenced directly without cloning. (iv) Mutants of the synthetic gene can be generated by substituting an appropriate set of oligonucleotides in the ligation/amplification mixture. The size of the PCR products obtained can be increased by increasing the length of the individual oligonucleotides without increasing the number or by increasing both the length and the number.

The error rates and the errors introduced by *Taq* polymerase have been well documented in several reports (10–12). The error rate depends on reaction conditions, number of starting molecules, and the sequence. Conditions for high-fidelity DNA synthesis by *Taq* polymerase have also been defined (10). The main concern in gene synthesis is the possible rearrangement of oligonucleotides due to spurious ligations when several oligonucleotides are ligated simultaneously. Another contributing factor for the error rate is that the oligonucleotides themselves may contain a small population of heterogeneous sequences despite extensive purifications. This problem is common to any gene synthesis methodology involving synthetic oligonucleotides. Cloning and sequencing of the PCR products showed that several clones contained the correct sequences while a few that contained incorrect sequences were mostly deletions. Base substitutions contributed to ~20% of the errors. Since the errors introduced by the *Taq* enzyme have been shown to be base substitutions and as most of the observed errors were deletions, the errors could be more due to the heterogeneity of oligonucleotides than the fidelity of DNA synthesis during PCR.

Strategy 2. PCR-Mediated Gene Synthesis Involving Assembly of Oligonucleotides Representing only One of the Strands

A further modification of this PCR-mediated gene synthesis strategy is discussed in this section. In the PCR-mediated gene synthesis strategy discussed above it is necessary to synthesize oligonucleotides corresponding to both strands. Depending on the size of the gene to be synthesized, this might require several oligonucleotides to be synthesized. Therefore, we investigated an alternate approach involving oligonucleotides corresponding to only one of the strands. In this method the PCR is carried out on a mixture containing oligonucleotides representing only one of the strands and short oligonucleotides that are complementary at the junction of these template strand oligonucleotides and two outer primers. There is no need to kinase or ligate the oligonucleotides. This approach was successfully applied to the synthesis of genes coding for human and porcine colipases. The design of oligonucleotides representing one of the strands of the gene and the bridging oligonucleotides is shown in Fig. 3. A possible mechanism by which the gene is generated is shown in Fig. 4. The initial step involves extension of the bridging oligonucleotides, P2 and P3, as well as one of the outer primers, P4. In the following steps, the extended strands generated from P2, P3, and P4 get further extended by annealing to their complementary strands using the complementarity present at the junction. It is necessary to have the outer primers P1 and P4 to amplify the gene once one of the complete strands is formed. The synthesis of two colipase genes was accomplished using this strategy. In this particular example, three oligonucleotides varying in length from 90 to 110 bases were designed. The bridging oligonucleotides chosen were 20 mers having a 10-base overlap on either side. The rationale for choosing the 20 mer was that the same oligonucleotides could be used for both human and porcine colipase genes. Because of the 10-base overlap, it was necessary to use an annealing temperature of 40°C in the initial PCR amplifications to allow for efficient binding and extension of the bridging oligonucleotides. Once one of the strands representing the full-length gene was formed, the normal PCR conditions could be employed. The PCR amplifications were therefore done first under low annealing temperature for 10 cycles containing a mixture of the oligonucleotides representing one of the strands, the two bridging oligonucleotides, and the outer primer P4 followed by 20 cycles of PCR under normal conditions (ca. 94°C for denaturation, 55°C for annealing, and 72°C for extension) with the addition of 1 μM of the amplification primers P1 and P4. Alternatively, the initial reaction mixture contained 1 μM of P1 and P4; 25 nmol of oligonucleotides 1, 2, 3; and 25 nmol of the bridging oligonucleotides. The thermal cycler was programmed to connect the first-step PCR containing an annealing temperature of 40°C after 10 cycles with a second-step PCR containing the normal conditions for 20 cycles. Yet another variation of this approach is that the bridging oligonucleotides could be used to ligate oligonucleotides 1, 2, and 3 and this ligation mixture can be PCR-amplified under normal conditions to generate the full-length gene. This strategy requires the oligonucleotides 2 and 3 to

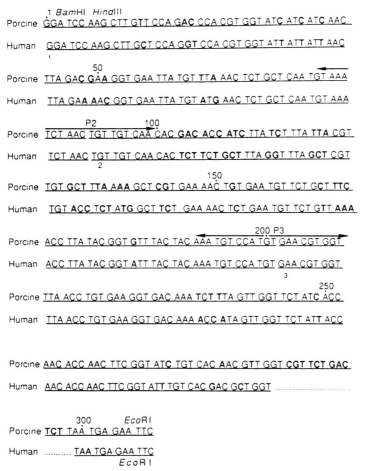

Fig. 3 DNA sequences of porcine and human colipase genes: the coding strands
of the genes are shown. The differences in bases are shown in bold letters. The length
of oligonucleotides is indicated by the continuous underline. They are numbered at
the beginning of each oligonucleotide below the human sequence. The gaps in the
underline indicate the ending of one oligonucleotide and the beginning of the other.
Bases are numbered on top of the porcine sequence. Overbars above the porcine
sequence show the region is spanned by the bridging oligonucleotides, P2 and P3.
The restriction sites at the ends of the genes are also indicated. The sequences of
P1 and P4 primers for the porcine gene were as follows: P1, 5′ GGATCCAAGCTTGT-
TCCAGA 3′; P4, 5′ GAATTCTCATTAAGAGTCAG 3′. The primer sequences for
the human gene were: P1, 5′ GGATCCAAGCTTGCTCCAGG 3′; P4, 5′ GAATTCT-
CATTAACCAGCGT 3′. Reproduced from ref. 6 © 1992 by Eaton Publishing.

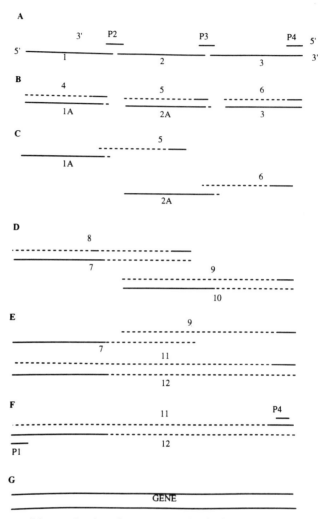

FIG. 4 A possible mechanism for gene synthesis from PCR of oligonucleotides comprising only one of the strands. The template strand oligonucleotides are numbered 1, 2, and 3. The two bridging oligonucleotides are labeled P2 and P3. P1 and P4 are the two outer primers. The extended strands are given new numbers, 1A, 2A, 4, 5, 6, etc. In the first step (B), the bridging oligonucleotides, P2, P3, and the primer P4 are extended. In step C, extended strands 5 and 6 anneal to the strands 1A and 2A using the partial complementarity at one of the ends. In step D, further extension of these strands takes place. Step E leads to the formation of full-length strands. Step F shows the PCR amplification of the gene using the primers P1 and P4. Other mechanisms not shown are also possible. Reproduced from ref. 6. © 1992 by Eaton Publishing.

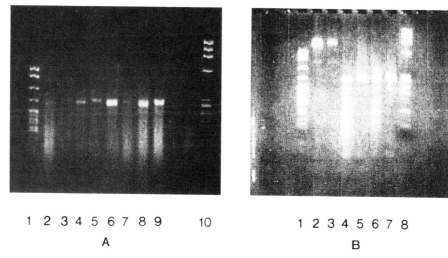

FIG. 5 Agarose gel electrophoresis of PCR reaction mixtures. The template for the PCRs contains equimolar concentration (25 nM) of oligonucleotides 1, 2, and 3 coding for the gene and the bridging oligonucleotides P2 and P3. This template mixture was labeled "N". Other oligonucleotide components are indicated as appropriate. Each pair of lanes represents results of amplification of human and colipase genes, respectively. (A) Lanes 2 and 3: Amplification of human and porcine colipase genes, respectively, from the template "N" and outer primers P1 and P4 using a single-step PCR. Normal PCR conditions (annealing temperature of 55°C) were used from the first PCR cycle. Lanes 4 and 5: Two-step PCR containing an initial 10-cycle PCR followed by a 20-cycle PCR with the addition of 1 μM of primers P1 and P4. Template "N" and normal PCR conditions were used. Lanes 6–9: The template was a ligation mixture containing the oligonucleotides 1, 2, and 3 and the primers P2 and P3. A 20-cycle PCR was performed under normal conditions with 1 μM of primers P1 and P4. Lanes 1 and 10: Molecular weight markers MspI digest of pBR322 (bp in decreasing order: 622, 527, 404, 307, 243, etc.) and HaeIII digest of ϕX174 DNA (bp in decreasing order: 1353, 1078, 872, 603, 310, 271, 234, 194, 118, 72), respectively. (B) Lanes 2 and 3: Positive controls. Lanes 4 and 5: Two-step PCR on the template mixture "N" also containing outer primers P1 and P4 (25 nM) for the first 10 cycles. An annealing temperature of 40°C was used for this initial PCR. This was followed by another 20-cycle PCR with the addition of 1 μM of primers P1 and P4 under normal PCR conditions (annealing temperature of 55°C). Lanes 6 and 7: The two-step PCR in 4 and 5 was combined into a single-step as described under Materials and Methods. Lanes 1 and 8: Molecular weight markers MspI digest of pBR322 and HaeIII digest of ϕX174 DNA, respectively.

be kinased and ligated before amplification. Figure 5 shows the results of various conditions used for PCR. The conditions for PCR amplification are described below.

Oligonucleotides: 2–5 pmol each except the amplification primers, 1 μM in a total volume of 5 μl.
dNTPs: 500 μM each
Buffer: 50 mM KCl, 10 mM Tris–HCl (pH 8.0), 2.5 mM MgCl$_2$ and gelatin (100 μg/ml)
Enzyme: *Taq* polymerase, 2 to 5 units
Cycle conditions: First 10 cycles
Denaturation, 94°C, 1 min
Annealing, 40°C, 30 sec
Extension, 70°C, 45 sec
Next 20 cycles
Denaturation, 94°C, 1 min
Annealing, 55°C 30 sec
Extension, 70°C 45 sec

Cloning and Sequencing of PCR Products

The crude PCR reaction mixtures were directly cloned into the Invitrogen (San Diego, CA) cloning vector as suggested by the manufacturer with some modifications. Only one-third of the white colonies obtained contained the full-length product as analyzed by restriction enzyme mapping of the plasmid DNA. Other colonies contained shorter or longer inserts or no visible inserts at all. When the gene products were purified from a low-melting gel and then cloned, almost all the clones contained the correct size inserts. Two clones from each of the colipase genes were sequenced by double-stranded sequencing procedures. The cloning procedure used is as follows:

Dilute the PCR reaction mixture to a final concentration of 50 ng/μl.
Ligate 1 μl with 50 ng of Invitrogen pCR 1000 vector in a total volume of 10 μl at 12°C overnight.
Use 5 μl of the ligation mixture for transformation using the procedure supplied by the manufacturer (TA Cloning instruction manual, Version, 1.3 (Invitrogen, San Diego, CA)).
Use 100 μl of the final cell suspension to spread on the agar plate.
Pick the white colonies randomly and carry out double-stranded sequencing as described by Wang *et al.* (13).

Joining of DNA Fragments in Frame

An overlap extension method was developed by Higuchi *et al.* (7) and Horton *et al.* (8) for joining different DNA fragments in frame. We have developed a similar approach to join synthetic DNA fragments. These fragments could be part of a large gene or any two DNA fragments that need to be joined in frame. One of the strategies in this approach involves the use of primers containing the class IIS restriction enzyme recognition sequence, *Fok*I. A similar strategy was used by Lebedenko *et al.* (9) using primers containing another class IIS restriction enzyme, *Eco*3II. The use of *Fok*I enzyme allows the inclusion of additional restriction enzyme sequences within the same sequence as described below.

Principle of Method

If a large synthetic gene (>1000 bp) is to be made by the single-step ligation approach as described above, it may have to be made in fragments each of which can be generated by any one of the two strategies mentioned above. This is due to the practical limitation in the number of oligonucleotides that can be ligated in a single step. The PCR-generated fragments can then be joined together to generate the full-length gene. A strategy to join these fragments in frame is described in this section. This is accomplished by carring out PCR using primers that contain class IIS restriction enzyme recognition sequences. An example of this class of enzyme that was successfully used is *Fok*I.

The recognition sequence and the cleavage site for this enzyme are separated by 9 bases on one strand and 13 bases on another strand and the enzyme does not discriminate the base sequences in this region as shown below:

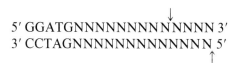

Because of lack of specificity in this region, we were able to introduce additional restriction sequences such as *Eco*RI and *Bam*HI. The sequences of the two PCR primers were chosen such that the cohesive ends produced after *Fok*I cleavage were complementary to the ends of the fragments to be ligated. This strategy was again successfully employed in joining three HRP gene fragments to generate the full-length gene. Each fragment was generated by a single-step ligation of several oligonucleotides. The middle fragment was generated by PCR from a single step ligation of oligonucleotides 13–26. The two primers used for amplifying the product contained the *Fok*I recognition sequences and either *Bam*HI or *Eco*RI sequences for cloning and sequencing purposes. The sequences of the primers are as follows:

5′ **AGGATG**CGGATCCCC***TTGG*** CTGGTGGTCCATCCTGGAGAG 3′

5′ **AGGATG**CGAATTCCC***CAAG*** TTACCGTTCAATGGACACAACCT 3′

The *Fok*I recognition sequences are shown in bold letters and the italicized bold letters are the cohesive 4-base sequences generated by the *Fok*I enzyme cleavage. The underlined sequences represent *Bam*HI and *Eco*RI recognition sequences and they facilitate cloning this fragment as an *Eco*RI–*Bam*HI fragment. The PCR amplification and *Fok*I treatment of this fragment yielded a 329-base pair (bp) sequence as shown below:

```
TTGGCTGGT---------------GTAA
GACCA--------------CATT GAAC
```

The third gene fragment was generated from a single-step ligation of oligonucleotides 27–40 followed by PCR amplification using primers containing the following sequences:

5′ **AGGATG**CGAATTCCCC***TTGT*** CTGCTTTGGTTGACTTCG 3′

5′ GGATCCGAGCTCTCATTAGGAGTTGGAGTTAACGAC 3′

Only one of the primers contains the *Fok*I recognition sequences because only that end of the fragment is to be joined to the second gene fragment. This fragment could also be cloned as an *Eco*RI–*Bam*HI fragment since the primers were designed with those recognition sequences also as shown by the underline. This fragment produced a 301-bp sequence after PCR amplification and treatment with *Fok*I as follows:

```
CTTGTCTGC-----------------GATCC
AGACG----------------CTAGG
```

Ligation of these two sequences produced a 630-bp fragment as shown below since they have a perfect 4-base complementary cohesive end.

```
TTGGCTGGT------------GTAACTTGTCTGC---------GATCC
GACCA-----------CATTGAACAGACG-------CTAGG
```

The first fragment was also generated in a similar fashion, treated with *Fok*I enzyme, and then ligated to this 630-bp fragment to yield the full-length gene. The three fragments could be ligated together in a single ligation reaction as long as the cohesive ends differ in their sequences as shown in the above example.

When there is no need to clone the individual fragments, the fragments could be synthesized and amplified to contain overlapping sequences with the fragments to be joined. These fragments can then be mixed and amplified with the two outermost fragments to produce the full-length product. This strategy was applied to the joining of the three HRP fragments to generate the full-length gene. Fragment 1 was synthesized from and amplification of oligonucleotides 1–14. Fragment 2 was produced using oligonucleotides 13–26 and fragment 3 was produced using oligonucleotides 25–40. Fragments 1 and 2 share oligonucleotides 13 and 14 and fragment 2 and 3 share oligonucleotides 25 and 26. Because of the complementarity in these shared oligonucleotides, PCR amplification using oligonucleotides 1 and 40 yielded the full-length gene. The gel electrophoresis results of joining the HRP gene from its fragments is shown in Fig. 6.

Procedure: Primer Design Containing FokI Recognition Sequences

The first 15 bases constitute the *Fok*I recognition-cleavage sequence and the rest should be complementary to the end of the target sequence. We recommend at least a 20-base complementarity to the target. The *Fok*I recognition sequence is preceded by at least 1 additional random base to ensure recognition and cleavage of the product. The bases between the recognition and cleavage sequences can be random or contain other restriction sequences. Examples are provided in the discussion above.

Carry out PCR amplification of the fragments as described above. Ethanol precipitate and dissolve in 18 μl buffer containing 20 mM KCl, 10 mM Tris–HCl (pH 7.5), 10 mM MgCl$_2$, 10 mM 2-mercaptoethanol and bovine serum albumin (100 μg/ml). Add 2 units of *Fok*I enzyme and incubate for 2 hr at 37°C. Electrophoreses on a 4% (w/v) NuSieve gel (low-melting), cut the product band, melt, extract with phenol and precipitate with ethanol. Finally dissolve in 10 μl of 1× TE. Ligate 5 μl of the fragments in a total volume containing 2 units of T4 DNA ligase by incubating at room temperature for 2 hr. Carry out electrophoresis on a 5-μl aliquot on a 4% NuSieve gel. Cut the appropriate size band and use for cloning.

Conclusions

The use of PCR in gene synthesis has several advantages over conventional procedures. It avoids the need for several sequential ligation and purification reactions required for the synthesis of large genes. The quantity of oligonucle-

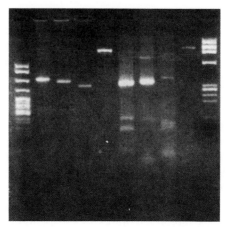

1   2   3   4   5   6   7   8   9   10

FIG. 6   Joining of HRP gene fragments in frame by PCR using primers containing *Fok*I restriction enzyme recognition sequences and fragments containing overlapping sequences. PCR products were analyzed on a 4% agarose gel. Lanes: 1, *Msp*I digest of pBR322 DNA; 2, ligation and PCR amplification of HRP oligonucleotides 1–14 (group 1); 3, ligation and PCR amplification of HRP oligonucleotides 13–26 (group 2); 4, ligation and PCR amplification of HRP oligonucleotides 27–40 (group 3); 5, ligation of PCR products from HRP groups 1, 2, and 3 after *Fok*I treatment; 6, ligation and amplification of HRP oligonucleotides 13–26 using oligonucleotides 13 and 26 as primers; 7, ligation and amplification of HRP oligonucleotides 25–40 using oligonucleotides 25 and 40 as primers; 8, ligation and amplification of HRP oligonucleotides 1–14 using oligonucleotides 1 and 14 as primers; 9, PCR amplification of ligation and PCR amplification mixtures of oligonucleotides 1–14, 13–26, and 25–40 using HRP oligonucleotides 1 and 40; 10, *Hae*III digest of ϕX174 DNA. Reproduced from ref. 5.

otide required is essentially very small and is especially helpful when long oligonucleotides are used (≥100 bases long). The entire gene can be assembled using 1–5 ng of oligonucleotides. It is also obvious that the time and effort needed in this approach are significantly less compared to that of non-PCR-mediated approaches. Large genes can be synthesized rapidly and in sufficient quantities. The strategy involving single-step ligation of all the overlapping oligonucleotides followed by PCR has been used for the synthesis of approximately a 1000-bp gene. This approach can be used for even larger genes by increasing the length or the number used or by increasing both the length and the number of oligonucleotides. An alternate approach would be to apply the strategy of joining the DNA fragments by PCR along with

Strategy 1. Large gene fragments ($\geq$1000 bp) could be synthesized by single-step ligation followed by PCR and the fragments could be fused in frame as described above. This has been illustrated with the synthesis of the horseradish peroxidase gene from three of its intermediate fragments.

A more attractive approach for PCR-mediated gene synthesis is described in Strategy 2. This approach has several advantages over Strategy 1. It requires fewer oligonucleotides. The oligonucleotides need not be phosphorylated and ligated before PCR. This approach is particularly well suited to the task of synthesizing a family of closely related genes as shown using the examples of human and porcine colipase genes. We have not extended this strategy to larger genes as yet.

A major concern in gene synthesis as well as PCR approaches that result in generating structural gene sequences is the fidelity of the sequences. This concern is due to the fact that synthetic oligonucleotides can contain a small percentage of heterogeneous population of sequences despite extensive purifications and that the *Taq* enzyme is prone to sequence errors depending on the conditions of PCR. We have used conditions that promote high fidelity of synthesis and the sequencing data of the genes provide the confirmation. Vent polymerase (New England Biolabs, Beverly, MA) has been reported (14) to have high fidelity in PCR due to its $3'-5'$ proofreading exonuclease activity and it is worthwhile to compare its performance with the *Taq* enzyme. We have found that the Invitrogen TA Cloning vector was useful in cloning the PCR products directly. The colipase genes were successfully cloned and sequenced.

References

1. K. B. Mullis, H. A. Erlich, N. Arnheim, G. T. Horn, R. K. Saiki, and S. J. Charf, U.S. Patent 4,683,195 (1987).
2. P. J. Dillon and C. A. Rosen, *BioTechniques* **9,** 298 (1990).
3. R. Ciccarelli, P. Gunyuzlu, J. Huang, C. Scott, and F. T. Oakes, *Nucleic Acids Res.* **21,** 6007 (1991).
4. K. Jayaraman, J. Shah, and J. Fyles, *Nucleic Acids Res.* **17,** 4403 (1989).
5. K. Jayaraman, S. A. Fingar, J. Shah, and J. Fyles, *Proc. Natl. Acad. Sci. U.S.A.* **88,** 4084 (1991).
6. K. Jayaraman and C. Puccini, *BioTechniques* **12,** 392 (1992).
7. R. Higuchi, B. Krummel, and R. Saiki, *Nucleic Acids Res.* **16,** 7351 (1988).
8. R. M. Horton, H. D. Hunt, S. N. Ho, J. K. Pullen, and L. R. Pease, *Gene* **77,** 61 (1989).
9. E. N. Lebedenko, K. R. Birkh, O. V. Plutalov, and Yu. A. Berlin, *Nucleic Acids Res.* **19,** 6757 (1991).

10. K. A. Eckert and T. M. Kunkel, *Nucleic Acids Res.* **18,** 3739 (1990).
11. J. M. Clark, *Nucleic Acids Res.* **16,** 9677 (1988).
12. A. Hemsley, N. Anaheim, M. D. Toney, G. Cortopassi, and D. J. Galas, *Nucleic Acids Res.* **17,** 6545 (1989).
13. L. M. Wang, D. K. Weber, T. Johnson, and A. Y. Sakaguchi, *BioTechniques* **6,** 839 (1988).
14. P. Mattila, J. Korpela, T. Tenkanen, and K. Pitkanen, *Nucleic Acids Res.* **18,** 4967 (1991).

Section IV

Quantitative PCR

[8] Quantitative PCR: Analysis of Rare Mitochondrial DNA Mutations in Central Nervous System Tissues

Nay Wei Soong and Norman Arnheim

Utility of PCR in Quantitative Applications

Although the sensitivity of PCR has rendered it the method of choice in the detection of low amounts of nucleic acid target, its utility as a quantitative tool has been slower in gaining credibility. The ability of PCR to make rare sequences detectable also makes it extremely challenging to extrapolate the amounts of initial input template molecules from the measured amounts of product molecules after many cycles of amplification. In the past few years a number of PCR strategies based on different methodological and technical approaches have been adopted for the semiquantitative or quantitative analysis of nucleic acids. These strategies deal with the basic problem of making the amplification process as predictable as possible. Because of the exponential nature of PCR, even minor variations in efficiency can lead to large deviations at the end of the reaction that will confound the quantitative relationship between product and initial template. An understanding of the theoretical and technical aspects of the kinetics of PCR product accumulation is imperative to designing quantitative PCR experiments. The next section deals with this topic. A few of the quantitative PCR techniques that have been employed in various applications are briefly reviewed to highlight the approaches that have been adopted.

Kinetics of PCR Product Accumulation

In PCR each cycle consists of denaturing the target DNA, annealing of primers, and their extension along the template DNA via a thermostable DNA polymerase. Each newly synthesized DNA segment serves as a template in subsequent cycles resulting in the exponential amplification of the original target DNA. There are three distinguishable phases of PCR. During the exponential phase, the target DNA is amplified at a nearly constant exponential rate. Thereafter, in the later cycles, the synthesis rate drops dramatically and enters a quasi-linear phase, eventually reaching a plateau phase where no further amplification takes place. Plateau in PCR can be defined as the attenuation in the rate of the exponential product accumulation and can be due to a number of factors. These are limiting concentration and thermal inactivation of the DNA polymerase, reduction in denaturation efficiency due to the increase in Tm of the DNA duplex with concentration, and progressive reduction in the efficiency of the primer–template annealing due to increasing reannealing of product strands.

Because of these factors, it is difficult to predict the behavior of the reaction at the quasi-linear or plateau phase. However, the accumulation of products in the exponential phase can be modeled by the equation

$$N = n(1 + E)^k \qquad\qquad (1)$$

where N is the number of molecules at the end of the reaction, n is the number of template molecules, k is the number of cycles, and E is the average efficiency. E has a theoretical maximum of 1 where all the template molecules are copied at each cycle. The value of E declines during multiple cycles of amplification as the reaction proceeds past the exponential phase. There is a linear relationship between the logarithm of the amount of starting template n, and the logarithm of the final amount of the specific, amplified product N.

$$\log N = \log n + k \log(1 + E). \qquad\qquad (2)$$

A plot of log N against log n for a fixed number of cycles should therefore generate a line with a slope of 1. For this to be true, E has to remain fairly constant over k numbers of cycles, although E does not necessarily have to have a value of 1. If the value of E is decreasing substantially with each cycle as the reaction progresses past the exponential phase, it will generate a plot with a slope significantly less than 1.

Brief Review of Quantitative PCR Techniques

Semiquantitative Analysis

Semiquantitative techniques are simplified approaches that provide for rough comparisons of levels of a particular sequence between different samples. Any differences in the PCR signals of the target sequence may be due to differences in the amount of total DNA added. Thus, samples must first be normalized before comparison of PCR signals can be performed. This can be done by adding identical amounts of total DNA determined spectrophoto- metrically to the reactions or alternatively by amplifying another endogenous sequence whose levels are relatively invariant. Thus, samples can first be adjusted by dilution such that they give the same intensity of signals for the "normalizing" endogenous sequence. These same dilutions are then amplified for the target sequence whose signal intensities should reflect the relative amounts of target among the samples as long as the amplifications are still exponential.

An assay of limiting dilutions of samples using PCR has also been used to obtain semiquantitative results. Rough relative estimates of differences in levels of target can be obtained by amplifying serial dilutions of the different samples and comparing the different dilutions at which the signals from the samples become undetectable. For example, if starting from equivalent concentrations of total DNA, the PCR signal from sample A disappears at 10^{-2} dilution while that from sample B disappears at 10^{-6} dilution, then sample B would possess roughly 10^4-fold more of the target sequence than sample A. We initially used this technique to compare the levels of a rare mitochondrial DNA deletion in different tissues (see below).

Poisson Dilution

Another approach entails amplifying multiple replicates of samples at very high dilutions under conditions that permit single molecule detection and counting the number of reactions that do not give a signal. Using the null class of the Poisson distribution, the frequency of negative reactions can be used to calculate the concentration of the target in the sample (1).

Although, these approaches are conceptually simple in theory, it has several drawbacks. Because exponential amplification occurs only within a limited range of starting template DNA, a dilution method may be very imprecise when samples containing highly variable amounts of target DNA are examined. Furthermore, because many PCR replicates per sample are required to quantitate the amount of the target sequence by Poisson distribution analysis, this approach is expensive, time-consuming, and impractical when many samples need to be examined (2).

Coamplification of Target with Independent, Internal Standard

A number of quantitative PCR methods have used coamplification of the target nucleic acid with a relatively invariant endogenous mRNA or a known amount of exogenous template target sequence. Chelly *et al.* (3) compared the levels of reverse-transcribed (RT) dystrophin mRNA to that of the endogenous "housekeeping" gene aldolase mRNA by coamplifying through increasing numbers of cycles. Quantitation was performed in the exponential phase of the process and the results normalized with respect to the levels of the aldolase transcript. In a later report, Chelly *et al.* (4) used exogenously added total RNA of a different species containing a specific mRNA absent from the sample of interest as the internal, normalizing sequence. Rappolee *et al.* (5) employed known concentrations of an exogenous RT RNA as internal standards to quantitate mRNA of low copy number. Pang *et al.* (6) described a reliable means of relative quantitation between different samples that employs a simultaneous, yet independent coamplification of a genomic DNA sequence (β-globin) indicative of cellular DNA content of the sample together with the target sequence, human immunodeficiency virus-1 (HIV-1) DNA. Addition of cloned target molecules establishes a standard curve for the quantitation of the HIV-1 sequence. An internal RNA sequence was also used in the quantitation of MDR1 (multidrug resistance) transcripts (7). The resolving power of this approach can be quite impressive (8).

Quantitative PCR demands high reproducibility of the overall reaction from tube to tube. Coamplification of standard and target in the same tube circumvents this requirement because any fluctuation in the amplification efficiency in a tube should be reflected in the amplification of both sequences. A decrease in the amplification efficiency of the target should be offset by a corresponding decrease in the amplification efficiency of the coamplified standard. However for this procedure to be valid, several requirements have to be met: (i) The amplification of both target and standard must be independent and not interfere with each other. Interference might be expected if both sequences share a common primer(s) or have significant homology. (ii) Measurements must be performed in the exponential phase of the amplification of both the target and standard. (iii) Both target and standard should be amplified with the same efficiency. (iv) Both sequences should also be present in comparable abundance to ensure similar amplification kinetics (9). This usually means that a dilution series of the standard has to be coamplified with the target to ensure that the appropriate range is encompassed.

Competitive Coamplification of Target with Internal Standard

Competitive PCR techniques have been applied successfully to quantitate absolute amounts of target nucleic acids. In this approach the specific target and a synthetic internal standard are coamplified in the same reaction using the same set of primers. The target and standard amplification products are designed so that they can be distinguished from each other by size or differential susceptibility to restriction endonucleases. Wang *et al.* (10) developed a synthetic, internal standard containing primer sequences for multiple genes that yielded amplicons with different sizes from target templates. A similar approach was employed by Siebert and Larrick (11). Gilliand *et al.* (12) used standards that differed minimally from the target by having either a small intron or an altered internal restriction enzyme site.

Since the target and standard templates compete for the same primers, they should behave with identical kinetics. This was investigated thoroughly by Bouaboula *et al.* (13) for a variety of different systems. The most appealing aspect of competitive PCR is that if true competition between target and standard exists, then both the coamplified products should accumulate in a parallel manner throughout *both* the exponential and nonexponential phases of amplification since both are affected equally by the changing amplification parameters. Thus the proportion of target to standard templates is maintained throughout the reaction. The technique is cycle-independent and can be run well into the plateau phase to accumulate enough material for easy detection and measurement. Quantitation is achieved by titrating an unknown, but constant amount of target with a dilution series of known amounts of standards. The amount of standard which gives a signal equivalent to that of the unknown defines the amount of the target (14).

Extrapolation to Cycle Zero

A method that does not require the use of any standards was employed by Wiesner *et al.* (15) to quantitate the copy number of rat mitochondrial DNA in different tissues. This approach involves measuring the accumulation of the product in successive cycles. A linear regression of a semilogarithmic plot of log N (product) versus k (cycle number) during the exponential phase allowed one to determine the amount of initial target by extrapolating to the y intercept at cycle zero.

Use of External Standards

In many quantitative PCR procedures, the standards can be amplified in separate reaction tubes and the data used to create standard curves. The amount of target in different samples can then be quantitated by comparing the amplification signals of the samples to the standard curves. Many applications of this approach make use of external, heterologous standards such as the relatively invariant β_2-microglobulin or β-actin for normalization between samples but this can only give comparative values (16, 17). Hoof *et al.* (18) utilized known amounts of MDR1 mRNA transcribed from a cDNA clone as the external standard for a RT-PCR assay for the same mRNA from tissue samples.

In theory, since the same sequences are being amplified in both the sample of interest and the external standard, the efficiency of amplification should be the same in both tubes. However, in practice, a number of factors must be considered when using this approach:

1. Since the amount of final reaction product is a function of the exponential amplification of the initial copy numbers, minor differences in amplification efficiency may lead to very large and unpredictable differences in the final product yield. In particular, tube to tube differences may depend on sample preparation, purity of template, the presence of inhibitors, and machine performance. As a consequence, especially if the amount of starting template is small, any differences generated in the first few PCR cycles may dramatically influence the quantitative analysis of reaction products (2).

2. Since the reactions are not competitive, care must be taken to ensure that quantitation is performed during the exponential phase of the PCR (16).

In conclusion, although these various strategies demonstrate that the quantitative power of PCR can indeed be exploited, the potential problems that may be encountered have to be considered in adapting a particular strategy for an application.

Mitochondrial DNA Mutations and Aging

In our laboratory, we are interested in the role of mutations of the mitochondrial DNA (mtDNA) in aging. Mitochondria are cytoplasmic organelles that produce most of the cellular ATP through a process known as oxidative phosphorylation (OXPHOS). Human mitochondria possess their own DNA which is a 16,569-bp double-stranded circle, coding for a significant part of the OXPHOS system. Each cell may contain thousands of copies of mtDNA (19) which are almost exclusively inherited maternally.

It is believed that mtDNA is especially prone to genetic damage due to (i) its proximity to the OXPHOS system which is thought to be a main site of oxygen-free radical generation, (ii) the absence of histone protein protection, and (iii) the relatively limited DNA repair capabilities of mitochondria. Mitochondria DNA has a high sequence evolution rate estimated at 10–20 times that of single-copy nuclear genes. There is extensive sequence polymorphism among individuals and populations (20). Thus mutations in mtDNA OXPHOS genes are very probable and deleterious mutations do occur. The past few years have seen the accumulation of much data linking mutations in mtDNA to many neurological and neuromuscular diseases ranging from mild myopathies to severe multisystem disorders (19, 21, 22). These mutations can be point mutations in coding genes, mutations in tRNA genes, and large-scale deletions and insertions. Depending on the disease, affected individuals may possess pure populations of mutant mtDNA (homoplastic) or a mixture of mutant and wild-type mtDNA (heteroplasmic). Diseases involving point mutations in coding genes (e.g., Leber's hereditary optic neuropathy; LHON) and tRNA genes (myoclonic epilepsy and ragged red fibers; MERRF) usually have a maternal mode of inheritance.

Mitochondrial DNA deletions have been found to cause the majority of cases of Pearson's Syndrome and ocular myopathies which range in severity from mild chronic progressive external ophthalmoplegia (CPEO) to severe Kearn's–Sayre Syndrome (KSS). Patients suffering from these diseases generally harbor a single type of deletion although the size and position of the deletion may vary among patients. The proportion of deleted mtDNA in muscle ranges from 20 to 80% and the deletions range in size from 1.3 to 7.6 kb (23, 24). They spare both mtDNA replication origins but may remove some tRNA and coding genes. Most of the deletion breakpoints occur within direct repeats ranging in size from 5 to 28 bp. The deletion found most frequently, in about 50% of the cases, the so-called "common deletion" (mtDNA^{4977}), removes 4977 bp of mtDNA making up part or all of seven protein reading frames. This particular deletion is flanked by 13-bp direct repeats (23, 25–27).

Since all deleted molecules within an individual appear to have the same deletion, it is apparent that they result from the clonal expansion of a single molecular event. In contrast to maternally transmitted diseases, the diseases associated with mtDNA deletions are often sporadic. The patients generally have no previous history of the disorders. In these individuals, the syndromes are probably caused by new mtDNA deletions that arose during oogenesis or early development (28).

Several salient points arising from what is known about the association of mtDNA and diseases led us to the hypothesis that these mutations might also be present in normal individuals and possibly accumulate with age. There is considerable evidence that the efficiency of OXPHOS declines with age. This has been proposed to be due to the accumulation of somatic mtDNA mutations in normal individuals that progressively cripple the ATP-synthesizing capacity of the mitochondria (29–32). Age-related increases of abnormal forms of mtDNA have been detected in senescent rodents by electron microscopy (33, 34). Since the mtDNA deletions that cause disease are usually sporadic events, they might also be expected to occur in normal individuals. In individuals afflicted with mtDNA diseases, the mutant mtDNA population is quite significant and can be detected readily without sensitive or selective methods. However, early studies using Southern hybridizations had failed to detect mutant mtDNA in normal controls (35–37). This failure to detect mutant mtDNA may have been due to lack of sensitivity. Cells typically contain thousands of copies of mtDNA. Thus, the signal of a few mutant mtDNA may easily escape detection in the midst of the overwhelming majority of wild-type mtDNA. Based on these arguments, we decided to look for the possible presence of mtDNA mutations in tissues from normal individuals. However the irrevocable identification and molecular characterization of mutant mtDNA in normal human tissue had to await the advent of PCR.

PCR Assay for Mitochondrial DNA[4977] Deletion

Short Cycle Assay

The mtDNA[4977] deletion removes almost 5 kb of mtDNA between two 13-bp repeats. Two primers were designed to lie just outside the 13-bp repeats. The PCR assay relies on the deletion to bring two primers sufficiently close together to enable efficient amplification (MT1A and MT2; Fig. 1). This "widely spaced primer PCR" strategy was used successfully to detect

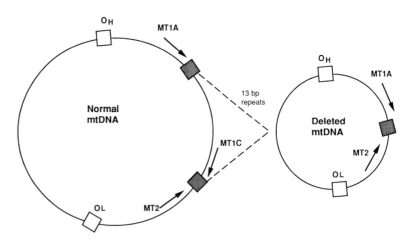

Fig. 1   The schematic shows how a 4977-bp deletion between two 13-bp repeats brings primers MT1A and MT2 close together to enable preferential amplification to take place under short cycle times. Primers MT1C and MT2 amplify a section of undeleted, wild-type mtDNA.

mtDNA^{4977} deletions in ocular myopathy patients (36, 38). However, it was expected that the mtDNA^{4977} deletion, if present at all in normal individuals, would be at much lower levels amidst a high background of wild-type mtDNA molecules. Thus a more selective PCR protocol was required.

Our laboratory (39) has been able to achieve this by significantly limiting the PCR cycle times used by other groups. The use of short cycle times preferentially amplifies the deleted molecules over the nondeleted wild-type molecules presumably because in the wild-type mtDNA, the short cycle times do not allow extension of each primer through the roughly 5 kb of intervening sequence. Thus, exponential amplification cannot take place. However, when the deletion removes this segment of DNA, the primers are brought close enough together that each primer can be extended through the binding sites for the apposing primer, a prerequisite for PCR. When DNA from adult heart muscle is amplified using a long PCR cycle time, a 5-kb product is detected corresponding to the amplified region in the undeleted mtDNA. When the total PCR cycle time is shortened 10-fold, the 5-kb product is no longer visible. Instead, a shorter product corresponding to the region amplified from deleted mtDNA^{4977} molecules appears. This is confirmed by restriction mapping and sequencing. Various tests provide evidence that these deletion products have an *in vivo* origin and are not PCR artifacts (39, 40).

Semiquantitative Comparisons of Mitochondrial DNA^{4977}

Any differences in deletion signals from PCR of different samples may be due to varying amounts of total mtDNA added to the reaction. Therefore, in order for a valid comparison of mtDNA^{4977} levels to be made between different samples, they first have to be normalized for total mtDNA content. This is done by using another set of primers (MT1C and MT2, Fig. 1) to amplify a region of wild-type mtDNA of similar size to the deleted product. The signals of the different samples from this control reaction are visually compared on ethidium bromide-stained 2% agarose gels. Samples which give more intense signals are diluted and the control reaction is performed again. Normalization is achieved through this iterative process of adjusting the DNA concentration of different samples such that they produce roughly equal intensities of wild-type PCR signals. PCR is then performed on the normalized samples using the deletion-specific primers (MT1A and MT2). A semiquantitative comparison of the relative mtDNA^{4977} levels between different samples can then be made. Typically, deletion-specific PCR are run for 30 cycles while control PCR for wild-type mtDNA are run for 15 cycles; the differences in cycle numbers reflect the rare occurrence of mtDNA[4977] molecules. Figure 2 illustrates the results of this semiquantitative comparison between different regions of an adult human brain (41) and shows that these regions can differ quite markedly in the levels of mtDNA[4977].

An estimate of the proportion of mtDNA[4977] relative to wild-type mtDNA can be obtained by using the method of limiting dilutions discussed earlier. Control and deletion PCR are performed separately on serial dilutions of a DNA sample using the same number of cycles. Comparison of the different dilutions at which the control and deletion signals become undetectable gives an idea of the proportion of mtDNA[4977] present. Using this procedure on adult heart DNA, we found that the limiting dilution for the detection of wild-type mtDNA was 1000 times less concentrated than the limiting dilution for the detection of mtDNA[4977] (39). Thus, there appears to be 1 mtDNA[4977] molecule for every 1000 wild-type mtDNA molecules in this tissue. It is assumed that the efficiencies of the deletion and control PCRs are similar since the sizes of the amplified regions are similar (324 bp for control product versus 303 bp for the deletion product).

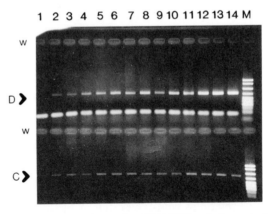

FIG. 2 Semiquantitative comparison of mtDNA[4977] levels in central nervous system tissue from a 57-year-old female. PCR products were detected by ethidium bromide staining. Each lane contains two wells (w). PCR product from samples amplified using primers specific for undeleted genomes were loaded into the lower wells and are shown at the position marked C. PCR products from the same samples but amplified with deletion specific primers were loaded into the upper wells and are shown at position D. Lanes 1–2, cerebellar gray and white matter. Lanes 3–4, cervical spinal cord white and gray matter. Lane 5, olfactory bulb. Lane 6, thalamus. Lanes 7–8, frontal cortex white and gray matter. Lanes 9–10, temporal cortex white and gray matter. Lane 11, hippocampus. Lane 12, putamen. Lane 13, caudate. Lane 14 substantia nigra. M, molecular weight marker. From Soong et al. (41).

Using this semiquantitative technique, low but detectable levels of mtDNA[4977] were found from nondiseased adults. Deleted mtDNA from fetal samples could only be detected after an increased number of cycles indicating that they are present at even lower levels. This suggests that there is a significant accumulation of deleted molecules with age (39). A wide survey of different tissues revealed that those with high metabolic rates and low mitotic activity tend to have higher levels of mtDNA[4977] (40).

Quantitative Assay for Mitochondrial DNA[4977]

Although the above method allows a rough comparisons between samples to be made, it is nonetheless limited in its quantitative value. Therefore, a more refined, efficient, and precise method of quantitation was sought.

Besides the obvious requirements for the assay to be accurate, reproducible, and sensitive, there are other operational considerations to be made in the final design. First, we are interested in measuring the relative ratio of mtDNA[4977] to wild-type mtDNA. Quantitation of the absolute amounts of wild-type and deleted mtDNA (in micrograms or copy number) is not necessary.

Second, we expect to be assaying large numbers of tissue samples. Therefore, it is preferable to keep the labor intensiveness of the assay as low as possible without compromising reliability. The smaller the number of reactions that have to be performed to assay one particular sample, the more manageable the experiment will be.

Third, as multiple experiments have to be conducted over different time periods, it is essential that quantitative data be comparable between experiments. Thus, there must be some mechanism to ensure the interexperimental as well as intraexperimental consistency of the data.

It is obvious that coamplifications of both mtDNA[4977] and wild-type mtDNA cannot be performed in the same tube because the wild-type mtDNA is in overwhelming excess. Both coamplification approaches (with independent standards and competitive PCR) require the standards to be of comparable abundance with the target sequence. It might be possible to quantitate the abundance of mtDNA[4977] and wild-type mtDNA separately with reference to a third, independent sequence. However, it seems superfluous to include this intermediate reference whose amplification kinetics and abundance would have to be investigated closely. The adoption of a competitive PCR approach is very appealing because of its robustness to plateau effects. However, it would involve construction of separate competitive templates for both deleted and wild-type mtDNA. If the distinction between target and competitive products were to be made by restriction enzymes, there are also inherent risks of errors arising from incomplete digestion and heteroduplex formation during the analysis of PCR products. Moreover, an exact measurement of the absolute amount of standards is imperative but susceptible to systematic errors. Both these co-amplification approaches require multiple PCR titrations of each sample and are therefore labor intensive.

Volkenandt *et al.* (42) have described a modification of the co-amplification technique using an endogenous gene as reference that required only a single titration per sample. But again, it requires comparable abundance of reference and target sequences. Furthermore, conditions have to be worked out carefully to ensure similar PCR efficiencies of both amplifications. Simultaneous amplifications have been shown to result in premature attenuation of the exponential phase of PCR (16) presumably because of competition for PCR reagents. The probability of spurious amplifications also increases with the addition of more primers.

Although the approach of extrapolation to zero cycle (15) has some advantages and seems reliable in their hands, it requires accurate determinations of the specific activities of the labels used and multiple readings are needed to obtain a good linear regression. We are also uncomfortable with the extrapolation process through a large cycle range as this can potentially exacerbate errors caused by a few 'off' points (8).

The use of external standards run separately has some very attractive features:

1. Only one set of external standards needs to be run with any number of samples for each particular PCR. This represents a fixed "overhead" as compared to the other techniques where multiple titrations have to be performed for each individual sample.

2. Since the control and deletion PCRs are compared to their own separate standards, the efficiencies of both need not be similar and conditions can be optimized separately for each PCR. This is useful as different cycle numbers can be used for control (wild-type) and deletion amplifications.

3. Absolute quantitation of the standards is not required. The levels of mtDNA[4977] and wild-type mtDNA in a sample can be derived as dilutions with respect to the appropriate deletion and control external standards. To obtain the proportion of mtDNA[4977]/wild-type mtDNA of a sample, only the relative concentrations of the deletion and control standards need to be known (see External Calibration of Standards). This ratio of mtDNA[4977]/wild-type mtDNA is immediately informative and meaningful.

4. Using the same batch of standards at different times means that data are directly comparable between different experiments performed at different times.

However, strict precautions and quality control criteria also need to be implemented and built into the design of the assay to directly address the concerns associated with using external standards (discussed above under Use of External Standards).

Design of Quantitative Assay Using External Standards

Tube to Tube Variability in Reactions

As a check of the performance of our thermal cyclers (Perkin-Elmer Cetus Norwalk, CT and MJ Research), preliminary control and deletion PCRs are performed. Master mixes of reagents, template and enzyme are prepared and aliquoted into multiple reaction tubes. The reaction tubes are then allocated randomly to the machine wells. Amplification is performed for 15 cycles (control) and 30 cycles (deletion). Products are then analyzed visually on ethidium bromide-stained agarose gels. No significant or systematic difference in product intensities was observed. It should be noted that the amounts of template added did not result in the PCRs entering the plateau phase. The preparation of PCR master mixes and the use of a specific machine for each experiment can limit intertube variability in the PCRs (43).

As a further precaution, we ran 2 aliquots of each sample for both control and deletion PCRs. This was done as two different dilutions of the same sample. Since the ratio of mtDNA^{4977}/wild-type DNA is independent of dilution, the two readings should give consistent results. Samples whose duplicate dilutions give significantly different ratios are reanalyzed.

Inhibitors in Sample DNA Preparations

We test for inhibitory effects on sample DNA preparations by performing preliminary PCRs on serial dilutions of the DNA. Signals should decrease with increasing dilution unless inhibitors are present, in which case signals actually increase with increasing dilution because the inhibitors are diluted out. Occasionally, such samples are encountered. Thus, only dilutions of sample DNA which give the expected decrease in signal intensities are used for final quantitation.

Preparation of External Standards

External standards are prepared from purified control and deletion amplification products as described under Methods and Materials. Volkenandt et al. (42) expressed concerns that the exogenously added standard templates may be more efficiently amplified over the target gene. They attributed this to a much less-complicated tertiary structure of the standard compared with genomic DNA. However, when the target cDNA is compared to a vector DNA standard or when the genomic DNA is first digested with a restriction enzyme, the problem is minimized. Since our target molecule itself is a 16.5-kb circular DNA that has probably been nicked or sheared in the process of extraction, differences in amplification efficiencies between standards and targets due to tertiary effects are probably insignificant.

As a precaution against degradation, contamination, and loss of standards through adherence to vessel walls during prolonged storage, the samples are diluted in solutions of *Escherichia coli* tRNA as carrier. These dilutions are then distributed into smaller volumes and stored at $-20°C$. Individual aliquots are used when necessary, minimizing handling of the rest of the standard stock.

Definition of Exponential Range

The use of external standards requires that quantitation be performed during the exponential phase of the reaction. In our early experiments with tissue samples, we had attempted to derive normalized ratios by dividing the signals obtained from deletion PCR (Del) at 30 cycles with that obtained from the control PCR (Con) for wild-type mtDNA at 15 cycles using ^{32}P end-labeled primers. The use of radiolabeled primers enables sensitive quantitation of products before the exponential range has been exceeded. From our experience, it seems that when the products become clearly visible by ethidium bromide staining, the PCR is at or on the verge of surpassing the exponential range. These Del/Con ratios should be independent of dilution. However, for some samples the ratios varied widely with dilution. A log–log plot of deletion or control counts versus dilution revealed that there is a linear relationship between log counts and log dilution. However, for those samples whose ratios are not constant with dilution, the slopes of the deletion plots are significantly less than 1. When the experiment was repeated with smaller cycle numbers, the same plots yielded slopes close to 1. In this case, the Del/Con ratios are consistent across different dilutions.

In the cases where the slopes of the deletion plots are less than 1, the deletion PCR exceeded the exponential phase before the control PCR. Thus, control product accumulates more rapidly than the deletion product. This situation is exacerbated with increasing concentrations of the sample leading to smaller ratios of Del/Con. When the deletion PCR cycle numbers are decreased, the reactions are kept in the exponential phase and the deletion and control products accumulate with similar kinetics, maintaining the Del/Con ratios across sample dilution. These early experiments show that linearity itself is not an adequate condition for defining the exponential phase of the reaction. A more stringent indicator is that the slope of the plot should be close to 1 as predicted by Eq. (2).

We therefore sought to define the range of dilutions for both our deletion and control external standards over which amplification is exponential. Operationally, this is determined as the range over which a plot of log counts versus log dilutions give a good linear fit with a slope close to 1. The ranges are optimized for 15 cycles of control amplification and 30 cycles of deletion amplification. These cycle numbers are found from earlier experiments to give good, quantifiable signals for most genomic DNA samples.

First, 10-fold serial dilutions of the external standard stocks are used as templates over a 10 log range. This allows the different phases of the amplification to be clearly distinguishable (Fig. 3 shows the plot for the deletion standards). The second step consists of amplifying 2-fold serial dilutions encompassing the suggested exponential phase. The range of dilutions which gives a slope closest to 1 can thus be determined with better resolution. The exponential dilution "window" for deletion amplification using 30 PCR cycles is thus defined as ranging from 10^{-6} down to $1/256 \times 10^{-6}$. The window for control amplification using 15 PCR cycles ranged from 10^{-3} down to $1/128 \times 10^{-3}$. The 2-fold difference in the ranges (256-fold for deletion PCR versus 128-fold for control PCR) reflects small disparities in background noise and amplification efficiencies. By spectrophotometric measurements, we estimate that this corresponds to a maximum of 6.2×10^7 input molecules for control amplification and a maximum of 10^4 input molecules for deletion amplification. These ranges are reproducible and agree well with the 2–3 log ranges obtained by other investigators (44–47). Thus, theoretically, we can quantitate differences in mtDNA^{4977}/wild-type mtDNA ratios over a 3.3×10^4 (128×256) range.

Quantitation of Samples

Preliminary deletion and control PCR with unlabeled primers are performed on dilutions of DNA samples. The product signals on ethidium bromide stained gels are then visually compared with those generated by amplification of the most concentrated standard dilution in the exponential window (10^{-3} for control, 10^{-6} for deletion). The samples are then diluted if necessary such that the amplification signals do not exceed that of the most concentrated standard dilution. Two different dilutions of each sample DNA that conform to this criterion are then used for quantitation, to ensure that amplification remains in the exponential phase. Aliquots of these sample DNA dilutions are then amplified with ^{32}P end-labeled primers in both control and deletion PCRs. Both series of standards are amplified in parallel with the samples. The products are run in an 8% (w/v) acrylamide gel and the specific deletion or control product bands counted using a Phosphorimager. The counts generated by each sample are then used to obtain the equivalent dilution of the standard stock that would have given the same signal from the appropriate

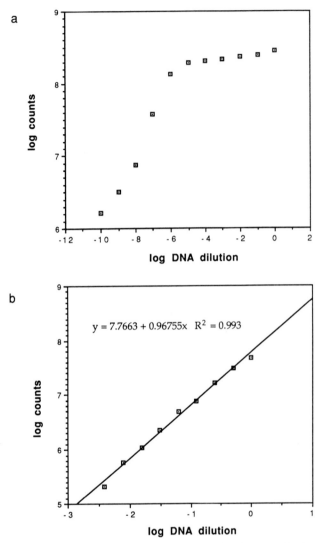

FIG. 3   Definition of the exponential range for the deletion standards. (a) PCR of
$10\times$ serial dilutions. The plot shows that the exponential range is confined between
10^{-6} and 10^{-9}. This is investigated more closely in (b) using two-fold serial dilutions.
The slope and fit is shown in this plot.

standard curve. The ratio of the equivalent dilution for the deletion standards to that for the control standards can then be used to derive the ratio of mtDNA^{4977}/wild-type mtDNA. The quantitative process is illustrated in Fig. 4.

All standard curves are inspected for conformity to the conditions that the slope should be close to 1 and for good linear regression fit. This check should warn of any significant interreaction variation in amplification effi-

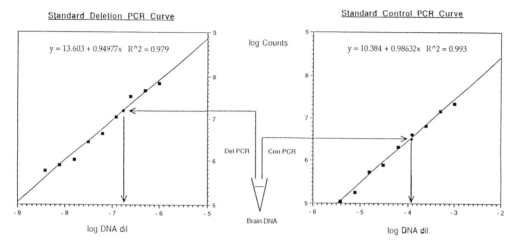

FIG. 4   Calculation of the ratio of mtDNA^{4977} to total mtDNA. Two standard calibration curves which relate the dilution of the standard template to the amount of incorporated radioactivity are shown. The standard curve specific for mtDNA^{4977} uses known dilutions of a 303-bp template (deletion) and similarly the calibration curve for undeleted mtDNA uses known dilutions of a 324-bp template (control) (see Methods and Materials). For each standard curve, the linear regression and correlation coefficient (R^2) are included. In the example shown, the deletion (Del) and control (Con) PCR signals for the caudate sample from Case 1 (41) are extrapolated from the respective standard curves to obtain the dilution of the standard templates which would have given an equivalent signal. From the deletion curve, a value of -6.75 for the Del PCR is obtained from the x axis. The antilogarithm of this value is taken to give an equivalent dilution of 1.76×10^{-7}. Similarly for the control curve, a value of -3.93 for the Con PCR is obtained which gives an equivalent dilution of 1.18×10^{-4}. Dividing the Del dilution by the Con dilution gives 0.149 %. At identical dilutions, the control standard is 5.4× more concentrated in amplifiable templates than the deletion standard (See Relative Calibration of Standard Curves). This value is therefore factored in to give a final ratio of 0.027% (0.149/5.4). Note that the value for the caudate sample of Case 1 shown in Table I (0.023%) represents the average of two replicates. From Soong *et al.* (41).

ciencies. Each experiment typically consists of 30 pairs of assay reactions for tissue samples and 10 serial dilutions for each of the control and deletion external standards.

Relative Calibration of Standard Curves

To convert the ratio of equivalent dilutions to the ratio of $mtDNA^{4977}$/wild-type mtDNA, the relative concentration of the control standard to the deletion standard must be known exactly. This is derived by the following experiment. Eight two-fold dilutions of both control and deletion standards starting from 10^{-3} dilution of each stock are amplified separately with their respective primers for 15 cycles. To avoid differences in specific activities, only the common primer, MT2, is end-labeled. The same lot of labeled MT2 is used for both PCRs. Log plots of both PCR series are made to ensure that the amplifications are in exponential phase. The ratio of counts of the control PCR to that of the deletion PCR is derived for each dilution. The average of the eight ratios works out to 5.4. Thus, for an equivalent dilution of control and deletion standards, the control standard would be 5.4 times more concentrated. This value is factored into the ratio of equivalent dilutions for each sample to obtain the ratio of $mtDNA^{4977}$/wild-type mtDNA. In an identical experiment performed nearly a year later, a very close value of 5.2 was obtained.

Regional Variation in Mitochondrial DNA^{4977} Levels in Adult Brain

We applied our quantitative assay to a study of the regional variation of $mtDNA^{4977}$ levels in different regions of the brain (41). Ten to twelve regions from each of six adults and one neonatal brain were assayed. The brains were procured and assayed over a period of nearly a year although all the regions from any one brain were assayed together. Table I shows a representative subset of the data. Mitochondrial DNA^{4977} levels varied from a low of 0.00011% in the cerebellar gray matter of a 39-year-old individual to a high of 0.46% in the substantia nigra of an 82-year-old individual, a range of 4000-fold. There was a definite pattern of mosaicism among the regions of each adult brain. However, the regions from the neonatal autopsy all had very low deletion levels which averaged 0.0004% and lacked the adult distribution pattern. Adult regions which had high deletion levels are characterized by high dopamine metabolism. Significant correlations of deletion levels with age were also detected in some of the regions.

A parallel study by Corral-Debrinski et al. (48) also produced the same observations of age correlation and regional variability using a dilution PCR

TABLE I   mtDNA^{4977}/Wild-Type mtDNA Ratios (%) for Adult Human Brain Areas

Area	Case 1: 39 years	Case 2: 45 years	Case 3: 57 years	Case 4: 60 years	Case 5: 70 years	Case 6: 82 years
Substantia nigra	0.00304	0.0447	0.362	0.324	0.363	0.459
Caudate	0.0234	0.0307	0.214	0.283	0.0564	0.252
Putamen	0.000993	0.0198	0.114	0.230	0.0591	0.189
Parietal gray matter	0.00347	0.00822	0.0230	0.0138	0.0572	0.0207
Frontal gray matter	0.00333	0.00926	0.0154	0.0129	0.0205	0.0281
Cerebellar white matter	0.000218	0.000355	0.00135	0.00696	0.00398	0.0119
Cerebellar gray matter	0.000105	0.000292	0.000640	0.00112	0.000492	0.00129

approach. Separate amplifications using different serial dilutions of sample DNA were performed for deleted and total mtDNA and the products quantitated using laser densitometry. The decline in PCR products for each dilution series was fit to a sigmoid curve. The ratio of the DNA dilutions that reduced the PCR product intensities of the deletion mtDNA curve and the total mtDNA to the same extent was used to calculate the relative levels of the mtDNA^{4977} deletion. Although the data sets between the Soong et al. (41) and Corral-Debrinski et al. (48) studies overlapped significantly, the highest observed values in the latter study were 12% for the putamen of the oldest individuals (86 and 94 years). This could reflect differences in methodology or interindividual variation, the latter being quite plausible because of the small sample sizes in both studies.

A comparison of mtDNA^{4977} levels in the substantia nigra from control and Parkinson's disease (PD) brains was performed to determine if these deletions could contribute to the pathogenesis of PD (49). The authors used mixtures of known proportions of deleted and control templates to generate a standard curve. The observed proportions after amplification did not correspond to the known initial proportions probably as a result of nonexponential amplification. The samples were coamplified for both deleted and wild-type mtDNA and the ratios of the signals compared to this standard curve were used to correct for these discrepancies. Using this method, no significant difference was found in the mtDNA^{4977} levels between control and PD substantia nigra. The corrected values obtained, however, were much lower than those of comparable regions from the Corral-Debrinski et al. (48) and our study (41).

The quantitation of mtDNA[4977] presents a special situation where the normalizing sequence (wild-type mtDNA) is in vast excess over the target sequence. The three studies above adopt different approaches to this problem. We amplified for deleted and wild-type mtDNA separately using different cycle numbers but with the same dilution of sample DNA. Corral-Debrinski et al. (48) also adopted separate amplifications but used different dilutions of the sample at the same cycle numbers. Mann et al. (49) coamplified for both sequences but had to correct for the data using an experimentally constructed standard curve. The case here with the quantitation of the relative levels of the mtDNA[4977] deletion may be analogous to situations where relative quantitation is required of a very rare mRNA transcript, an extremely low viral DNA load, or a small pool of cells harboring a somatic mutation within a heterogenous population. The choice of any quantitative PCR strategy would have to depend on the operational requirements of the application and must be tempered by an understanding of its potential limitations.

Methods and Materials

PCR Analysis

PCR is carried out in 50-μl volumes in 1× PCR buffer (50 mM KCl, 10 mM Tris–HCl, pH 8.3, 2.5 mM MgCl$_2$, 0.1 mg/ml gelatin). The primer and nucleotide concentrations are 1 and 187.5 μM per dNTP, respectively. Deletion-specific PCR are performed using primers MT1A and MT2 while control PCR for wild-type mtDNA are performed using primers MT1C and MT2. The sequences and the regions they correspond to on the mtDNA sequence map (50) are listed below.

MT1A: GAATTCCCCTAAAAATCTTTGAAAT, nucleotides 8224–8247.
MT2: AACCTGTGAGGAAAGGTATTCCTGC, nucleotides 13,501–13,477.
MT1C: AGGCGCTATCACCACTCTTGTTCG, nucleotides 13,176–13,198.

Both deletion and control PCRs are performed under the same PCR conditions except for cycle numbers and the amount of Taq (Thermus aquaticus) polymerase used. An initial denaturation step of 3 min at 92°C is used. Cycling is carried out with a 20-sec denaturation segment at 92°C followed by a single annealing and extension segment of 20 sec at 60°C. A final extension step of 72°C for 3 min is performed at the end of the appropriate number of cycles. Deletion PCR is typically carried for 30 cycles with 2 units of Taq polymerase while control PCR is typically carried out for 15 cycles using 1 unit of *Taq* polymerase. One microliter of template DNA is used for all reactions.

DNA Extraction from Tissues

The tissues are frozen immediately after removal and thawed just prior to DNA isolation. Differences in the integrity of the isolated DNA will not affect the PCR assay as we are measuring the relative levels of mtDNA[4977] to total mtDNA by PCR of a very small target region. Thus, the amplification should not be adversely affected if the average size of the DNA is above the size of the expected PCR products. Thawed samples are digested in 1–2 ml of a solution containing 10 mM Tris–HCl (pH 8.0), 25 mM EDTA, 0.5% sodium dodecyl sulfate (SDS), and 0.3 mg/ml proteinase K. The samples are incubated for 48–72 hr at 37°C with agitation. Phenol/chloroform extraction is followed by ethanol precipitation. The DNA precipitate is resuspended and stored in TE (10 mM Tris, 0.1 mM EDTA, pH 7.8).

Purification of Deleted and Control PCR Products

For the construction of standard curves for deletion and control PCR systems, the respective PCR products are purified as a source of templates for the amplification reactions. Aged heart DNA is used as template for these preparative PCRs. Each of the deleted and control reactions are performed and electrophoresed on 8% polyacrylamide gels separately. The product bands are excised, electroeluted, and concentrated by centrifuging through a Centricon-10 (Amicon). Thus stock solutions of both purified deleted and control products are obtained and stored at −20°C.

End Labeling of Primers

Primers are end-labeled with [γ-^{32}P]ATP to specific activity of 2.5×10^5 cpm/μg by T4 polynucleotide kinase (IBI, New Haven, CT or United States Biochemical, Cleveland, OH). Unincorporated nucleotides are removed by spinning through P4 columns. Primer lots prepared in this way are of approximately 10× concentration for PCR and are diluted directly into the PCR mix.

Quantitation of PCR Signals

PCRs are run using both primers end-labeled. A total of 10% of each reaction is electrophoresed through 8% polyacrylamide gels. The gel is then dried and the counts from each signal band are quantitated with a Molecular Dynamics PhosphorImager after 15–24 hr exposure.

References

1. P. Simmonds, P. Balfe, J. F. Peutherer, C. A. Ludlam, J. O. Bishop, and A. J. L. Brown, *J. Virol.* **64,** 864 (1990).
2. M. Clementi, S. Menzo, P. Bagnarelli, A. Manzin, A. Valenza, and P. E. Varaldo, *PCR Methods Appl.* **2,** 191 (1993).
3. J. Chelly, J.-C. Kaplan, P. Maire, S. Gautron, and A. Kahn, *Nature (London)* **333,** 858 (1988).
4. J. Chelly, D. Montarras, C. Pinset, Y. Berwald-Netter, J.-C. Kaplan, and A. Kahn, *Eur. J. Biochem.* **187,** 691 (1990).
5. D. A. Rappolee, D. Mark, M. J. Banda, and Z. Werb, *Science* **241,** 708 (1988).
6. S. Pang, Y. Koyanagi, S. Miles, C. Wiley, H. V. Vinters, and I. S. Chen, *Nature (London)* **343,** 85 (1990).
7. K. E. Noonan, C. Beck, T. A. Holzmayer, J. E. Chin, J. S. Wunder, I. L. Andrulis, A. F. Gazdar, C. L. Willman, B. Griffith, D. D. von Hoff, and I. B. Roninson, *Proc. Natl. Acad. Sci. U.S.A.* **87,** 7160 (1990).
8. M. B. Lubin, J. D. Elashoff, S.-J. Wang, J. I. Rotter, and H. Toroda, *Mol. Cell. Probes* **5,** 307 (1991).
9. F. Ferre, *PCR Methods Appl.* **2,** 1 (1992).
10. A. M. Wang, M. V. Doyle, and D. F. Mark, *Proc. Natl. Acad. Sci. U.S.A.* **86,** 9717 (1989).
11. P. D. Siebert and J. W. Larrick, *BioTechniques.* **14,** 244 (1993).
12. G. Gilliland, S. Perrin, K. Blanchard, and H. F. Bunn, *Proc. Natl. Acad. Sci. U.S.A.* **87,** 2725 (1990).
13. M. Bouaboula, P. Legoux, B. Pessegue, B. Delpech, X. Dumont, M. Piechaczyk, P. Casellas, and D. Shire, *J. Biol. Chem.* **267,** 21830 (1992).
14. M. Becker and K. Hahlbrock, *Nucleic Acids Res.* **17,** 9437 (1989).
15. R. J. Wiesner, J. C. Ruegg, and I. Morano, *Biochem. Biophys. Res. Commun.* **183,** 553 (1992).
16. L. D. Murphy, C. E. Herzog, J. B. Rudick, A. T. Fojo, and S. E. Bates, *Biochemistry* **29,** 10351 (1990).
17. K. M. Mohler and L. D. Butler, *Mol. Immunol.* **28,** 437 (1991).
18. T. Hoof, J. R. Riordan, and B. Tummler, *Anal. Biochem.* **196,** 161 (1991).
19. A. E. Harding, *Trends Neurosci.* **14,** 132 (1991).
20. R. L. Cann, M. Stoneking, and A. C. Wison, *Nature (London)* **235,** 31 (1987).

21. D. C. Wallace, *Annu. Rev. Biochem.* **61,** 1175 (1992).
22. M. Zeviani and C. Antozzi, *Brain Pathol.* **2,** 121 (1992).
23. C. T. Morales, S. DiMauro, M. Zeviani, A. Lombes, S. Shanske, A. F. Miranda, H. Nakase, E. Bonilla, L. C. Werneck, S. Servidei, I. Nonaka, Y. Koga, A. Spiro, A. K. W. Brownell, B. Schmidt, D. L. Scotland, M. Zupanc, D. C. DeVivo, E. A. Schon, and L. P. Rowland, *N. Engl. J. Med.* **320,** 1293 (1989).
24. E. A. Schon, R. Rizzuto, C. T. Moraes, H. Nakase, M. Zeviani, and S. DiMauro, *Science* **244,** 346 (1989).
25. D. R. Johns and O. Hurko, *Genomics* **5,** 623 (1989).
26. S. Mita, R. Rizzuto, C. T. Moraes, S. Shanske, E. Arnaudo, G. M. Fabrizi, Y. Koga, S. DiMauro, and E. A. Schon, *Nucleic Acids Res.* **18,** 561 (1990).
27. J. Poulton, *BioEssays* **14,** 763 (1992).
28. D. C. Wallace, *Trends Genet.* **9,** 128 (1993).
29. D. Harman, *Am. Geriatr. Soc.* **20,** 145 (1972).
30. J. Miquel, A. C. Economos, J. Fleming, and J. E. Johnson, *Exp. Gerontol.* **15,** 575 (1980).
31. A. W. Linnane, S. Marzuki, T. Ozawa, and M. Tanaka, *Lancet* **1,** 642 (1989).
32. J. Muller-Hocker, *Brain Pathol.* **2,** 149 (1992).
33. L. Piko and L. Matsumoto, *Nucleic Acids Res.* **4,** 1301 (1977).
34. K. J. Bulpitt and L. Piko, *Brain Res.* **300,** 41 (1984).
35. I. J. Holt, A. E. Harding, and J. A. Morgan-Hughes, *Nature (London)* **331,** 717 (1988).
36. J. M. Shoffner, M. T. Lott, A. S. Voljavec, S. A. Soueidan, D. A. Costigan, and D. C. Wallace, *Proc. Natl. Acad. Sci. U.S.A.* **86,** 7952 (1989).
37. Y. Goto, I. Nonaka, and S. Horai, *Nature (London)* **348,** 651 (1990).
38. D. R. Johns, S. L. Rutledge, O. C. Stine, and O. Hurko, *Proc. Natl. Acad. Sci. U.S.A.* **86,** 8059 (1989).
39. G. A. Cortopassi and N. Arnheim, *Nucleic Acids Res.* **18,** 6927 (1990).
40. G. A. Cortopassi, D. Shibata, N. W. Soong, and N. Arnheim, *Proc. Natl. Acad. Sci. U.S.A.* **89,** 7370 (1992).
41. N. W. Soong, D. R. Hinton, G. A. Cortopassi, and N. Arnheim, *Nat. Genet.* **2,** 318 (1992).
42. M. Volkenandt, A. P. Dicker, D. Banerjee, R. Fanin, B. Schweitzer, T. Horikoshi, K. Danenberg, P. Danenberg, and J. R. Bertino, *Proc. Soc. Exp. Biol. Med.* **200,** 1 (1992).
43. R. Makino, T. Sekiya, and K. Hayashi, *Technique* **2,** 295 (1990).
44. D. E. Kellog, J. J. Sninsky, and S. Kwok, *Anal. Biochem.* **189,** 202 (1990).
45. S. Oka, K. Urayama, Y. Hirabayashi, K. Ohnishi, H. Goto, K. Mitamura, S. Kimura, and K. Shimada, *Biochem. Biophys. Res. Commun.* **167,** 1 (1990).
46. M. Holodniy, D. A. Katzenstein, S. Sengupta, A. M. Wang, C. Casipit, D. H. Schwartz, M. Konrad, E. Groves, and T. C. Merigan, *J. Infect. Dis.* **163,** 862 (1991).
47. F. Ferre, A. Marchese, P. C. Duffy, D. E. Lewis, M. R. Wallace, H. J. Beecham, K. G. Burnett, F. C. Jensen, and D. J. Carlo, *AIDS Res. Hum. Retroviruses* **8,** 269 (1992).

48. M. Corral-Debrinski, T. Horton, M. T. Lott, J. M. Shoffner, M. F. Flint, and D. C. Wallace, *Nat. Genet.* **2,** 324 (1992).
49. V. M. Mann, J. M. Cooper, and A. H. V. Schapira, *FEBS Lett.* **299,** 218 (1992).
50. S. Anderson, A. T. Bankier, B. G. Barrell, M. H. L. De Bruijn, A. R. Coulson, J. Drouin, I. C. Eperon, D. P. Nierlich, B. A. Roe, F. Sanger, P. H. Schreier, A. J. H. Smith, R. Staden, and I. G. Young, *Nature (London)* **290,** 457 (1981).

[9] PCR-Aided Transcript Titration Assay: Competitive PCR for Evaluation of Absolute Levels of Rare mRNA Species

Michael Becker-André

Introduction

Conventional methods for monitoring quantitative changes in individual mRNAs are based on hybridization-mediated detection of nucleic acid targets. These techniques rely on the principles of either mix-phase hybridization or solution hybridization both of which have detection limits in the range of 10^6 target molecules (1). Another approach using the polymerase chain reaction (PCR) has been employed to amplify specifically the target itself to allow direct quantification (2–4). Because of its extraordinarily high sensitivity PCR technology is now widely used to detect low-abundance nucleic acid targets such as viral DNA or mRNA. To apply PCR technology to mRNA analysis, the target mRNA has to be converted into cDNA by reverse transcription (RT-PCR) (5, 6). However, using PCR for quantitative evaluations of specific DNA or mRNA targets has been difficult for several reasons. Within the exponential phase of the amplification reaction the extent of amplification (Y) is theoretically proportional to the amount of input target (A) according to the equation

$$Y = A(1 + R)^n,$$

where R is the efficiency (between 0 and 1) and n the number of cycles performed. The equation reflects the correlation between the number of input target nucleic acid molecules and the amount of target-specific PCR product accumulated after a given number of synthesis cycles. However, even slight differences in the R value, reflecting the efficiency of the synthesis reaction, can dramatically influence the amount of amplification product accumulated during the reaction. A difference in efficiency makes extrapolation to the initial amount of starting target unreliable (7). In other words, quantitative PCR requires almost unobtainably high reproducibility of the overall reaction from test tube to test tube and from sample to sample. A solution to this problem is the addition of reference nucleic acid molecules to the sample.

The reference nucleic acid molecules are thus coamplified together with the target molecules of interest using the same oligonucleotide primer pair. This PCR format, referred to as "competitive PCR" (7, 8), corrects for potential reaction differences and varying amplification efficiencies. The reference nucleic acid can be a synthetic cDNA competitor derived from the sequence of the target. Competitive PCR has been successfully applied to the quantification of several mRNA molecules (7, 9). In these examples mRNA was first converted into cDNA by reverse transcription using either oligo(dT) or random oligonucleotide primers. However, possible variations in reverse transcription efficiencies were not addressed. A preferable solution to this problem is the addition of an RNA competitor which is coreverse-transcribed along with the mRNA targets. The competitor RNA can be a synthetic, unrelated, RNA transcript (10, 11) or a synthetic RNA transcript derived from the target's sequence (12–17). If an unrelated transcript is used as the reference, potential differences in the amplification efficiencies of the target and the reference molecules may skew the titration results. Establishing calibration curves is therefore essential and can be done using either kinetic measurements (10, 18–21) or by a titration series (22, 23). On the other hand, if a synthetic RNA derived from the target mRNA is used as the reference, the efficiency of amplification can be assumed to be identical for the target. Thus the target-derived reference templates allow a direct calculation of initial templates present from the ratio of end products observed. To best approximate this assumption, the reference RNA should differ from the target sequence by only a small mutation. Examples of possible mutations are an internal deletion of a few nucleotides (16, 17), insertion of an unrelated sequence (14, 15), or insertion of a unique restriction site (12, 13). A reference molecule made by deletion mutation must be sufficiently smaller than the target to allow a clear discrimination of target- and reference-specific PCR products. At the same time the reference molecule must be sufficiently similar in size to the target to compete efficiently with the target molecules in the RT-PCR reactions. The PCR-aided transcript titration assay (PATTY) is a competitive PCR format designed for the quantification of specific mRNAs using an *in vitro*-generated reference RNA for coreverse transcription and coamplification. In this article I present a state-of-the-art technical protocol for performing PATTY. In the protocol, I describe a number of improvements and refinements of the originally published method.

Principle of PCR-Aided Transcript Titration Assay

The principle steps of PATTY are schematically represented in Fig. 1. Identical aliquots of an RNA master sample are spiked with different known

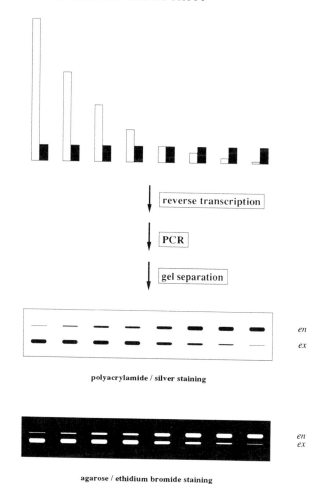

reverse transcription

PCR

gel separation

en
ex

polyacrylamide / silver staining

en
ex

agarose / ethidium bromide staining

FIG. 1   Scheme illustrating the technical principle of PATTY. An RNA master sample is subdivided in a series of aliquots containing unknown, yet identical, amounts of the target mRNA (■) to be quantified. Titration of these target molecules with decreasing amounts of internal reference RNA (□), reverse transcription, amplification to approximately equivalent amounts of DNA (PCR), and analysis by gel electrophoresis (gel separation) result in a series of double bands. The upper band represents DNA fragments derived from the target mRNA (*en*, endogenous); the lower band represents DNA derived from the reference RNA (*ex*, exogenous). The amplified DNA fragments can be separated, because the reference RNA sequence contains a small deletion rendering the resulting DNA fragments shorter than those originating from the target mRNA.

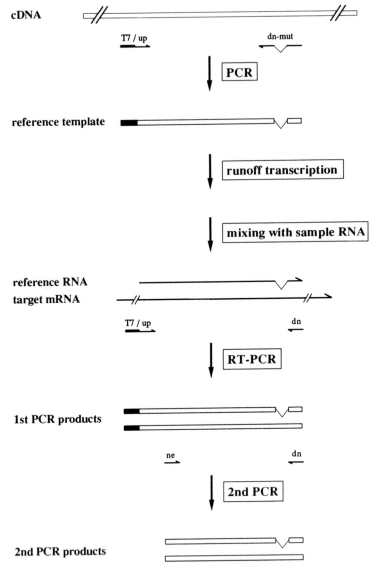

Fig. 2   Outline of the salient molecular steps in PATTY. Creation of the mutant cDNA template (>0.3 kbp) is done by PCR using a mutant downstream oligonucleotide primer ("dn-mut"; 35-mer) that introduces a deletion of 5–15 bp close to one end and using an upstream oligonucleotide primer ("T7/up") that introduces the bacteriophage T7 RNA polymerase promoter (17 bp). Synthesis of the reference RNA is performed by *in vitro* transcription off the PCR product using T7 RNA polymerase. The reference RNA is spiked into RNA samples for coreverse transcrip-

amounts of a reference RNA. This reference RNA is an *in vitro*-synthesized transcript identical to a portion of the target mRNA to be quantified. The reference RNA serves as a standard for the amount of specific target mRNA present in the RNA sample. The different mixtures of target and reference RNA are subjected to cDNA synthesis and PCR using specific primers. The amplification step allows easy detection and analysis of the PCR products. The ratio of target-type and reference-type DNA fragments in the resultant PCR products reflects the ratio of the corresponding RNA species present in the sample. In the case where equal or nearly equal amounts of both types of DNA fragments are detected, the amount of specific target mRNA originally present is assumed to equal the amount of reference RNA added.

The molecular events occurring during the PATTY protocol are depicted schematically in Fig. 2. The template for the deletion mutant reference transcript is generated by PCR starting with cDNA from the target mRNA of interest. One of the oligonucleotide primers (dn-mut) introduces a deletion into the PCR product. The other oligonucleotide primer (T7/up) fuses the PCR product to the promoter sequence of the T7 RNA polymerase. The resulting DNA fragment is used in a runoff transcription reaction to synthesize the reference RNA. Reverse transcription PCR is performed on the mixed populations of target mRNA and dilutions of reference transcripts. To amplify the total amount of DNA product synthesized, a second, heminested, PCR is carried out. The final products are then analyzed by gel electrophoresis.

The reference RNA contains a deletion of 5 to 15 nucleotides close to one end. This deletion allows discrimination of the reference RNA-specific PCR-amplified DNA products from those originating from the endogenous target mRNA by virtue of their size difference. The PCR-generated DNA fragments can be analyzed directly by gel electrophoresis. Because the difference in size constitutes only 5% or less of the overall length, conventional agarose gel electrophoresis is inappropriate. Separation of the two bands requires the use of an electrophoresis medium with a high resolving power such as 6% polyacrylamide. Incorporation of radiolabeled nucleotides during PCR allows detection and quantification of the bands by autoradiogra-

---

tion and coamplification (RT-PCR and second PCR) together with the target mRNA to yield DNA fragments (*ex* in Fig. 1) that can be discriminated from those originating from the target mRNA (*en* in Fig. 1) by virtue of different gel mobility. The oligonucleotide primers T7/up (37-mer) and dn and ne (20-mers) used for RT-PCR and the second PCR, respectively, are shown paralleling their annealing sites within the templates.

phy. For safety reasons, however, the PCR products might be preferably visualized by a nonradioactive procedure such as silver staining. Alternatively, the PCR products can be separated on an agarose support with a high-resolution capacity as demonstrated by MetaPhor agarose (FMC Bio-Products, Rockland, ME). The latter method is simple to employ but does not provide as good a resolution as electrophoresis in a polyacrylamide gel (24).

Materials and Reagents

Oligonucleotides

Oligonucleotides are prepared on an Applied Biosystems 380 B automated synthesizer. Following synthesis, they are deprotected by incubating at 55°C for 6 hr in ammonium hydroxide, cooled on ice, and desalted on a Sephadex G-50 (medium grade) column equilibrated with 10 mM Tris–HCl, pH 8.0/1 mM EDTA (TE buffer), diluted to 25 pmol/ml in TE buffer, and stored in aliquots at 4 or −20°C. Primers are designed using Primer Designer software (Scientific & Educational Software, State Line, PA; 1990). Special care is taken to ensure that there is no 3' complementarity between primer pairs.

Enzymes

Polymerase chain reaction is performed using Vent DNA polymerase purchased from New England Biolabs (Beverly, MA). *In vitro* transcription is performed via T7 RNA polymerase (Boehringer-Mannheim, FRG) on purified PCR fragments using an RNase inhibitor from Pharmacia (Piscataway, NJ). RNase-free DNase is from Boehringer-Mannheim. Reverse transcription is performed using Moloney murine leukemia virus (M-MLV) reverse transcriptase from Life Technologies (Gaithersburg, MD).

The following solutions are required for RNA and DNA manipulations:

Quartz-distilled water and water treated with diethyl pyrocarbonate (DEPC)

Transcription buffer (5×): 200 mM Tris–HCl (pH 8.0), 40 mM $MgCl_2$, 10 mM spermidine, 250 mM NaCl (Life Technologies)

PCR buffer (10×) (Vent reaction buffer; according to the supplier's specification)

The following nucleotide solutions in water: 10 mM dNTP; 10 mM NTP
TE buffer: 10 mM Tris–HCl (pH 8.0), 1 mM EDTA
Ammonium acetate (4 M), pH 5.4

Gel Electrophoresis

Analysis of PCR fragments is performed on native 2% agarose gels in 1×
TAE buffer containing 0.1–0.2 μg/ml ethidium bromide. Analysis of *in vitro*
synthesized runoff transcripts is performed on standard formaldehyde gels
(24). Separation of target- and reference-specific PCR-generated DNA fragments is done in denaturing 6% polyacrylamide (PA) gels in 0.5× TBE buffer
or in native 3.5% MetaPhor agarose gels in 1× TBE (FMC BioProducts,
Rockland, ME). For the preparation of the polyacrylamide gels follow the
instructions given in the "Guidelines for Quick and Simple Plasmid Sequencing" (edited by Boehringer-Mannheim).
  The following solutions are required for gel electrophoretic analyses:

TAE buffer (50×): 2 M Tris–acetate (pH 8.0), 100 mM EDTA
TBE buffer (10×): 1 M Tris base, 830 mM boric acid, 10 mM EDTA
Formamide loading buffer: 98% (w/v) deionized formamide, 10 mM
  EDTA (pH 7.5), 0.2% (w/v) bromophenol blue, 0.2% (w/v) xylene
  cyanol
Loading buffer (10×) for native agarose gel electrophoresis: 0.2 M EDTA
  (pH 7.5), 25% Ficoll (type 400, Pharmacia), 0.2% (w/v) bromophenol blue
Loading buffer for denaturing formaldehyde–agarose gel electrophoresis: combine 50 μl deionized formamide, 20 μl 37% formaldehyde
  solution, 10 μl 10× running buffer (i.e., MOPS) (24), 1 μl bromophenol
  blue (saturated solution in water), and 0.5 μl ethidium bromide (10
  mg/ml). Prepare freshly before use
Acrylamide stock (40%, w/v): dissolve 95 g acrylamide (Fluka, Buchs,
  Switzerland) and 5 g N,N'-methylenebisacrylamide (Fluka) in a final
  volume of 250 ml H$_2$O, filter through a 0.45-μm membrane filter, and
  store in the dark at 4°C
PA premix: dissolve 420 g urea (ultrapure, Fluka) and 145 ml 40%
  acrylamide stock in final 950 ml H$_2$O, stir with 5 g of mixed bed ion-
  exchange resin for 30 min at room temperature, and store in the dark
  at 4°C
Ammonium persulfate (Sigma, St. Louis, MO): prepare a 10% solution
  in H$_2$O and store in the dark at 4°C
N,N,N',N'-Tetramethylethylenediamine (TEMED) (Sigma)

Cross-linker: dilute before use 15 μl γ-methacryloxypropyltrimethylsilane (Sigma) and 15 μl glacial acetic acid in 5 ml ethanol (industrial grade)

Repellent: 5% solution of dichlorodimethylsilane in chloroform; store in fume hood

Acetic acid (10% solution in water)

Silver stain impregnation solution: dissolve 1 g $AgNO_3$ in 1 liter deionized water ($\approx$6 mM) and add 1.5 ml 37% formaldehyde solution; prepare just before use

Silver stain developing solution: dissolve 30 g $Na_2CO_3 \cdot H_2O$ in 1 liter deionized water ($\approx$0.25 M) and add 1.5 ml 37% formaldehyde solution and 20 μl 0.1 M $Na_2S_2O_3$; prepare just before use; cool down to 4°C

The dimension of the cast PA gel is 20 cm $\times$ 20 cm $\times$ 0.4 mm. The cross-linker is applied to the larger glass plate, allowed to dry for a few minutes, and washed extensively with water. The glass plate is wiped dry with an ethanol-soaked paper towel. The smaller or notched glass plate is treated with repellent and allowed to dry for a few seconds. The glass plate is washed extensively with water and wiped dry. Especially new glass plates or those not used for several weeks should be cleaned with chromosulfuric acid before coating. After electrophoresis and drying of the gel, the glass plates can be recovered for reuse by soaking in water and simply scraping off the rehydrated gel.

Methods

Creation of Mutant cDNA Template by PCR

The mutant cDNA template contains a small deletion (5–15 bp) that is introduced via PCR (Fig. 2) using the mutant downstream oligonucleotide primer dn-mut. This primer (35-mer) is derived from the nucleotide sequence of the target spanning a region of 40–50 nucleotides and creating an internal deletion of 5–15 nucleotides. The deletion is situated at position 20 downstream of the 5' end of the primer. The upstream primer, T7/up, is chimeric in sequence origin: its 3' half is derived from the target sequence (20 nucleotides); its 5' half is derived from the bacteriophage T7 RNA polymerase promoter (17 nucleotides). The overall size of the reference DNA template should be close to the size of the target mRNA or at least 0.3 kbp.

Procedure

Set up a PCR mixture with the following composition:

H_2O	83 μl
PCR buffer (10×)	10 μl
dNTP (10 mM)	2 μl
Mutant oligonucleotide primer (dn-mut; 50 pmol)	2 μl
Upstream oligonucleotide primer (T7/up; 50 pmol)	2 μl
Plasmid containing the cDNA of the mRNA target (uncut; 1 ng)	1 μl
Vent DNA polymerase (1 unit)	0.5 μl

Twenty-five PCR cycles are performed with the following profile: 94°C (1 min), 45°C (2 min), and 72°C (1 min per 1 kb). About 5% of the product is analyzed on a 2% agarose gel. After phenol/chloroform extraction the product is precipitated with 20 μg glycogen (Boehringer-Mannheim), 1 vol 4 M ammonium acetate, pH 5.4, and 4 vol ethanol; pelleted by centrifugation at 14,000 rpm for 10 min at 4°C; and redissolved in 10 μl DEPC-treated water at about 0.2–0.4 $\mu g/\mu l$.

Synthesis of Reference RNA by in Vitro Runoff Transcription

The PCR-generated mutant DNA fragment serves as a template for *in vitro* transcription via T7 RNA polymerase. It contains the T7 RNA polymerase-specific promoter introduced by the T7/up oligonucleotide primer (Fig. 2).

Procedure

Set up an *in vitro* transcription reaction mixture of the following composition:

DEPC-treated water	17.5 μl
PCR-generated mutant cDNA template (0.5–1 μg)	2 μl
Transcription buffer (10×; Boehringer-Mannheim)	2.5 μl
NTP (10 mM)	1 μl
Dithiothreitol (DTT; 1 M)	1 μl
RNase inhibitor (20 units)	0.5 μl
T7 RNA polymerase (10 units)	0.5 μl

Incubate the reaction mixture at 37°C for 30 min, add 1 μl RNase-free DNase, and incubate at 37°C for 10 min. Purify the reference RNA phenol/chloroform extraction, precipitate with ethanol, and redissolve the reference

RNA in 100 μl DEPC-treated water. Quantitate the reference RNA by OD$_{260/280}$ measurement. Mix 5 μl of the reference RNA with 2 volumes loading buffer for denaturing formaldehyde gel electrophoresis, heat the mixture to 68°C for 5 min, chill on ice, and directly analyze on a formaldehyde agarose gel (24).

Reverse Transcription and Polymerase Chain Reaction

Using the downstream oligonucleotide primer, dn, the transcripts are converted into first-strand cDNA via reverse transcriptase (Fig. 2). Primer dn is an oligonucleotide (20-mer) derived from the target sequence. Primers dn and dn-mut share the sequence downstream of the deletion site. For the sake of convenience, the reaction is carried out in the PCR buffer in the presence of Vent DNA polymerase. The reverse transcription reaction is set up in a microtiter plate and performed in an appropriate thermocycler. After the reverse transcription is completed the samples are directly treated for PCR without any further manipulation. For quantification of RNA samples, typically 10–100 ng of total RNA is taken for each RT-PCR well and spiked with 10-fold dilutions of reference RNA.

Procedure

Pipette into individual wells of a thermostable microtiter plate 1 μl reference RNA (for example, a 10-fold dilution series in DEPC-treated water, beginning with 10 pg and ending with 100 ag) and using a multipipettor add to each sample 20 μl of the master mix with the following composition:

H$_2$O	15.3 μl
PCR buffer (10×)	2 μl
dNTP (10 mM)	0.5 μl
Upstream primer (T7/up, 10 pmol)	0.5 μl
Downstream primer (dn, 10 pmol)	0.5 μl
DTT (1 M)	0.1 μl
RNase inhibitor (1–3 units)	0.1 μl
Total RNA (10–100 ng)	1 μl

Overlay the mixtures with 30 μl light mineral oil (Sigma), place into the thermocycler block, raise the temperature to 90°C for 1 sec, and cool down as quickly as possible to 20°C or lower. Then add 5 μl 1× PCR buffer containing 100 units M-MLV reverse transcriptase, 1–3 units RNase inhibitor, and 0.2 units Vent DNA polymerase to each sample beneath the oil phase to give a final volume of 25 μl. The pipetting work can be enormously facilitated by using an electronic multichannel pipettor (e.g., Stratagene, La Jolla, CA). Shift the temperature of the thermocycler block to 42°C and incubate for 30 min. Stop reverse transcription by shifting the temperature to 94°C for 2 min and carry out the amplification through 40 PCR cycles with the following profile 94°C (30 sec), 50°C (1 min), and 72°C (1 min per 1kb). This temperature profile has been optimized using a Techne PHC3 apparatus (Princeton, NJ). Another thermocycler might require a different profile.

Second Polymerase Chain Reaction

The second PCR enhances the sensitivity and the specificity of PATTY. The nested primer (ne) is an oligonucleotide (20-mer) whose sequence is derived from the amplified DNA target. Its position is 3' of the upstream primer starting DNA synthesis in the same direction (Fig. 2). The distance to the downstream primer dn should be at least 15 times the size of the discriminative deletion of the reference template giving PCR products at least 0.2 kbp in size. Smaller sizes will increase the difference in length between mutant and authentic templates causing considerable differences in amplification efficiency (26). Larger fragment sizes will make separation of the amplification products by virtue of their gel mobility differences difficult.

Procedure

After RT-PCR withdraw 5 μl of each PCR sample and dilute into 200 μl H_2O. Have the 200-μl H_2O samples in the wells of a polystyrene microtiter culture plate. Use for this transfer again an electronic multichannel pipettor. Mix by pipetting up and down several times. Pipette into the wells of a fresh thermostable microtiter plate 20 μl of fresh PCR mixture with the following composition:

H_2O	16.4 μl
PCR buffer (10×)	2 μl
dNTP (10 mM)	0.5 μl
Nested primer (ne; 10 pmol)	0.5 μl
Downstream primer (dn; 10 pmol)	0.5 μl
Vent DNA polymerase (0.2 units)	0.1 μl

Add 5 μl of the diluted RT-PCR products into the respective wells and overlay the mixtures with 30 μl light mineral oil. Carry out the amplification through 35 PCR cycles with the following profile: 94°C (30 sec), 50°C (1 min), and 72°C (1 min per 1 kb).

Analysis of Amplified DNA Fragments for Quantitative Discrimination

Separation of the PCR products is performed either in 6% denaturing poly-acrylamide gels or in 3.5% MetaPhor agarose gels (FMC BioProducts). If polyacrylamide is used, detection of the DNA is achieved by using a silver staining procedure (26, 27). If agarose is used, the DNA fragments are visualized by ethidium bromide-mediated fluorescence in UV light.

Polyacrylamide Gel Electrophoresis

After completion of the second PCR take 2 μl of each sample and mix with 20 μl formamide loading buffer. Heat the samples to 80–90°C for 2 min and quick-chill on ice. Load 1 μl on a 0.4-mm-thick 6% denaturing polyacrylamide gel (the same as used for separation of nucleotide sequencing reactions). Carry out the electrophoresis at 30 V/cm until the xylene cyanol blue dye has migrated about 15 cm. Remove the siliconized glass plate. Submerse the gel, together with the glass plate to which it is covalently bound, in 10% acetic acid for 15 min. Rinse the gel with deionized water from a tap for 2 min to remove urea. Submerse the gel in the silver stain impregnation solution for 40–60 min. Briefly rinse the gel with deionized water (10 sec). Submerse the gel in cold silver stain developing solution until the DNA bands appear (3–5 min). Stop the silver stain development by submersing the gel in 10% acetic acid (5 min). Rinse the gel with deionized water for 1 min. Dry the gel in an oven at 80–100°C for 1 hr. Analyze the dried gel by laser densitometry. Figure 3A shows a representative example (27a).

Make sure not to overdo the silver staining. Stop the development when DNA bands begin to become clearly visible. The silver staining procedure exhibits a rather narrow dynamic range, being prone to a nonlinear response to DNA quantity.

Agarose Gel Electrophoresis

After completion of the second PCR take 2–8 μl of each sample, mix with 1 μl loading buffer (for native agarose gel electrophoresis), and add H_2O up to 10 μl final volume. Load the samples on a 3.5% MetaPhor agarose gel (FMC BioProducts) supplemented with 1× TBE buffer and 0.2 μg/ml ethidium bromide (both in gel and running buffer). Carry out electrophoresis at 5–8 V/cm for 2–3 hr. Visualize the DNA bands on a UV light transilluminator. Photograph the stained gel. Determine the ratios of the absorbance values

A

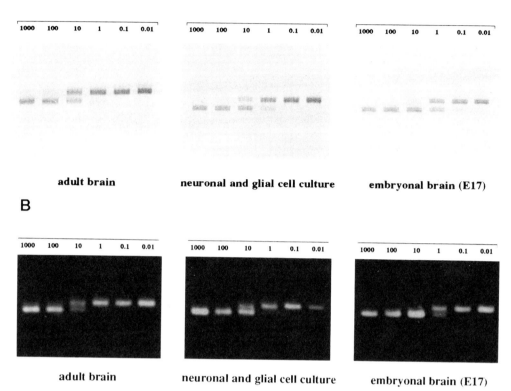

B

FIG. 3   A typical PATTY experiment. Samples containing 0.1 μg total RNA isolated from total rat brain, cultured rat brain neurons and glial cells, and rat fetal brain, respectively, and different amounts of deletion-mutated rat RZRβ-specific reference RNAs (337 nucleotides in size; deletion of 4 nucleotides) were subjected to PATTY to titrate endogenous RZRβ mRNA (27a). The amounts of reference RNAs added to the six identical RNA sample aliquots before RT-PCR were according to a 10-fold dilution series starting with 1 pg and ending with 10 ag. Amplified products (103 bp/ 99 bp) were resolved either on 6% polyacrylamide and visualized by the silver staining technique (A) or on 3.5% MetaPhor agarose (FMC BioProducts) and visualized by ethidium bromide-mediated fluorescence in UV light (B). In this particular experiment the size difference between target and reference sequence was extremely small with only 4 base pairs of a total of 103 base pairs leading separation in MetaPhor agarose to its resolution limits.

of the relevant pairs of bands in view of the concentration of the reference RNA spiked into the original samples. Figure 3B shows a representative example.

Comments

The competitive PCR assay described in this chapter provides a sensitive method for quantification of rare mRNA species. All the manipulations of the PATTY procedure are carried out *in vitro* using standard laboratory equipment and a thermocycler. An *in vitro*-generated reference RNA derived from the mRNA target is included before the reverse transcription reaction step to address several potential problems. Due to the presence of the reference RNA, uncertainties about cDNA synthesis rates are avoided while sample-to-sample variations in the reverse transcription process are internally corrected. In contrast to other methods, PATTY does not require any calibration of the RT-PCR process, since the reference and the target molecules are almost identical (with the minor caveat of a 5–10% difference in overall size). Creation of the reference RNA is straight forward because it is independent of any cloning manipulations. The use of *in vitro* transcripts as competitors, however, requires careful manipulations in an RNase-free environment. Similarly, the amplification process through two rounds of PCR requires strict exclusion of any source of contamination.

The evaluation of target mRNA levels using competitive PCR or PATTY is based on the quantitative discrimination of target- and reference-specific DNA fragments. Gel electrophoretic separation of the two types of DNA fragments is possible because of their different electrophoretic mobilities. Quantification of the corresponding double band patterns is done by measurement of signal intensities according to the specific readout of the analysis system employed. If PATTY is performed with radiolabeled nucleotides, the PCR products can be directly detected by autoradiography, by scintillation counting, or by radioanalytic imaging systems. Autoradiography provides an image of signal intensities that can be quantitated by densitometry. However, it should be kept in mind that X-ray films respond linearly to radiation only over a limited range of signal intensities. If available, a radioanalytic imaging system like a phosphoimager with software to quantitate the signals would be superior (11). This system displays linear signal response characteristics over a wide range of signal intensities.

If PATTY is performed nonisotopically, the PCR products have to be visualized by indirect methods. Here, I have described two methods: (i) Silver staining of DNA fragments separated in polyacrylamide gels provides sensitivity and resolution comparable with an autoradiography of radiolabeled PCR products (26, 27). The dehydrated silver-stained gel is subjected to densitometry without further treatment. Similar to autoradiography, care should be taken to keep the system in the range of linear response. Loading of different sample amounts of a given PCR-amplified titration series may be required. (ii) Ethidium bromide staining of DNA fragments separated on agarose with high resolution (for example, MetaPhor agarose) (24) provides both sensitivity and resolution that are somewhat inferior to electrophoresis in polyacrylamide and detection by silver staining. However, the analysis is extremely easy to perform. The gel is photographed under UV light and the negative is subjected to conventional densitometry. This DNA detection gives linear signals only over a range of one order of magnitude. As with the radiolabeled PCR products, an image analysis system (for example, a video densitometer that scans the gel by positive fluorescent emission) (29) would be advantageous as it provides a means of precise signal quantification.

An attractive alternative for the quantification of the PCR products has been described by Porcher et al. (30). The authors modified the competitive PCR reaction by using fluorescent oligonucleotide primers. Separation and quantification of the PCR products was then performed on an automated DNA sequencer. Electrophoretic separation of the DNA products and laser-detected fluorescence quantification of them are accomplished simultaneously. If an automated sequencing machine is available, this approach provides a protocol which can be routinely and reproducibly employed for a large number of samples.

The rationale for estimating the number of nucleic acid molecules in a given biological specimen is to obtain information about changes in the cellular expression of the target gene. However, a meaningful interpretation of absolute quantification requires normalization to a fixed biological parameter. Normally this parameter is the amount of total RNA isolated. If only minute amounts of total RNA are available, their exact mass can be evaluated by the following method. An aliquot of each RNA sample is analyzed by dot-blot hybridization using a cDNA encoding the 18S rRNA as specific probe (31). A dilution series of known quantities of an RNA sample should be included to serve as a standard. The hybridization signal intensities of the various sample RNAs are compared with those of the standard RNA dilution series. A representative example is shown in Fig. 4. The recovery of target mRNA during the purification process could be controlled by addition of known amounts of an unrelated ^{35}S-labeled RNA standard to the biological specimen (32). The recovery standard should interfere neither with the quantification of total RNA (the ^{35}S isotope is a mild β-particle emitter; its radiation can be absorbed by a thin plastic film without substantially reducing the signal of the hybridized ^{32}P-labeled 18S cDNA probe) nor with PATTY (the unrelated standard probe will not be amplified).

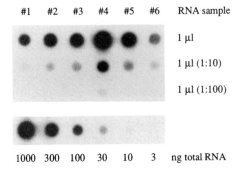

FIG. 4   Estimation of total RNA amounts by dot-blot hybridization. Different RNA samples and 10-fold and 100-fold dilutions of them were dot-blotted onto a nitrocellulose membrane using standard methods. For calibration, a dilution series of a total RNA sample of known concentration was included as indicated. All RNA samples were from various rat organs. The RNA was cross-linked by UV light irradiation and hybridized to a radiolabeled murine 18S rDNA probe. Since the 18S rRNA consistently accounts for about 40% of the total RNA mass it lends a measure for quantification of total RNA.

In general, PATTY offers a sensitive assay for the quantification of specific mRNAs to be performed in any laboratory with standard equipment. With PATTY, a coamplification strategy insensitive to experimental errors due to internal controls in the form of near-identical competitor templates is used. Analysis through separation in gel electrophoretic media appears the method of choice for scientific purposes. For high throughput analyses (for example, clinical studies), however, a combination with a hybridization step would be desirable to facilitate the analytical process (22, 33).

Acknowledgments

I thank Dr. J. F. DeLamarter for careful reading of the manuscript and C. Hebert for photographic assistance. I am grateful to Dr. I. Grummt (DKFZ, Heidelberg) for providing the mouse 18S ribosomal cDNA clone.

References

1. M. Becker-André, *Methods Mol. Cell. Biol.* **2,** 189 (1991).
2. R. K. Saiki, S. Scharf, F. Faloona, K. B. Mullis, G. T. Horn, H. A. Erlich, and N. Arnheim, *Science* **230,** 1350 (1985).

3. R. K. Saiki, D. H. Gelfand, S. Stoffel, S. J. Scharf, R. Higuchi, G. T. Horn, K. B. Mullis, and H. A. Erlich, *Science* **239**, 487 (1988).

4. K. B. Mullis and F. A. Faloona, *in* "Methods in Enzymology" (R. Wu, ed.), Vol. **155**, p. 335. Academic Press, Orlando, FL, 1987.

5. D. A. Rappolee, D. Mark, M. J. Banda, and Z. Werb, *Science* **241**, 708 (1988).

6. J. W. Larrick, *Trends Biotechnol.* **10**, 146 (1992).

7. G. Gilliland, S. Perrin, K. Blanchard, and H. F. Bunn, *Proc. Natl. Acad. Sci. U.S.A.* **87**, 2725 (1990).

8. P. D. Siebert and J. W. Larrick, *Nature (London)* **359**, 557 (1992).

9. P. D. Siebert and J. W. Larrick, *BioTechniques* **14**, 244 (1993).

10. A. M. Wang, M. V. Doyle, and D. F. Mark, *Proc. Natl. Acad. Sci. U.S.A.* **86**, 9717 (1989).

11. R. H. Scheuermann and S. R. Bauer, *in* "Methods in Enzymology" (R. Wu, ed.), Vol. **218**, p. 446. Academic Press, San Diego, 1993.

12. M. Becker-André and K. Hahlbrock, *Nucleic Acids Res.* **17**, 9437 (1989).

13. J. H.-C. Lin, B. Grandchamp, and N. G. Abraham, *Exp. Hematol.* **19**, 817 (1991).

14. S. Menzo, P. Bagnarelli, M. Giacca, M. Manzin, P. E. Varaldo, and P. E. Clementi, *J. Clin. Microbiol.* **30**, 1752 (1992).

15. S. Diviacco, P. Norio, L. Zentilin, S. Menzo, M. Clementi, G. Biamonti, S. Riva, A. Falaschi, and M. Giacca, *Gene* **122**, 313 (1992).

16. M. Piatak, K.-C. Luk, B. Williams, and J. D. Lifson, *BioTechniques* **14**, 70 (1993).

17. M. Becker-André, *in* "Methods in Enzymology" (R. Wu, ed.), Vol. **218**, p. 420. Academic Press, San Diego, 1993.

18. T. Hoof, J. R. Riordan, and B. Tümmler, *Anal. Biochem.* **196**, 161 (1991).

19. R. J. Wiesner, *Nucleic Acids Res.* **20**, 5863 (1992).

20. T. Kinoshita, I. Imamura, N. Hirokazu, and K. Shimotohno, *Anal. Biochem.* **206**, 231 (1992).

21. R. Duchmann, W. Strober, and S. P. James, *DNA Cell Biol.* **12**, 217 (1993).

22. T. Jalava, P. Lehtovaara, A. Kallio, M. Ranki, and H. Söderlund, *BioTechniques* **15**, 134 (1993).

23. V. Zachar, R. A. Thomas, and A. S. Goustin, *Nucleic Acids Res.* **21**, 21017 (1993).

24. M. Becker-André, FMC Corporation, *Resolutions Newsl.* **9**(3) (1993).

25. J. Sambrook, E. F. Frisch, and T. Maniatis, "Molecular Cloning: A Laboratory Manual," 2nd ed. Cold Spring Harbor Lab., Cold Spring Harbor, NY, 1989.

26. M. Becker-André, *in* "Reverse Transcription PCR" (J. W. Larrick and P. D. Siebert, eds.). Simon and Schuster, Englewood Cliffs, Nd, 1995.

27. R. C. Allen, G. Graves, and B. Budowle, *BioTechniques* **7**, 736 (1989).

27a. C. Carlberg, R. Hooft van Huijsduijnen, J. F. Staple, J. F. DeLamarter, and M. Becker-André, *Mol. Endocrinol.* **8**, 757–770 (1994).

28. B. J. Bassam, G. Caetano-Anollés, and P. M. Gresshoff, *Anal. Biochem.* **196**, 80 (1991).

29. M. Clementi, S. Menzo, P. Bagnarelli, A. Manzin, A. Valenza, and P. E. Varaldo, *PCR Methods Appl.* **2**, 191 (1993).

30. C. Porcher, M.-C. Malinge, C. Picat, and B. Grandchamp, *BioTechniques* **13,** 106 (1992).
31. I. Grummt and H. J. Gross, *Mol. Gen. Genet.* **177,** 223 (1979).
32. M. F. Gaudette and W. C. Crain, *Nucleic Acids Res.* **19,** 1879 (1991).
33. H. Kohsaka, A. Taniguchi, D. D. Richman, and D. A. Carson, *Nucleic Acids Res.* **21,** 3469 (1993).

[10] Comparative Evaluation of Quantitative PCR Methods

Sanjiv Sur, Gerald J. Gleich, Mark E. Bolander, and Gobinda Sarkar

Introduction

Over the past few years, considerable evidence in the literature indicates an association between increased expression or production of interleukin 5 (IL-5) and occurrence of eosinophilia *in vivo*. In early experiments, it was shown that mice constitutively expressing the IL-5 gene have much higher eosinophil numbers in the blood and other organs (1, 2). For example, antibody to IL-5 suppressed blood and tissue eosinophilia in parasitized mice (3) and administration of antibody to the IL-5 receptor inhibited eosinophilia in IL-5 transgenic mice (4). Subsequently, studies performed in human diseases characterized by eosinophilia showed elevated IL-5 levels in the bronchoalveolar lavage (BAL) fluids (5–7) or blood (8, 9). In patients with allergic asthma, the numbers of cells expressing IL-5 mRNA were increased in the bronchial biopsies and BAL cells compared to those of normal subjects (10, 11). Further, allergen challenge in atopic patients and in patients with asthma resulted in an increase in the number of cells expressing IL-5 mRNA (12–14). Thus, considerable evidence indicates that IL-5 is an important cytokine in eosinophilic disorders. For further research related to these diseases, there is need for a simple, accurate, rapid, and cost-effective method of IL-5 gene quantitation.

We desired to evaluate quantitatively IL-5 gene expression in the BAL cells of patients with asthma. For this purpose, we sought to utilize a method that was sensitive, accurate, rapid, and easy to execute. Quantitative polymerase chain reaction (PCR) following transcription of mRNA to cDNA is a sensitive method for evaluating cytokine mRNA expression in cells. There are two general methods of quantitative PCR, competitive and noncompetitive. In the competitive method, a reference DNA molecule with nearly identical sequence homology to the test DNA competes with the test cDNA for PCR amplification in the same tube (15). The competitive method is generally regarded as the "gold standard" of quantitative PCR because it is thought to eliminate tube to tube variation and is therefore considered accurate (15). The method has been widely applied to quantitate RNA and DNA; applications have included assessment of hepatitis C virus RNA levels (16),

Methods in Neurosciences, Volume 26

147

bone Gla protein mRNA (17), and acquired immunodeficiency syndrome (AIDS) virus levels (18–20). In the second general approach (noncompetitive PCR), the test cDNA molecule and various concentrations of a homologous reference DNA molecule are amplified in separate tubes and therefore do not compete with each other for amplification (21, 22). This method has not been used extensively because it is thought to be less accurate than the competitive method. The advantages and disadvantages of the competitive and noncompetitive methods are summarized in Table I.

Because both methods have strengths and weaknesses, we decided to compare them with a model system before choosing one for our studies. Our results suggest that the values obtained by the two methods are very comparable.

Materials and Methods

AmpliTaq and DNA thermal cyclers are from Perkin–Elmer Cetus (Norwalk, CT). Oligonucleotides are synthesized on an Applied Biosystems DNA synthesizer (Foster City, CA).

TABLE I   Comparison of Competitive and Noncompetitive Methods of PCR Quantitation

Characteristic	Competitive method	Noncompetitive method
Requirement of unique reference molecule for every gene being quantitated (time consuming)	Yes	No
Amount of test cDNA required	Large	Small
Number of samples quantified per assay	Few	Many
Labor intensive	Yes	No
Cost	High	Relatively low
Effect of tube to tube variation in PCR product	Considered none	Considered significant
Accuracy	Considered "gold standard"	Accuracy not well-defined
Heteroduplex formation	Possible	Not possible
Ease of using duplicate test samples	Difficult	Easy
Ease of obtaining statistical values	Difficult	Easy

Overall Strategy for Comparing Methods

The overall goal of the present study is to compare the noncompetitive and competitive methods of quantitative PCR. For this purpose, two reference molecules (mutant type or MT and wild type or WT) corresponding to interleukin 5(IL-5) cDNA are generated. The actual concentrations of DNA in the calibrating solutions of MT and WT are determined by titrating the intensity of bands visualized in ultraviolet light in an ethidium bromide-stained agarose gel against known concentrations of ϕX174/*Hae*III DNA markers (Promega Corporation, Madison, WI). These reference molecules (MT and WT) also serve a dual role of the first (MT) and second (WT) test DNA molecules. A third test molecule is generated by reverse transcription of mRNA from NS1 cells, a transfected mouse cell line expressing human IL-5 mRNA (a generous gift from Dr. S. Narula, Schering-Plough Corporation, Kenilworth, NJ). The two methods (competitive and noncompetitive) of quantitative PCR are applied to determine the number of IL-5 DNA copies (molecules) in these three test molecules, utilizing MT and WT as reference molecules (concentration known). The values determined by these two methods are compared to each other and to the actual concentrations.

Generation of Test and Reference Molecules

The MT is generated as a mutant segment corresponding to wild-type IL-5 cDNA. The restriction enzyme map of the wild-type IL-5 cDNA has two *Rsa*I (GTAC) restriction enzyme sites. One of these *Rsa*I sites (R2) was mutated by altering one base (G to T) and novel *Hind*III and *Bam*HI sites were introduced 5' to the mutated *Rsa*I site, utilizing the megaprimer mutagenesis protocol (see Fig. 1) (23). The megaprimer method was selected because it represents one of the simplest methods of creating site-specific changes in a target DNA (23). Introduction of *Bam*HI and *Hind*III sites into MT resulted in incorporation of 12 novel nucleotides. It was thought that while abolition of R2 may be sufficient to distinguish the wild-type from MT target DNA, incorporation of 12 bases would allow two additional means of differentiation between WT and MT, first, on the basis of size of the amplified products without restriction enzyme digestion and, second, on the basis of size after digestion with either *Bam*HI or *Hind*III.

To generate the MT IL-5, briefly, a PCR with primers A and C (see Fig. 1 for schematic location of these primers with respect to IL-5 cDNA and Table II for primer sequences) was performed on 1 ng of cloned IL-5 cDNA template (primer C has a sequence which abolishes one *Rsa*I site, R2, and adds a *Hind*III and a *Bam*HI novel restriction enzyme sites) to yield AC. Restriction

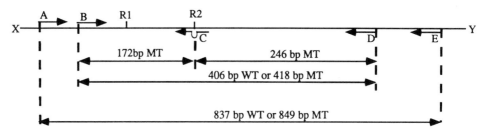

Fig. 1   Schematic plot of primers used. XY is an IL-5 cDNA template. The location of primers A to E and the expected product sizes after PCR are shown on this template. R1 and R2 are the two *Rsa*I restriction enzyme sites on IL-5 cDNA. Primer C has a mutated R2 and two novel restriction enzyme sites (*Hind*III and *Bam*H1). Primers A and C were used in a PCR with template XY to yield AC, and AC having mutated *Rsa*I and two novel restriction enzyme sites, *Hind*III and *Bam*HI. AC was used as a megaprimer along with E in a PCR to yield a 849-bp mutant type IL-5 DNA (MT). Primers A and E were used with XY template in a PCR to yield large amounts of a 837-bp wild-type IL-5 DNA (WT). For both methods of quantitation, a nested PCR was performed with primers B and D. This yielded a 418-bp MT (if the 849-bp MT was used as template) or 406-bp WT (if the 837 bp WT or IL-5 cDNA from NS1 cell line was used as template).

enzyme digestion of gel-purified AC with *Hind*III and *Bam*HI yielded expected restriction fragments (data not shown). Purified AC is used in a PCR as a megaprimer along with primer E and 1 ng of cloned IL-5 cDNA template to yield an 849-bp MT, the first reference molecule. Large amounts of MT are generated by performing a PCR with primers A and E (see Fig. 1) with MT template. Digestion of MT with *Rsa*I and *Bam*HI produced expected restriction fragments of DNA, confirming that the mutations had been introduced successfully (data not shown).

TABLE II   Interleukin 5 Primer Sequences

A (sense with a 23 base T7 sequence 5' to the primer sequence)
    5' TAATACGACTCACTATAGGGAGAGCCAAAGGCAAACGCA 3'
B (sense)
    5' ATGAGGATGCTTCTGCA 3'
C (antisense with mutated *Rsa*I site and novel *Hind*III and *Bam*H1 sites)
    5'GAATAGTCTTTCCACAGTAAGGATCCAAGCTTCCCCTTGCACAG 3'
D (antisense)
    5' CTCAACTTTCTATTATCCAC 3'
E (antisense with a 12-base dT sequence 5' to the primer sequence)
    5' TTTTTTTTTTTTGAACAGTTGTCTATTTTTG 3'

An 837-bp segment corresponding to the wild-type IL-5 cDNA (WT) is generated by PCR amplification of 1 ng of cloned IL-5 cDNA template with primers A and E. Another test molecule is generated by reverse transcription of mRNA from NS1 cells, a transfected mouse cell line expressing human IL-5 mRNA. Total cellular RNA is extracted from 10^6 NS1 cells utilizing RNAzol (Tel Test B Inc., Friendswood, TX). The mRNA in the total cellular RNA is reverse-transcribed to first-strand cDNA with AMV reverse transcriptase and oligo(dT).

Quantitation by Competitive PCR

The MT is quantitated using WT as a reference molecule. For this purpose, templates in the PCR consist of a constant volume (1 μl) of MT along with 1 μl of variable concentrations of WT (12.3, 3.7, 1.2, 0.37, 0.12, and 0.04 attomol/ml). A nested PCR is performed utilizing primers B and D (see Table II for primer sequences and Fig. 1 for schematic location of these primers with respect to IL-5 cDNA) along with 1 μl of [^{32}P]dATP (800 Ci/mmol, Amersham Corporation, Arlington Heights, IL) to radiolabel the PCR products. A 22-cycle PCR is performed in a DNA thermal cycler using 94°C for 1 min, 50°C for 2 min, and 72°C for 3 min. In our study, the primers B and D yielded a 406-bp WT (WT template) and 418-bp MT (MT template) after PCR.

After the PCR amplification of these two templates, *Bam*HI restriction enzyme digestion is performed on the products. For this purpose, 7 μl of PCR product, 1 μl 10× buffer, and 80 units (2 μl) of *Bam*HI (Boehringer-Mannheim, Indianapolis, IN) are incubated at 37°C for 2 hr. One aliquot of this digested product is analyzed by agarose gel electrophoresis (2.5% agarose) followed by autoradiography of the dried gels.

Another aliquot of the digested product is spiked with an unlabeled mixture of the 406-bp WT and *Bam*HI digestion product of the 418-bp MT (digestion yields 246- and 172-bp segments). This spiked product is also subjected to agarose gel (2.5%) electrophoresis. The DNA bands are localized by visualizing under ultraviolet light, excised, and counted in a β scintillation counter (Tm Analytic, Elk Grove Village, IL).

The ratio of WT (406 bp) to MT (the sum of counts localized to the 246- and 172-bp digestion products of MT) bands is determined. This ratio is plotted against the input concentration of WT. The concentration of WT at which MT/WT = 1 is determined from this curve. When the ratio of wild and mutant bands is 1, the input concentration wild-type IL-5 cDNA is the same as IL-5 mutant cDNA (12). The values determined by this method are compared to the actual concentration.

Quantitation of test molecules WT and IL-5 cDNA from NS1 cells are also performed using MT as a reference molecule. Briefly, a constant volume of WT in different tubes along with serial dilutions of MT are coamplified by the PCR. The amplified products are digested by *Bam*HI and subjected to agarose gel electrophoresis. The ratio of counts localized to the 406-bp (WT) band to the sum of counts localized to 246- and 172-bp (MT) bands is determined. This ratio is plotted against the input concentration of MT and the concentration of MT at which this ratio of WT/MT is 1 is determined. This is the input concentration of WT. Likewise, to determine the concentration of IL-5 cDNA in cDNA from NS1 cells, a constant volume (1 μl) of NS1 cDNA and variable concentrations of MT are coamplified by PCR. The concentration of MT at which the counts localized to 246- and 172-bp (MT) bands are equal to the counts localized to 406 bp (IL-5 cDNA from NS1 cells) is the input concentration of NS1 cDNA. These data are expressed as IL-5 cDNA copies per 10^6 NS1 cells.

Quantitation by Noncompetitive PCR

To quantify MT, serial dilutions of 1 μl of duplicate samples of the reference molecule WT (12.3, 3.7, 1.2, 0.37, 0.12 and 0.04 attomol/ml) are amplified in separate tubes. Duplicate samples of the test molecule MT are also amplified in separate tubes. Primers B and D are used in a 22-cycle PCR. The PCR products are radiolabeled as above and subjected to agarose gel electrophoresis. These radiolabeled PCR products are spiked with unlabeled WT or MT, localized under UV light, excised, and counted in a β scintillation counter. A standard curve is generated by plotting the Cerenkov counts localized to 406-bp region (WT reference DNA) against the input concentration of WT. The counts localized to the 418-bp MT (test DNA) are also determined and plotted against the standard curve generated by WT to determine the concentration of MT.

To quantify WT and IL-5 cDNA from NS1 cells by noncompetitive PCR, duplicate samples of 1 μl WT and 1 μl of various concentrations of MT (same as that used for competitive PCR above) are amplified in separate tubes in a 22-cycle PCR. The PCR products are radiolabeled as above. A standard curve is generated by plotting the counts localized to 418 bp (MT) against the input concentration of MT. The counts localized to the 406-bp WT (test DNA) are plotted against the standard curve generated by MT to determine the concentration of WT. This experiment is repeated once to determine reproducibility. The mean $\pm$ SD of four values is determined from these two experiments. The ability of this method to discriminate threefold differences in the initial concentration of test WT is tested by also analyzing

WT/3, equal to one-third the concentration of WT. Likewise, to quantitate the third test molecule (first-strand cDNA from NS1 cells), duplicate samples of 1 μl of NS1 cDNA and 1 μl of various concentrations of MT are amplified in separate tubes. This experiment is also repeated once. Like WT/3, NS1/3 (equal to one-third concentration of NS1) is also tested.

Results

Our initial strategy was to distinguish WT and MT by *Rsa*I restriction enzyme digestion of PCR products after coamplification of WT and MT. *Rsa*I digestion of the WT-amplified product yielded three products of 78, 158, and 167 bp. *Rsa*I digestion of the MT-amplified product yielded two products, 167 and 250 bp. Because both WT and MT yielded 167-bp products, this approach could not be used to distinguish the two. Further, the 158-bp WT product could not be distinguished from the 167-bp products on the basis of size in a 2.5% agarose gel. This left the 78-bp product as a marker for WT and the 250-bp product as a marker for MT. Because the size and sequence of these products are quite different and because the 78-bp fragment incorporated relatively few counts above background (data not shown), this strategy of distinguishing WT from MT was not pursued further. These observations prompted exploration of a second alternative to distinguish WT from MT: *Bam*HI digestion of PCR products. This method successfully distinguished WT and MT and was used in the competitive PCR described below.

Quantitation by Competitive PCR

A constant volume of MT and 1 μl of various concentrations of WT (12.3 to 0.04 attomol/ml) in six tubes (lanes 1–6, Fig. 2) were coamplified by the PCR. Another tube (lane 7, Fig. 2) only had 1 μl of MT (and no WT). PCR was performed with primers B and D and in the presence of [α-^{32}P]dATP. Twenty-two cycles of amplification were carried out. After PCR, an aliquot of the products were digested with *Bam*HI. Figure 2 shows the autoradiogram of the restriction enzyme (*Bam*HI) digestion products analyzed by agarose gel electrophoresis. The restriction enzyme digestion yielded two segments of 246 and 172 bp corresponding to the 418-bp MT. A 406-bp segment corresponding to WT is produced by amplification of WT with the same set of primers (B and D). The intensity of bands corresponding to MT increases progressively (lanes 2 through 7) with the concomitant decrease in the intensity of the band corresponding to WT (this inverse relationship between

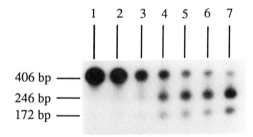

FIG. 2   Competitive PCR to determine the concentration of MT. Autoradiography of the *Bam*HI restriction enzyme-digested PCR products was performed in a model experiment for quantitation of MT. A constant volume (1 μl) of MT was added to seven PCR tubes (lanes 1 to 7). One microliter of variable concentrations of WT was also added to six tubes (lane 1, 12.3; 2, 3.7; 3, 1.2; 4, 0.37; 5, 0.12; 6, 0.04; 7, 0 attomol/ml). PCR was performed with primers B and D. These primers yield a 418-bp MT and a 406-bp WT. [^{32}P]dATP was used to radiolabel the PCR products. After PCR, the products were digested with *Bam*HI restriction enzyme. An agarose gel (2.5%) electrophoresis was performed on the digested products followed by autoradiography. *Bam*HI digestion of the 418-bp MT resulted in the generation of 246 and 172-bp bands.

WT- and MT-specific bands in competitive PCR has been demonstrated previously) (15).

Figure 2 also shows an unexpected band in the 406-bp region of lane 7. Because the PCR reagents were not contaminated with WT (data not shown), the possibility of partially digested MT was suspected. To test this hypothesis, the PCR product from lane 7 was digested with 10-fold more enzyme for a 3-fold longer incubation period. Further, *Bam*HI from another company was also tested (Promega Corporation, Madison, WI). Both approaches failed to digest this product (data not shown). When another aliquot of the product in lane 7 was digested with *Rsa*I using the same protocol as that used for *Bam*HI, digestion was complete. This suggested that the reaction conditions for *Bam*HI digestion were not the problem. These observations led us to conclude that the MT preparation itself has a small contamination of WT that probably occurred during synthesis of MT. This is possible because the original MT and WT molecules are 837 and 849 bp, respectively, which cannot be separated from each other by agarose gel purification. The presence of WT and MT molecules could form heteroduplexes which are resistant to *Bam*HI digestion (heteroduplex formation during competitive PCR has been observed previously) (17). Interestingly, this amount of heteroduplex formation did not alter the linear relationship between the ratio of WT/MT to the input concentration of WT ($r = 0.99$, $p = 0.0002$), indicating that quantitation is still valid. For the purpose of calculations, the radioactive counts corresponding to 406 bp region of lane 7 (Fig. 2) was subtracted from all other lanes.

Figure 3 shows a graph of the ratio of the WT/MT Cerenkov counts plotted against the input concentration of WT. The ratio of the counts of the WT/MT PCR products correlated to the input concentration of WT ($r = 0.99$, $p = 0.0002$). The point on the curve where WT/MT ratio is 1 corresponds to a WT concentration of 1.0 attomol/ml (15). This is the predicted input concentration (before PCR) of the MT test molecule. Utilizing the Avogadro's number (6.023×10^{23} molecules/mole), this is the same as 6.02×10^5 copies (molecules) per ml.

Utilizing a strategy similar to that outlined above for the competitive PCR, the concentration of WT test molecule determined was 3.3 attomol/ml or 19.9×10^5 copies/ml. Likewise, the amount of IL-5 cDNA from NS1 cells (third test molecule) was 2.3×10^6 copies per 10^6 NS1 cells.

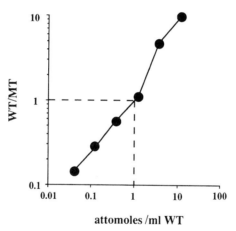

FIG. 3   Calculation of input concentration of MT by competitive PCR. Following agarose gel electrophoresis of the *Bam*HI digestion products, the 406-bp (WT) and the 246-bp + 172-bp (MT) bands were excised and their radioactivity determined. The counts corresponding to the 406-bp DNA in lane 7 in Fig. 2 were subtracted from the 406-bp counts of the other lanes (see text for explanation). The input concentration of WT (before PCR) was plotted against the radioactivity of WT to MT. The ratio of radioactivity of the WT to MT correlated to the input concentration of WT ($r = 0.99$, $p = 0.0002$). The concentration of WT at which the WT to MT radioactivity ratio was 1 (1 attomol/ml) is the predicted input concentration (before PCR) of MT (test).

Quantitation by Noncompetitive PCR

For the quantitation of test molecule MT by this procedure, the WT and MT bands were excised after agarose gel electrophoresis and their Cerenkov counts determined. Figure 4 shows the counts of WT plotted against the input concentration of WT to generate a standard curve. The counts of the WT bands correlated to the input concentration of WT ($r = 0.96$, $p = 0.003$), indicating its usefulness as a standard curve. The concentration of the test molecule MT determined was 1.1 attomol/ml or 6.7×10^5 copies/ml.

The noncompetitive quantitation of WT yielded a concentration of 3.1 ± 0.77 attomol/ml or $18.7 \pm 4.6 \times 10^5$ copies/ml (mean $\pm$ SD of four values from two experiments). The value of WT/3 was 1.2 attomol/ml or 7.3×10^5 copies/ml (mean of two values). Likewise, evaluation of cDNA from NS1 cells (third reference molecule) by this method yielded values of $2.1 \pm 0.4 \times 10^6$ copies/10^6 cells (mean $\pm$ SD of four values from two experiments).

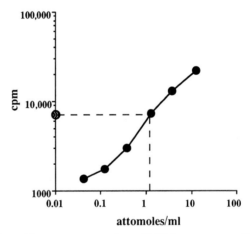

Fig. 4   Calculation of input concentration of MT by noncompetitive PCR. Various concentrations of WT (12.3, 3.7, 1.2, 0.37, 0.12, 0.04, 0 attomol/ml) and a test sample of MT were amplified in a 22-cycle PCR. After agarose gel electrophoresis, the bands were excised and their radioactivity determined. The counts of the WT bands correlated to the input concentration of WT ($r = 0.96$, $p = 0.003$). A standard curve was generated by plotting the counts of the WT bands against the input concentration of WT. The counts of MT were read against this standard curve and the concentration of IL-5 mutant cDNA determined was 1.1 attomol/ml (6.7×10^5 copies per ml).

Comparison of Competitive and Noncompetitive PCR

The major goal of this investigation was the comparison of the two methods of quantitation with a model system. For this reason, the sample sizes of the reference and test molecules and PCR conditions were kept unchanged wherever applicable. In addition, the two methods were carried out at the same time in the same thermal cycler, e.g., if some slots in the thermal cycler were used for one method at a given time, other slots were used for the second method. Therefore, the intrinsic nature of the two methods of quantitation remained as the only variable. The values of the three test molecules obtained by competitive and noncompetitive methods of quantitative PCR are summarized in Table III. The values of the three test molecules (MT, WT, and cDNA from NS1 cells) determined by the competitive method are comparable to the noncompetitive method. Further, the values of MT and WT determined by these two methods are comparable to the actual concentration.

Discussion

Considerable emphasis has been paid to the competitive method of quantitative PCR because this method is internally controlled and is thought to have the ability to reduce tube to tube variation of PCR products (15). This method, however, has several limitations as listed in Table I. A second method of quantitative PCR is the noncompetitive procedure. In contrast to the competitive method, this method is relatively simple and rapid. However, the accuracy of the noncompetitive method, relative to the competitive method (the gold standard method) is not known.

In the present study, we compared the two methods of quantitative PCR utilizing three test molecules and two reference molecules. The values of the MT and WT test molecules determined by the competitive method were

TABLE III   Comparison of Competitive and Noncompetitive PCR

Sample	Competitive method	Noncompetitive method	Actual concentration[a]
MT (copies $\times$ 10^5/ml)	6.2	6.7	6.2
WT (copies $\times$ 10^5/ml)	19.9	18.7 ± 4.6	22.7
NS1 cDNA (IL-5 cDNA copies $\times$ 10^6/10^6 cells)	2.3	2.1 ± 0.4	

[a] The concentrations of stock solutions of the test molecules MT and WT were determined by comparing the intensities of ethidium bromide staining of bands in an agarose gel to that of a set of known concentrations of ϕX174 DNA digested with HaeIII. These values were multiplied by the dilution factor to determine the actual concentrations.

comparable to the actual concentrations, thus validating the accuracy of the competitive method (and demonstrating technical competence in executing this method). The values of the MT and WT test molecules determined by the noncompetitive method were also comparable to those determined by the competitive method. This indicates that the two methods yield very comparable values for such pure molecules. The reliability of the noncompetitive method in evaluating concentration of a molecule from a mixture of a large number of different cDNA molecules was also tested by determining the concentration of IL-5 cDNA copies in NS1 cells by the two methods; again the values were comparable. These data indicate that the noncompetitive method of evaluation of cDNA concentration yields values comparable to the competitive method.

A previous report suggested that the principal drawback of noncompetitive PCR was that duplicate samples do not yield comparable values (15). When we performed noncompetitive PCR with duplicate samples and used the mean of two values to generate a standard curve, the results were comparable to competitive PCR. Obtaining duplicate values in noncompetitive PCR is relatively easy (in contrast to competitive PCR where obtaining duplicate values is considerably more difficult) and enables one to generate a mean of duplicate or triplicate values. Another potential approach for reducing the tube to tube variation in noncompetitive PCR (or any PCR) is to use the new second-generation DNA thermal cyclers that claim to eliminate virtually such variation. At least one of these new DNA thermal cyclers has 96 slots, which can also overcome the problem of the reduced number of samples that can be quantitated if duplicates are used in noncompetitive PCR.

We are not aware of any report comparing the two methods of PCR quantitation with the same reference molecules. The presumed unreliability of the noncompetitive method may be due to use of nonhomologous reference molecules, performing PCR at different times in a thermal cycler, or failure to use duplicate samples. Our data suggest that the tube to tube variation may be insignificant if duplicate samples and highly homologous reference molecules are used in noncompetitive PCR. The highly significant correlation between input DNA and output PCR product in the noncompetitive method ($r = 0.96$, $p = 0.003$) adds credence to the reliability of noncompetitive PCR in our study. In addition, the value of WT/3 (7.3×10^5 copies/ml) was remarkably close to the actual concentrations (7.4×10^5 copies/ml), indicating the ability of this method to discriminate threefold differences in test molecule concentrations.

It is important to realize that neither of these methods can yield absolute values, although such claims have been reported for the competitive method (20, 24). The term "absolute value" should signify something that does not change under any conditions. There are a number of reasons which make absolute quantitation by quantitative PCR theoretically difficult. Important among those are that: (i) the accuracy of both methods of quantitation reflects the accuracy of the method used for initial quantitation of the reference molecule. Because the two commonly used methods of reference DNA quantitation (optical density and/or second comparison of band intensities on an agarose gel against various concentrations of a DNA standard) have an inherent margin of error, the values determined by quantitative PCR, in theory, will also reflect this error. (ii) Because of differences in template size, the rates of cDNA synthesis (when quantifying RNA) of the reference molecule and its cognate in the test molecule, in theory, probably are never the same. (iii) In PCR quantitation of RNA, only a small segment of the RNA molecule is amplified. The segment being amplified may well be represented by both intact and degraded RNA, irrespective of whether oligo(dT) or random hexamers are used in cDNA synthesis. Keeping these limitations in mind, we suggest that it is premature to use the term "absolute value" in the context of quantitative PCR at present.

In summary, our data indicate that the values obtained by the noncompetitive method of quantitating IL-5 cDNA levels are comparable to those of the competitive method of quantitative PCR. The advantages of the noncompetitive method should, therefore, allow its application in quantitative evaluation of IL-5 gene expression in various disorders associated with eosinophilia. This method should be technically easier and faster to perform than the competitive method of IL-5 gene quantitation described previously (25). To determine if our observations from the model system utilizing IL-5 cDNA have more general implications, we suggest that similar comparisons of the two methods be performed with other genes.

Acknowledgments

We thank Linda H. Arneson for help in preparing the manuscript.

Supported in part by grants from the National Institutes of Health, AI 15231, AI 31155; and AI 07047; a Mayo Thompson Fellowship; and by the Mayo Foundation.

References

1. L. A. Dent, M. Strath, A. L. Mellor, and C. J. Sanderson, *J. Exp. Med.* **172,** 1425 (1990).
2. D. L. Vaux, P. A. Lalor, S. Cory, and G. R. Johnson, *Int. Immunol.* **2,** 965 (1990).
3. R. L. Coffman, B. W. P. Seymour, S. Hudak, J. Jackson, and D. Rennick, *Science* **245,** 308 (1989).

4. Y. Hitoshi, N. Yamaguchi, M. Korenaga, S. Mita, A. Tominaga, and K. Takatsu, *Int. Immunol.* **3,** 135 (1991).

5. C. Walker, E. Bode, L. Boer, T. T. Hansel, K. Blaser, and J.-C. Virchow, *Am. Rev. Respir. Dis.* **146,** 109 (1991).

6. J. B. Sedgwick, W. J. Calhoun, G. J. Gleich, H. Kita, J. S. Abrams, L. B. Schwartz, B. Volovitz, M. Ben-Yaakov, and W. W. Busse, *Am. Rev. Respir. Dis.* **144,** 1274 (1991).

7. T. Ohnishi, H. Kita, D. Weiler, S. Sur, J. B. Sedgwick, W. J. Calhoun, W. W. Busse, J. S. Abrams, and G. J. Gleich, *Am. Rev. Respir. Dis.* **147,** 901 (1993).

8. J. H. Butterfield, K. M. Leiferman, N. Gonchoroff, J. E. Silver, J. Abrams, J. Bower, and G. J. Gleich, *Blood* **79,** 688 (1992).

9. A. P. Limaye, J. S. Abrams, J. E. Silver, K. Awadzi, H. F. Francis, E. A. Ottesen, and T. B. Nutman, *J. Clin. Invest.* **88,** 1418 (1991).

10. Q. Hamid, M. Azzawi, S. Ying, R. Moqbel, A. J. Wardlaw, C. J. Corrigan, B. Bradley, S. R. Durham, J. V. Collins, P. K. Jeffrey, and A. B. Kay, *J. Clin. Invest.* **87,** 1541 (1991).

11. D. S. Robinson, Q. Hamid, S. Ying, A. Tsicopoulos, J. Barkans, A. M. Bentley, C. Corrigan, S. R. Durham, and A. B. Kay, *N. Engl. J. Med.* **326,** 298 (1992).

12. D. H. Broide, M. M. Paine, and G. S. Firestein, *J. Clin. Invest.* **90,** 1414 (1992).

13. A. M. Bentley, Q. Meng, D. S. Robinson, Q. Hamid, A. B. Kay, and S. R. Durham, *Am. J. Respir. Cell Mol. Biol.* **8,** 35 (1993).

14. A. B. Kay, S. Ying, V. Varney, M. Gaga, S. R. Durham, R. Moqbel, A. J. Wardlaw, and Q. Hamid, *J. Exp. Med.* **173,** 775 (1991).

15. G. Gilliland, S. Perrin, K. Blanchard, and H. F. Bunn, *Proc. Natl. Acad. Sci. U.S.A.* **87,** 2725 (1989).

16. H. Hagiwara, N. Hayashi, E. Mita, M. Naito, A. Kasahara, H. Fusamoto, and T. Kamada, *Hepatology* **17,** 545 (1993).

17. N. Araki, F. D. Robinson, and S. K. Nishimoto, *J. Bone Miner. Res.* **8,** 313 (1993).

18. M. Piatak, M. S. Saag, L. C. Yang, S. J. Clark, J. C. Kappes, K.-C. Luk, B. H. Hahn, G. M. Shaw, and J. D. Lifson, *Science* **259,** 1749 (1993).

19. D. T. Scadden, Z. Wang, and J. E. Groopman, *J. Infect. Dis.* **165,** 1119 (1992).

20. S. Menzo, P. Bagnarelli, M. Giacca, A. Manzin, P. E. Varaldo, and M. Clementi, *J. Clin. Microbiol.* **30,** 1752 (1992).

21. J. Singer-Sam, M. O. Robinson, A. R. Bellve, M. I. Simon, and A. D. Riggs, *Nucleic Acids Res.* **18,** 1255 (1990).

22. M. O. Robinson and M. I. Simon, *Nucleic Acids Res.* **19,** 1557 (1991).

23. G. Sarkar and S. S. Sommer, *BioTechniques* **8,** 404 (1990).

24. P. D. Seibert and J. W. Larrick, *Nature (London)* **359,** 557 (1992).

25. A. Guiffre, K. Atkinson, and P. Kearney, *Anal. Biochem.* **212,** 50 (1993).

Section V

Application of PCR in Mutation Detection

[11] Mutational Detection by Single-Strand Conformational Polymorphism

Nabeel Bardeesy and Jerry Pelletier

Introduction

The final proof that a candidate gene is responsible for a particular disease or developmental pathway is often the identification of mutant alleles in affected tissues or at the germline level in individuals with congenital defects. Until recently, rapid screening for mutations has been limited primarily to the detection of large-scale genetic changes due to a lack of sensitivity in the available technology. The possibility of quickly analyzing genes for more subtle changes has been greatly aided by the advent of polymerase chain reaction (PCR)-based techniques. All that is required for these procedures is knowledge of the sequence of the gene under study, and a source of nucleic acid from which the gene can be studied. It is in this context that we discuss technical aspects of mutational analysis from tissue samples, using the Wilms' tumor suppressor gene, WT1, as a model system. This review focuses on techniques that have worked in our laboratory for the analysis of gene mutations in Wilms' tumors, as well as their pitfalls and alternative strategies. It is hoped that the problems discussed herein will be useful in developing a mutational screen for any gene under study from any species.

Wilms' tumor (WT) is an embryonal malignancy of the kidney which affects ~1 in 10,000 children. It generally occurs in children under the age of 5 years and germline mutations within the WT1 gene, located at chromosome 11p13, are associated with predisposition to Wilms' tumors as well as developmental abnormalities of the urogenital system. A subset of WT1 mutations are associated with Denys-Drash syndrome, a constellation of Wilms' tumors, intersex disorders, and renal failure. The WT1 gene spans ~50 kbp and contains 10 coding exons, two of which are alternatively spliced to yield four mRNA species with an approximate length of 3.1 kb (1). Deletions of all or part of the WT1 gene are found in a small proportion of WTs. The genetics of WT is complex in that a subset of tumors appear to be caused by mutations in a separate gene located at chromosome 11p15. In addition, mapping of certain familial cases of the disease suggests the presence of a third locus; thus, only a proportion of tumors have WT1 involvement (1). The overall frequency with which WT1 is altered in WTs is not known since an extensive fine structural analysis of the entire WT1 gene in these tumors has thus far not been reported. For this to be accomplished it is necessary to employ a sensitive means of mutation detection which can rapidly scan large regions of DNA. Tumor specimens are frequently available only as paraffin-embedded blocks, so the means of analysis must also be of sufficient power to utilize these DNA sources.

Types of Mutational Analysis

The ultimate characterization of mutations in a gene relies on nucleotide sequencing (2, 3). This defines the exact site and nature of the alteration. If one is limited by sample size (e.g., a fairly rare tissue sample or unique developmental disease or animal mutant) then this is probably the method of choice to identify potential mutations. The main drawback is that it can be very time-consuming, although with recent automation, the amount of "hands-on" time has decreased. For the analysis of a large number of samples, this method becomes unreasonable; therefore, techniques have been developed to screen thousands of nucleotides for differences between wild-type and mutant genes. Some of these methods have been reviewed previously (4) and only those techniques which allow for a high throughput or high sensitivity are summarized in Table I (5–8). The goal of this article is to focus on one particular method which in our hands has allowed for the simple and rapid analysis of a large number of samples and has a high mutation detection rate: single-strand conformational polymorphism (SSCP) analysis.

Single-Strand Conformational Polymorphism

Single-strand conformational polymorphism relies on the ability of single-stranded nucleic acid to assume sequence-specific conformations (conformers) dependent on intramolecular hydrogen bonding, under nondenaturing conditions (6, 7). The resulting conformers have a characteristic electrophoretic mobility. The presence of sequence polymorphisms is expected to produce different conformers which are detected by a shift in electrophoretic mobility. The experimental scheme for SSCP analysis in current usage involves PCR amplification of a target sequence in the presence of a radiolabeled oligonucleotide followed by resolution on a nondenaturing polyacrylamide gel. This technique has been used effectively in the detection of subtle mutations in a wide range of studies.

TABLE I Screening Methods for Detection of Mutations[a]

Method	Position of mutation defined	Mutations detected (%)	Number of bases analyzed per reaction	Advantages	Disadvantages	Ref.
Sequencing	Yes	100	~400	Nucleotide change defined. Detects all mutations	Time-consuming	2, 3
Denaturing gradient gel electrophoresis (DGGE)	No	50–100	~1000	Large number of samples can be processed	Specialized equipment	5
Single-strand conformation polymorphism	No	70–90	200–300	Large number of samples can be processed. Simple and rapid	Limited length of DNA screened	6, 7
Chemical cleavage mismatch	Yes	?100	<1000	Potentially detects all mutations	Toxic reagents	8

[a] Methods developed for rapidly screening small mutations are tabulated. The appeal for SSCP analysis resides in its simplicity, power of analysis, and rapid sample through-put.

Isolation of Genetic Material

The isolation of nucleic acids from blood or tissue is fairly standard and most protocols in current use yield material of sufficiently high quality for analysis by Southern blotting or the PCR. The following procedures work well in our hands. Since these samples are subsequently analyzed by the PCR method, it is essential that appropriate steps be taken to avoid contamination from the investigator, pipetman, or reagents.

Isolation of DNA from Blood

1. When blood (5–10 ml) is to be shipped from a foreign institute, transport in yellow cap ACD tubes (Vacutainer 4816; Becton–Dickinson) at room temperature is sufficient to preserve the integrity of the white blood cells for several days, avoiding unnecessary shipping charges for material on dry ice. Tubes should be carefully packed in Styrofoam containers and sealed in plastic (in the event of breakage). On arrival, the specimens can be frozen or immediately processed.

2. Pour the blood into a 50-ml plastic conical centrifuge tube (Falcon), and add an equal volume of lysis buffer (50 mM HEPES, pH 8, 50 mM NaCl, 5 mM MgCl$_2$, 10% sucrose, 0.5% Triton X-100). Keep on ice for 10 min, inverting the tube occasionally to mix the buffer gently with the blood.

3. Centrifuge at 3000g for 10 min.

4. Pour off the supernatant into a clean tube and save. To the pellet, add 1.1 ml of 10 mM Tris–HCl, pH 8/1 mM EDTA (TE):EDTA (1 ml TE + 100 μl 0.5 M EDTA). Mix gently to loosen the pellet from the base of the tube. Put tube back on ice and carefully break up the pellet using a P1000 pipette tip.

5. Once the pellet has been disrupted and resuspended, add 0.25 ml of 20% sodium dodecyl sulfate (SDS). Incubate at 65°C for 10 min.

6. Add 50 μl 10 mg/ml proteinase K (BMC) and 50 μl of RNase A (10 mg/ml).

7. Incubate at 65°C for 90 min.

8. Add 4 ml of TE.

9. Extract two times with an equal volume of phenol which has been preequilibrated with 100 mM Tris–HCl, pH 8.0. We extract each time by slowly rotating the phenol/aqueous mixture for 30 min end-over-end on a wheel. The phases are separated by centrifugation at 5000g for 10 min. Generally, following each phenol extraction it is easiest to pipette out the organic phase, by inserting a 5-ml pipette with a wide tip into the bottom of the tube and pipetting up the phenol.

10. After the second phenol extraction, transfer the aqueous phase to a new 50-ml conical tube. The aqueous phase is extracted two times with an equal volume of preequilibrated phenol/chloroform, and finally two times with an equal volume of chloroform.

11. Add one-tenth volume of 3 M sodium acetate, pH 5.2 and 2.5 volumes of ethanol. Remove the DNA by spooling with a glass rod, dip into a solution of 70% ethanol, and transfer into an Eppendorf tube. (This step can be tricky and requires the investigator to "work" the nucleic acid off of the glass rod.) Allow the sample to air-dry for several hours or overnight. Resuspend in 400 μl of TE and quantitate by reading the absorbance at OD_{260}.

For the isolation of DNA from frozen tissue we use the following protocol. If the sample has been flash-frozen following its isolation, this procedure gives DNA of sufficiently high quality for Southern analysis. However, if the material was not immediately frozen, the nucleic acid will be fine for analysis by PCR, but unlikely to be useful for Southern blot analysis.

Isolation of DNA from Frozen Tissue

1. Using a prechilled pestle and mortar, grind a 1-cm^3 block of tissue into powder on dry ice. Transfer the powder into a 50-ml plastic conical tube containing 5 ml of 10 mM Tris–HCl, pH 8, 100 mM NaCl, 25 mM EDTA (TNE).

2. Add 50 μl proteinase K (10 mg/ml) (BMC).

3. Add 100 μl 10% SDS and swirl gently to mix.

4. Add 10 μl RNase A (DNase-free) (10 mg/ml).

5. Incubate by gently shaking at 37–50°C for 2 to 12 hr.

6. Extract twice with an equal volume of Tris–HCl, pH 8, (100 mM), equilibrated phenol. Extract and centrifuge as described in the previous protocol.

7. Repeat the extractions twice with equilibrated phenol/chloroform and twice with chloroform.

8. Add one-tenth volume 3 M sodium acetate, pH 5.2, and 2.5 volumes of ethanol to precipitate the DNA. Spool out the DNA with a glass rod or precipitate by centrifugation if very little material is recovered.

9. Wash in 70% ethanol, let air-dry, and resuspend in 400 μl TE. Quantitate by reading the absorbance at OD_{260}.

Access to archival material represents a rich resource for molecular genetic studies. This material is most often in the form of formaldehyde-fixed, paraffin-embedded tissue specimens. The nucleic acids contained in these specimens are of variable quality, often considerably degraded, and are contaminated with impurities from the fixation procedure. Nevertheless, the sensitivity of the PCR should permit analysis from most specimens. When PCR amplification is unsuccessful (for example when little DNA is available or it is of poor quality) the use of nested oligonucleotides frequently solves the problem. We have found that the protocols described by Wright and Manos (9) and Jackson *et al.* (10) generally yield material amenable for analysis by PCR. The best results are obtained when a paraffin block of sufficient size to yield about 50 mg of tissue is available; however, material from a single microscope slide is often sufficient.

Isolation of DNA from Paraffin-Embedded Tissues

1. Using a sterile scalpel blade, scrape ~50 mg of tissue into a sterile 1.5-ml microfuge tube and add 1 ml xylene. Incubate end-over-end for 2 hr at room temperature. Microfuge 3 min and discard supernatant. Repeat the xylene extraction, with a 30-min incubation.

2. Add 1 ml 100% ethanol, mix by inverting, and spin 3 min in a microfuge. Discard the supernatant. Repeat the ethanol wash.

3. Add 1 ml 70% ethanol, mix, and microfuge as above. Remove as much of the supernatant as possible and dry under vacuum.

4. Add 1 ml of digestion buffer (50 mM Tris, pH 8.5, 1 mM EDTA, 0.5% Tween 20) containing 200 μg/ml proteinase K per 100 mg of tissue. Incubate at 55°C for 1 hr then transfer to 37°C for 1 to 5 days (end-over-end incubation aids in the digestion of samples with large particulate matter). We aliquot the proteinase K to minimize the number of times this enzyme is thawed.

5. Boil 10 min, add more proteinase K (50 μg/ml), and digest for an additional 2 hr. This step ensures that DNA trapped in particulate matter is adequately liberated from proteins.

6. Add an equal volume of phenol/chloroform, vortex, centrifuge, and collect the upper aqueous phase. Back extract from the lower organic layer by adding an equal volume of TE, mix, centrifuge, and combine the aqueous phases.

7. Repeat the phenol/chloroform extraction.

8. Add one-tenth volume 3 M sodium acetate, pH 5.2, and 2.5 volumes of 100% ethanol, vortex, and precipitate for 1 hr at −70°C.

9. Pellet in a microfuge for 20 min at 4°C.

10. Add 500 μl 70% ethanol and microfuge 10 min.

11. Dry pellet under vacuum.

12. Resuspend the pellet in sterile water and analyze the suitability of the material for PCR analysis by setting up test reactions with serial dilutions of the samples (see below). Often, high concentrations of DNA inhibit the PCR reaction because of copurification of contaminants from the fixed tissue. When DNA from a small number of slides is being extracted, we omit the phenol/chloroform extraction and the ethanol precipitation to increase the nucleic acid yield.

For the isolation of RNA from snap-frozen tissue, we routinely use the guanidinium isothiocyanate method, as described by Sambrook *et al.* (11). We have found this to be the most reliable procedure for yielding high-quality RNA. When a large number of samples are processed, where time and number of manipulations become an issue, the following procedure yields RNA of sufficiently high quality for Northern blot analysis, but may have some contaminating genomic DNA. When amplifying across different exons by the PCR, this generally does not create a problem. This procedure is a modification of the method described by Auffray and Rougeon (12).

Isolation of RNA from Frozen Tissue by LiCl$_2$ Method

1. Prepare 3 M LiCl$_2$/6 M urea in diethyl pyrocarbonate (DEPC)-treated water and filter-sterilize through a 0.2-μm filter. This solution should be prepared fresh (i.e., <2 weeks old). If the contribution of water by the tissue will be significant, prepare a 4 M LiCl$_2$/8 M urea solution.

2. Take the frozen tissue and quickly drop it into 5–10 ml Li/urea solution. Homogenize (Brinkmann Kinematica AG) at full speed for 1 min, ensuring that the tissue quickly becomes uniformly solubilized. Perform the homogenization in a 30-ml Corex tube which has been previously baked at 80°C for at least 2 hr.

3. Let sit at 4°C overnight.

4. Centrifuge in a Sorval SS34 rotor at 10,000 rpm for 45 min. Remove as much lipid and supernatant as possible with a sterile Pasteur pipette. The lipid component will be at the surface of the centrifuged material. Remove this first, change Pasteur pipettes, and remove as much of the supernatant as possible. Avoid touching the pellet.

5. Resuspend the pellet in 4 ml fresh Li/urea by vigorous vortexing. Let sit on ice >1 hr.

6. Centrifuge in a Sorval SS34 rotor at 10,000 rpm for 45 min. Resuspend the pellet in 1 ml TE + 0.1% SDS. Extract once with preequilibrated phenol/chloroform and once with chloroform, and ethanol precipitate the nucleic

acid. Ensure that the RNA pellet is well-dissolved before attempting to phenol/chloroform extract.

7. Resuspend in 400 μl of sterile TE, and quantitate the nucleic acids by reading the absorbance at OD_{260}.

A variation of this method, incorporating the chaotropic agent—guanidinium isothiocyanate—can also be used to isolate RNA of excellent quality from tissue culture cells.

Isolation of RNA from Cell Lines by GITC/LiCl₂ Method

1. Wash cells (1 × 10 cm² dish) twice with sterile PBS.

2. Lyse by directly adding 1 ml of GITC buffer [5 M guanidinium isothiocyanate, 10 mM EDTA, 50 mM Tris–HCl, pH, 7.5, 8% (v/v) 2-mercaptoethanol] to the dish.

3. Transfer to a 15-ml Corex tube which has been previously baked for 2 hr at 80°C. Alternatively, a sterile 15-ml plastic snap cap tube can be used. Add 7 ml sterile 4 M LiCl₂, mix well, and incubate at 4°C overnight.

4. Centrifuge at 8000 rpm for 90 min in a Sorval SS-34 rotor at 4°C.

5. Resuspend the pellet in 5 ml of 3 M LiCl₂. Transfer to a new centrifuge tube.

6. Incubate on ice for 1 hr. Pellet the RNA by centrifugation at 8000 rpm for 90 min in a Sorval SS-34 rotor at 4°C.

7. Resuspend the pellet in 400 μl of solubilization buffer (0.1% SDS, 1 mM EDTA, 10 mM Tris–HCl, pH 7.5).

8. Vortex very well. Extract once with preequilibrated phenol, twice with phenol/chloroform, and once with chloroform.

9. Ethanol precipitate and resuspend in 100 μl sterile TE, and quantitate the nucleic acid by reading the absorbance at OD_{260}.

Reverse Transcription

A number of slightly different protocols give good results for reverse transcribing RNA. The protocol below is particularly useful for the reverse transcription of RNA with extensive stable secondary structure due to the denaturing properties of methylmercuric hydroxide (CH_3HgOH). For many templates, steps 1 and 2 can be replaced by heat denaturing at 65°C for 10 min followed by quickly cooling on 4°C ice/water.

1. Add 1–5 μg total RNA [or 0.1–0.5 μg poly(A)$^+$ RNA] to a 1.5-ml centrifuge tube. Add 1 μl 100 mM CH$_3$HgOH and incubate at room temperature for 10 min.

2. Add 2 μl 700 mM 2-mercaptoethanol and incubate at room temperature for 5 min (this step reduces the CH$_3$HgOH).

3. Add 100 ng oligonucleotide in a total of 13.6 μl, 4 μl 10× reverse transcription buffer, 6.4 μl 1.25 mM dNTPs, 1 μl RNasin (Promega), 1 μl 100 mM dithiothreitol (DTT), and 1 μl Moloney murine leukemia virus (M-MLV) reverse transcriptase. Incubate 2 hr at 37°C.

4. Add 60 μl water and store at −20°C. For PCR amplification, 1 μl of cDNA per 10 μl reaction volume usually works; however, in some cases this quantity must be titrated.

Gene Amplification by Polymerase Chain Reaction

In the PCR, the ability to amplify a particular DNA site specifically results from the use of two flanking oligonucleotide primers complementary to the target. For mutational analysis by single-strand conformational polymorphism, one oligonucleotide is generally radiolabeled to allow detection of small amounts of amplified products. This is achieved with [γ-^{32}P]ATP and T4 polynucleotide kinase. The following procedure, followed by direct amplification by the PCR, works well and reproducibly in our hands.

Kinasing PCR Oligonucleotide

In a 1.5-ml sterile Eppendorf tube, set up the following reaction:

10× PNK buffer (0.7 M Tris–HCl, pH7.6, 0.1 M MgCl$_2$, and 50 mM DTT)	2 μl
PCR oligonucleotide (0.1 μg/μl)	1 μl
[γ-^{32}P]ATP (3000 Ci/mmol)	5 μl
T4 PNK (10 U/μl)	1 μl
Water	11 μl
Total	20 μl

Leave at 37°C for 30 min. Add 20 μl water; store at −20°C in a shielded container until ready to use.

Polymerase Chain Reaction

$10\times$ PCR Mix [100 mM Tris–HCl, pH 8.4, 500 mM KCl, 15 mM MgCl$_2$; 0.1% gelatin, 0.1% Nonidet P-40, (NP-40) and 0.1% Tween 20]	2 μl
1.25 mM dNTPs	3.2 μl
Primer 1 (20 μM)	1 μl
Primer 2 (20 μM)	1 μl
^{32}P-labeled oligonucleotide	1 μl
Taq polymerase (0.2 U/μl)	1 μl
DNA (0.1 μg/μl)	1 μl
Water	9.8 μl
Total	20 μl

Cycle for 30–35 cycles. For SSCP analysis, most products will be under 400 bp, and we generally perform 1-min cycles.

Single-Stranded Conformational Polymorphism

Few changes to the basic protocol for SSCP analysis have been made since the inception of the original technique by Orita *et al.* (6, 7). Essentially, in this procedure the nucleic acid is denatured, generally by heating in a formamide-containing buffer, and loaded directly onto a nondenaturing poly-acrylamide gel. The DNA strands assume stable conformations once they have entered the gel. Parameters affecting sensitivity of the technique include the size of the PCR product generated, the temperature of electrophoresis, the presence of glycerol in the gel matrix, and the GC content of the PCR product (13). We process samples for SSCP analysis directly from the PCR described above as follows:

SSCP Analysis of PCR Products

1. Combine 100 ml 8% nondenaturing polyacrylamide gel mix [50:1, acryl-amide: bisacrylamide in 1X TBE (90 mM Tris/90 mM boric acid/2.5 mM EDTA)], 700 μl 10% APS, and 100 μl TEMED.

2. Pour the gel between siliconized sequencing plates and allow to poly-merize for 1 hr.

3. Preelectrophorese 30 min in 1$\times$ TBE buffer at 30 W in the cold room.

4. Take 2 μl of the amplified PCR sample and mix with 8 μl of formamide dye mix (95% formamide, 20 mM EDTA, 0.05% bromophenol blue, 0.05%

xylene cyanol FF). Place in a boiling water bath for 5 min; quickly transfer the tubes to icewater for 5 min. Prepare one sample in nondenaturing TBE loading buffer.

5. Electrophorese for 3–5 hr at 30 W in the cold room.

6. Dry the gel on filter paper and expose to Kodak (Rochester, NY) X-OMAT film at −70°C for 12–24 hr with an intensifying screen or at room temperature 24–36 hr (the latter gives a much sharper signal).

For the fine structure analysis of the WT1 gene, we have designed oligonucleotide primer pairs which allow us to amplify the WT1 coding, as well as the 5′ and 3′ untranslated regions (UTR). Using the SSCP assay (14), we have scanned the WT1 gene in sporadic tumors as well as in Denys-Drash patients for point mutations, small deletions, and rearrangements. Some of the regions we routinely analyze, as well as the resultant PCR–SSCPs across individual exons of WT1 from sporadic tumors are shown in Fig. 1.

There are a variety of parameters which influence the ability to detect a mobility shift. These are the surrounding sequence context of the mutation, the electrophoresis conditions, the presence of glycerol in the gel, and the size of the DNA fragment under analysis (13). In our hands, the type of mutation (transition versus transversion) does not influence the ability to detect a mobility shift. The sequence context in which a mutation is located can have striking influences on the shift detected by SSCP analysis. For these reasons, it is important to analyze both strands of the gene of interest when searching for mutations. This point is illustrated by the analysis of WT1 Exon 6 (Fig. 2). It is clear that one strand of the PCR product is more informative than the other for this particular analysis since shifts are obtained when oligonucleotide INT-9 is radiolabeled (Fig. 2), but not when the same samples are analyzed with radiolabeled oligonucleotide INT-10 (Fig. 1B). The sequence of the allele producing the altered shift has been previously defined and is a polymorphism found in normal individuals (data not shown).

Additionally, the composition, as well as temperature at which the gels are electrophoresed can significantly affect the quality of the results. This is illustrated in Fig. 3 where the same samples were electrophoresed at room temperature on an 8% polyacrylamide gel (50 : 1, polyacrylamide : bisacrylamide) (Fig. 3A), at 4°C on an 8% polyacrylamide gel (50 : 1, polyacrylamide : bisacrylamide) (Fig. 3B), or at 4°C on an 8% polyacrylamide gel (80 : 1, polyacrylamide : bisacrylamide) (Fig. 3C). For this region, the conditions in Fig. 3A give the clearest results. The presence of glycerol in the gels, as well as electrophoresis buffer (some individuals use 0.5× TBE), can also affect the number of different conformers observed, as well as number of mobility shifts detected (13). These must be determined empirically for each primer set to establish the most informative conditions. The optimal size

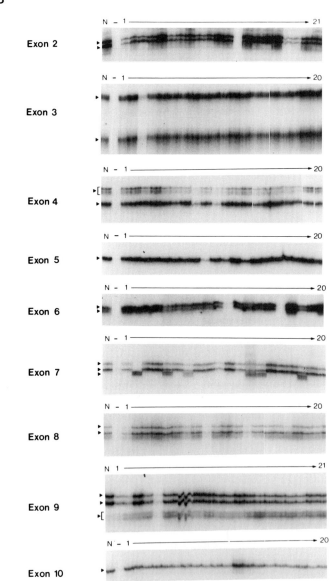

range for detection of base substitutions by SSCP is approximately 130–180 bp (13). Under these conditions, SSCP analysis detects mutations at a frequency of 80–95% (13). When amplifying across exons, we are limited in obtaining a lower size range by the size of the exon. When possible, we aim for PCR products of 150–250 bp. Products larger than this can be cleaved with restriction enzymes to yield shorter fragments for the SSCP analysis.

The ability to load more samples/gel would greatly increase the output of the method since the rate-limiting step is the gel analysis. We have used the small shark tooth combs from BRL enabling us to load up to 96 samples per gel, additionally we have loaded two sets of samples in the same lanes on a gel at staggered intervals (multiplexing). When multiplexing the samples, we offset the loading pattern to easily establish reference points in interpreting the autoradiographs. Since a single DNA strand can yield several con-

---

FIG. 1   Schematic diagram of the genomic organization of the WT1 gene and oligonucleotide primer pairs used to amplify the WT1 coding region. (A) Exon/intron structure of the WT1 gene. The 10 exons of the WT1 gene are represented by boxes. The open boxes represent the alternatively spliced exons, whereas the hatched boxes symbolize the four zinc fingers. The remaining WT1 exons are shown as blackened boxes. The ATG and TGA codons are in italics and indicate the start and stop sites of translation. Each exon is numbered and the position of the $(CA)_n$ polymorphic repeat within the 3' UTR is indicated. (B) PCR–SSCP analysis of Exons 2 through 10 of the WT1 gene in sporadic Wilms' tumors. Genomic DNA from sporadic tumors analyzed is indicated above the individual lanes. N, normal DNA; —, water control. The sequences of the oligonucleotide primer pair used in the amplification reactions are as follows: For Exon 2, A2 (5' CCGTCTTGCGAGAGCACC 3') and S2 (5' CTAATTTG-CTGTGGGTTAGG 3'); Exon 3, INT-16 (5' CAGCTGTCTTCGGTTC 3') and INT-15 (5' GGGTCTGCGTCTCGG 3'); Exon 4, INT-14A (5' CAGTTGTGTA-TATTTGTGG 3') and 106A (5' CCCTTTAAGGTGGCTCC 3'); Exon 5, INT-11 (5' CGCCATTTGCTTTGCC 3') and INT-12 (5' CCACTCCCCACCTCTTC 3'); Exon 6, INT-10 (5' CCTTTTTCCCTTCTTTG 3') and INT-9 (5' CCTTCCGCTGGGGC 3'); Exon 7, INT-6 (5' GCTTAAAGCCTCCCTTC 3') and INT-5 (5' CTTGAAC-CATGTTTGCCC 3'); Exon 8, INT-4 (5' GAGATCCCCTTTTCCAG 3') and INT-3 (5' GTGTCGACGGTCGTTAC 3'); Exon 9, INT-2 (5' CTCACTGTGCCCACATTG 3') and INT-1 (5' CAATTTCATTCCACAATAG 3'); Exon 10, INT-7 (5' CCTGTCTCTTTGTTGC 3') and 103 (5' GTCCCCGAGGGAGACCCC 3'). Oligonucleotides which were radiolabeled in the PCR are as follows: Exon 2, A2; Exon 3, INT-16; Exon 4, INT-14A; Exon 5, INT-11; Exon 6, INT-10; Exon 7, INT-6; Exon 8, INT-4; Exon 9, INT-1; Exon 10, Oligo 103. Following amplification, samples were electrophoresed on 8% polyacrylamide gels at 30 W at 4°C. Gels were dried and exposed to Kodak X-OMAT X-ray film for 12–24 hr at −70°C. Arrowheads indicate SSCP conformers.

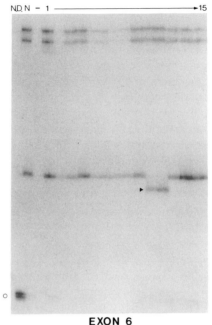

EXON 6

FIG. 2   PCR-SSCP Analysis of WT1 Exon 6 using oligonucleotide INT-9 as radiola-beled tracer. Analysis was performed as described in the text. The lane numbers refer to Wilms' tumor samples. ND, nondenatured; N, normal; –, water control. The arrowhead indicates mobility shifts detected with oligonucleotide INT-10. The open circle indicates the position of migration of undenatured, double-stranded DNA.

formers with different mobilities and intensities (see for example Exon 7, Fig. 1B), it is crucial to load a nondenatured control sample to determine the position of migration of the double-stranded nondenatured DNA hybrid. These parameters which we have established for analysis of the WT1 gene should be used only as a general guide when establishing specific conditions for another gene of interest.

Optimization of PCR

Primer Design

The proper design of oligonucleotide primers is critical for effective amplification by the PCR. Although a variety of computer programs are available to assist in this, we generally find that following a few simple guidelines is

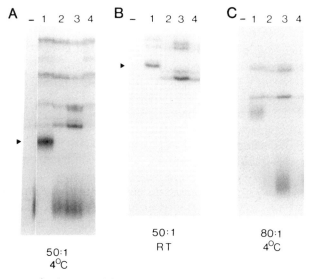

Fig. 3 Influence of gel composition on mobility shifts. Exon 7 of the p53 gene was amplified from four Wilms' tumors (1–4) with oligonucleotides D1 (5′ GTGTTGTCTCCTAGGTT 3′) and D2 (5′ CAAGTGGCTCCTGACCTGGA 3′). In the analysis presented, oligonucleotide D1 was radiolabeled. Following amplification, the PCR products were loaded on 8% polyacrylamide gels whose acrylamide/bisacrylamide ratio is indicated below the panel. The temperature at which electrophoresis was performed is also indicated below each panel. Mobility shifts are indicated by arrowheads. –, water control; RT, room temperature.

sufficient for choosing primers which work well. We generally aim to make 20 base pair primers with 50% G–C content. Additionally we aim to choose sequences with two guanines and/or cytosines at the 3′ ends to clamp the primer to the template.

Troubleshooting

The relatively small size of PCR product usually desired for SSCP analysis ensures that amplification will be accomplished easily. As seen in Fig. 1, the primer pairs covering the WT1 gene all yield specific PCR products amenable to SSCP analysis. It is usually sufficient to simply assess various annealing temperatures to optimize the PCR conditions. However, some regions, for example those with very high GC content, may require extra considerations. The addition of 10% DMSO to the PCR often increases the generation of specific products. Additionally, the concentration of $MgCl_2$ can be titrated in the PCR buffer (usually between 1.5 and 10 mM). Another parameter which can be adjusted is the concentration of DNA template; a very high concentration of DNA may lead to nonspecifically amplified products or the presence of a high concentration of an inhibiting contaminant in the DNA preparation may prevent amplification. This is demonstrated in Fig. 4 where DNA isolated from paraffin-embedded WTs show optimal amplification at differing DNA concentrations. Note the inhibition of PCR at high concentrations of samples B and C (Fig. 4). Vent polymerase (NEB), which has higher thermostability and processivity, can sometimes be used to amplify regions in which *Taq* polymerase fails. It should be noted that PCR products generated by Vent polymerase do not have deoxyadenosine 3' overhanging ends and thus cannot be cloned using a T vector (see below). A final aid to PCR amplification which we sometimes employ is Perfect Match (Promega), used at 0.1 U/10 μl reaction volume.

Contamination

A very frequent problem confronting investigators using PCR techniques is plasmid contamination of the reagents. A small amount of plasmid containing sequences to be amplified represents many more target sites for amplification versus very few sites in a similar concentration of genomic DNA. Therefore, a very small quantity of contaminating plasmid can effectively compete with amplification of a desired target in genomic DNA. In practice we find that

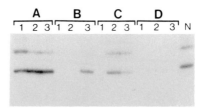

FIG. 4   Titration of DNA isolated from paraffin-embedded Wilms' tumor. DNA from paraffin-embedded WTs (samples A–D) was prepared as described in the text and Exon 11 of the p53 gene was amplified by the PCR with oligonucleotides G1 (5' GTCTCCTACAGCCACCTGAAG 3') and G2 (5' GGCTGTCAGTGGGGAACAA 3'). Tenfold dilutions of each specimen were performed: 1, 1×; 2, 0.1×; 3, 0.01×. *N* indicates amplification from DNA isolated from a normal individual. Samples were analyzed on 8% polyacrylamide (50:1, acrylamide:bisacrylamide) by electrophoresis at 30 W at 4°C for 3 hr.

a few common sense procedures are sufficient to avoid the problem of plasmid contamination of the PCR reagents. A separate set of dedicated Pipetman, reagents, and tubes should be kept exclusively for PCR and these should never be used with plasmids. Extreme care should be taken with the oligonucleotides as these are the most expensive of the reagents. We make diluted aliquots of the oligonucleotides and only open the stock solutions in areas remote from where plasmids are used (e.g., fume hoods or other labs). A control sample with no DNA added should be included with each set of PCRs to ensure the absence of contamination.

Time Considerations

Analysis with SSCP is a rapid means of detecting mutations and provides the possibility of analyzing a large number of samples simultaneously. Labeling the oligonucleotide takes minimal setup time and the reaction is allowed to proceed for 30 min. Setting up PCRs for 60 samples (the capacity of the thermal cyclers used in our laboratory) using the same oligonucleotide pairs takes about 30 min and 35 cycles of the PCR under typical cycling parameters takes about 4 hr. Preparing the samples in formamide buffer and loading the gel takes about 30 min and the gel takes about 3 hr for electrophoresis and 1 hr to dry under typical conditions. The investigator, therefore, reasonably can scan a region of ~200 bp in 60 samples in 1 day, with approximately 1.5–2 hr of "hands on" time. Analysis of the autoradiographs is very quick since one is looking for a pattern which deviates from the normal position of migration of most of the other samples. Therefore with about 2 weeks work, one can effectively analyze ~168,000 bp for mutations.

Cloning and Sequence Analysis of PCR Products

Once a sample is identified as having a mobility shift by the PCR–SSCP method, the investigator will generally seek to identify the altered DNA sequence. In our laboratory, we have accomplished this by both direct DNA sequencing and by cloning the PCR product into a plasmid followed by sequencing from the minipreparation DNA. Direct DNA sequencing has the advantage of saving time but it generally gives poorer quality data which may be difficult to analyze, particularly in the case of a heterozygous deletion where the sequence of alleles will overlap on the sequencing gel. Thus the sequencing ladder becomes unreadable above the site of mutation on the gel. However, direct sequencing may still be the method of choice when a very large number of samples are to be analyzed or when a particular, frequently occurring mutation is being screened for. A number of protocols have been established for direct sequencing from PCR products and the reader is referred to them for more details (15).

For most of our studies, we have chosen to first clone our PCR products before sequence analysis. We have found the extra time required by this approach is more than compensated for by the subsequent ease of analysis of the higher quality sequencing data. Generally, six clones are characterized to ensure coverage of both alleles.

Cloning of PCR Products

Our preferred method of cloning PCR products involves quaternary ammonium ion (QN) extraction of the DNA (16) from a low melting temperature agarose gel (QN extraction gives good yields for low-molecular-weight DNA although Geneclean may also produce satisfactory results). We generally exploit the presence of deoxyadenosine overhanging 3′ ends added cryptically by the *Taq* polymerase (17) to ligate the PCR product into a vector containing a complementary end (T-Vector) as described (17).

Amplification of the DNA Product

1. Set up a 50 μl PCR. Include a control reaction with no DNA added. Perform 30–35 cycles of the PCR.

2. Resolve the PCR products on a low-melt agarose gel (the fragments analyzed by SSCP will be in the 100 to 400 bp range so a 2–3% agarose gel is suitable).

3. Visual the PCR products with long-wavelength UV light and cut out the desired fragment with a sterile razor blade. Isolate the DNA as described below.

QN–Butanol Extraction of DNA

Prepare QN–butanol and QN–water as follows: Dissolve 1 g of hexadecyltrimethylammonium bromide (Fluka) in 100 ml *n*-butanol. Add 100 ml sterile water and 50 μl of Antifoam A (Sigma). Vigorously shake and allow the phases to separate overnight. Store at room temperature in a dark bottle. The QN–butanol is the top phase, whereas the QN–water is the bottom phase.

1. Note that this procedure works with low-temperature melting or Nu-Sieve agarose only. Weigh the gel slice and add a quantity of water such that the final agarose concentration is less than 1%. Melt the agarose slice at 65°C for 3–5 min. Add an equal volume of QN–butanol and QN–water. Vortex and spin briefly in a microfuge (2 min) full speed, at room temperature.

2. Transfer the butanol phase (upper) to a new Eppendorf, reheat the QN–water/agarose mixture to 65°C for 3–5 min, and reextract with an equal volume of QN–butanol.

3. Combine the two butanol phases and add one-fourth volume of 0.2 M NaCl, vortex, and briefly microfuge.

4. Transfer the aqueous phase (lower) to a new tube. Add an equal volume of chloroform, vortex, and place on ice for 5 min. Spin briefly and remove the upper aqueous phase to a new tube.

5. Add one-tenth volume 3 M sodium acetate and 2.5 volumes 100% ethanol. Place at −70°C for 15 min and collect the DNA by centrifugation for 15 min in a microfuge (centrifuging for 30 min increases the yield when only a small quantity of DNA is present).

Preparation of T-Vector

1. Digest 20 μg of pBluescript II plasmid (Stratagene LaJolla, CA) with *Eco*RV restriction enzyme. It is necessary to use a large excess of enzyme and an extended incubation to ensure complete digestion.

2. Gel-purify the linearized plasmid.

3. Resuspend the plasmid in 340 μl water and add 40 μl 10× buffer (500 mM KCl, 100 mM Tris–HCl, pH 8.3, 35 mM MgCl$_2$), 8 μl 10 mg/ml bovine serum albumin (BSA), 8 μl 100 mM dTTP, and 4 μl 5 units/μl *Taq* polymerase. Incubate 2 hr at 70°C. Under these conditions the *Taq* polymerase adds a single thymidine to the 3′ ends of the DNA fragment.

4. Add 400 μl phenol/chloroform, vortex, and centrifuge. Add to the aqueous phase 40 μl 3 M sodium acetate and 1 ml 100% ethanol and precipitate for 30 min at −70°C. Centrifuge 30 min at 4°C, wash the pellet with 70% ethanol, and dry under vacuum. Resuspend the vector in water at a concentration of 50 ng/μl.

We usually use the entire PCR product in each ligation reaction (10 μl total volume), together with 50 ng of T-vector. The ligation is allowed to proceed overnight at 16°C. The ligation mixture is used to transform competant bacteria for which blue/white colony selection is feasible. We sequence six clones for our studies and we find that screening minipreparations from 12 white colonies usually compensates adequately for false positives. Using the methodology described above, we nearly always clone in our first attempt a PCR product visible by ethidium bromide staining.

Summary

In addition to providing valuable information on the possible location of mutations within particular genes, PCR-SSCP is a powerful method for converting random DNA fragments to polymorphic markers for linkage analysis. In addition, once a given mutation is identified, a specific oligonucleotide primer can be designed such that the 3' most nucleotide discriminates between the wild-type versus mutant allele. In this fashion, a previously identified mutation can be easily retyped on a large number of samples. The ease of application of PCR-SSCP has rendered it invaluable to clinical diagnosis, analysis of archival material, and genetic mapping.

Acknowledgments

Many of the procedures we have described were established during postdoctoral training (JP) in the laboratory of Dr. David Housman (Massachusetts Institute of Technology, Cambridge) to whom I am indebted for advice, guidance, and encouragement. I am also grateful to several of my colleagues from that era, notably Drs. Alan Buckler and Vincent Stanton for their enthusiasm and contributions, directly and indirectly, to many of the procedures and ideas described herein. NB is supported by a studentship from the Medical Research Council of Canada. JP is an MRC scholar. Work presented and described in this review was funded by grants to JP from the National Cancer Institute of Canada and the Medical Research Council of Canada.

References

1. J. Pelletier, D. Munroe, and D. Housman, *in* "Molecular Genetics of Wilms' Tumor, Genome Analysis: Genes and Phenotypes" (K. E. Davis and S. M. Tilghman, eds.), Vol. 3, p. 135. Cold Spring Harbor Lab., Cold Spring Harbor, NY, 1991.
2. A. M. Maxam and W. Gilbert, *Proc. Natl. Acad. Sci. U.S.A.* **74,** 560 (1977).
3. F. Sanger, S. Nicklen, and A. R. Coulson, *Proc. Natl. Acad. Sci. U.S.A.* **74,** 5463 (1977).
4. R. G. H. Cotton, *Biochem. J.* **263,** 1 (1989).
5. S. G. Fischer and L. S. Lerman, *Cell (Cambridge, Mass.)* **16,** 191 (1979).
6. M. Orita, Y. Suzuki, T. Sekiya, and K. Hayashi, *Genomics* **5,** 874 (1989).

7. M. Orita, H. Iwahara, H. Kanazawa, K. Hayashi, and T. Sekiya, *Proc. Natl. Acad. Sci. U.S.A.* **86,** 2766 (1989).
8. R. G. H. Cotton, N. R. Rodrigues, and R. D. Campbell, *Proc. Natl. Acad. Sci. U.S.A.* **85,** 4397 (1988).
9. D. K. Wright and M. M. Manos, *in* "PCR Protocols: A Guide to Methods and Applications" (M. A. Innis, D. H. Gelfand, J. J. Sninsky, and T. J. White, eds.), p. 153. Academic Press, San Diego, 1990.
10. D. P. Jackson, J. D. Hayden, and P. Quirke, *in* "PCR: A Practical Approach" (M. J. McPherson, P. Quirke, and G. R. Taylor, eds.), p. 29. IRL Press, New York, 1992.
11. J. Sambrook, E. F. Fritsch, and T. Maniatis, (1989) "Molecular Cloning: A Laboratory Manual," 2nd ed. Cold Spring Harbor Lab., Cold Spring Harbor, NY, 1989.
12. C. Auffray and F. Rougeon, *Eur. J. Biochem.* **107,** 303 (1980).
13. V. C. Sheffield, J. S. Beck, A. E. Kwitek, D. W. Sandström, and E. M. Stone, *Genomics* **16,** 325 (1993).
14. R. Varanasi, N. Bardeesy, M. Ghahremani, M.-J. Petruzzi, N. Nowak, M. A. Adam, P. Grundy, T. Shows, D. Housman, and J. Pelletier, *Proc. Natl. Acad. Sci. U.S.A.* **91,** 3554 (1994).
15. U. Gyllensten, *in* "PCR Technology: Principles and Applications for DNA Amplification" (H. A. Erlich, ed.), p. 45. Stockton Press, New York, 1989.
16. J. Langridge, P. Langridge, and P. L. Bergquist, *Anal. Biochem.* **103,** 264 (1980).
17. D. Marchuk, M. Drumm, A. Saulino, and F. S. Collins, *Nucleic Acids Res.* **19,** 1154 (1991).

[12] Detection of Mutation in Yeast hsp60 Gene by PCR

A. Sanyal and G. S. Getz

Introduction

The biogenesis of mitochondria is widely studied in the yeast *Saccharomyces cerevisiae* because of its two important characteristics: ease with which it can be manipulated genetically and the ability to grow without mitochondrial function. Mitochondrial biogenesis involves the cooperation of two genomes: the nuclear genome, which encodes about 90% of the proteins engaged in the formation of mitochondria, and the mitochondrial genome, which contains the genes responsible for ribosomal and transfer RNA and the remaining mitochondrial inner membrane proteins (1). A number of approaches have been employed to identify the nuclear genes that encode proteins that participate in mitochondrial formation, structure, and function. Temperature-sensitive mutants, which are unable to grow on nonfermentable carbon sources at restrictive temperature, are useful to learn about such genes. These mutants can then be transformed with yeast genomic DNA library and functional complementation sought. Once the complementing gene is identified and its function established, it is often necessary to locate and define the mutation in the mutant gene. The resulting information helps to establish the relationship between the structure and function of the gene product in the mitochondria.

In 1987, Mueller *et al.* (2) described a series of temperature-sensitive mutants that resulted in a partial or total loss of mitochondrial RNA when grown at restrictive temperature. These mutants were encompassed by eight complementation groups. One of these mna2, which includes two alleles, mna2-1 and mna2-2, is the subject of this chapter. These two alleles can be complemented functionally by wild-type heat-shock protein 60 (hsp60) gene (3), the product of which is present inside the mitochondria as a 14-member homopolymeric complex and functions in the assembly and refolding of the proteins imported into mitochondria (4).

The polymerase chain reaction (PCR) has made a revolutionary impact on molecular biology research (5). Among its many applications, PCR has the potential to play a major role in determining the molecular basis of mutations. In this chapter we discuss how PCR was utilized to characterize the mutations in the hsp60 genes present in mna2-1 and mna2-2 instead

Methods in Neurosciences, Volume 26

of resorting to the more conventional approach of molecular cloning and sequencing of the mutant genes.

Experimental Methods

The task of identifying the mutation in the resident hsp60 gene of the mna2 mutants can be divided into the following steps: (a) isolation of the total yeast DNA from the mutants, (b) isolation of the different fragments of the gene using the polymerase chain reaction, and (c) sequencing of the PCR-amplified fragments.

Isolation of DNA

Yeast genomic DNA has been isolated from the mna2 mutants essentially by the procedure of Cryer et al. (6). The mutants mna2-1 and mna2-2 along with the wild-type strain D-273-10B are grown in media containing (w/v) 1% peptone, 1% yeast extract, 2% lactate, and 0.1% glucose to late log phase. The cells are harvested by centrifugation and washed once with 50 mM EDTA (pH 7.5) and then suspended in 50 mM EDTA (pH 9.0) containing 14 mM 2-mercaptoethanol. The suspension is incubated at room temperature for 15 min. The cells are reharvested and suspended in 1 M sorbitol containing 0.1 M EDTA (pH 7.5), and Zymolyase (100T from ICN Cleveland, OH) is added to a final concentration of 100 μg/ml and incubated at 37°C for 90 min. The spheroplasts are recovered by centrifugation at 3500 rpm for 5 min at 4°C in a Sorvall centrifuge (RC2B, SS-34 rotor). The spheroplasts are then suspended in 0.15 M NaCl containing 0.1 M EDTA (pH 8.0). Proteinase K is added to this suspension to a final concentration of 100 μg/ml. Sodium dodecyl sulfate (SDS) is then added to a final concentration of 1%. The lysate is incubated at 37°C for 3 hr, heated to 60°C for 30 min, and then cooled to room temperature. The lysate is extracted three times with phenol/chloroform (1 : 1, v/v) mixture followed by a single extraction with chloroform alone. The DNA is precipitated by adding two volumes of 100% ethanol to the aqueous phase, harvested by centrifugation, washed with 70% ethanol, and eventually dissolved in TE (10 mM Tris–HCl, pH 8.0, and 1 mM EDTA).

For the remaining two steps, i.e., isolation of the different fragments of hsp60 from the yeast genomic DNA and their sequencing, we follow the method of Stoflet et al. (7). This method has been designated genomic amplification with transcript sequencing (GAWTS). It involves (i) amplification of the gene from the genomic DNA by polymerase chain reaction using two oligonucleotides one of which contains the T7 phage promoter, (ii) transcription of the amplified gene from the phage promoter, and (iii) sequencing of the resulting transcript by reverse transcriptase, using internal oligonucleotides as primers and following the method of chain termination with dideoxynucleotides.

Oligonucleotide Primers

Oligonucleotides, used for polymerase chain reaction as well as for reverse transcriptase-mediated sequencing, are synthesized on an Applied Biosystems 380B DNA synthesizer. These primers are chosen based on the published hsp60 sequence (8).

Isolation of the Fragments of hsp60 Gene by PCR

PCR is done using the Thermocycler (Ericomp, Inc., San Diego). For each sequencing reaction two primers, flanking the fragment to be amplified, are used and one of the primers contains the T7 promoter. The volume of the reaction is 30 μl, which contains 10 mM Tris–HCl, pH 8.3, 1.5 mM MgCl$_2$, 0.01% (w/v) gelatin, 300 ng yeast genomic DNA, 30 pmol of each primer, 50 mM KCl, 250 μM of each dNTP, and 2.5 U of *Taq* DNA polymerase. Initially the DNA is denatured at 94°C for 3 min and then 30 cycles are performed with annealing at 55°C for 90 sec, elongation at 72°C for 4 min, and denaturation at 94°C for 1 min. Final elongation is done at 72°C for 7 min. Following PCR, 10 μl of the reaction mix is analyzed by agarose gel electrophoresis. After ascertaining that the amplification has been satisfactorily achieved, the remaining reaction mix is used for the next step.

Transcription

Each of the PCR-isolated fragments contain the T7 promoter at one end. This allows for transcription prior to sequencing of the resulting single-stranded RNA. A 20-μl transcription reaction mixture contains 3 μl of the amplified DNA fragment, 40 mM Tris- HCl, pH 7.5, 6 mM MgCl$_2$, 2 mM spermidine, 10 mM NaCl, and 500 μM each of NTP, 1.6 U of RNasin (Promega, Madison, WI), 10 mM dithiothreitol(DTT), and 10 U of T7 RNA polymerase. Samples are incubated at 37°C for 2 hr. In some examples the synthesis of the transcript is confirmed by including 50 μCi of [^{32}P]UTP (400 Ci/mmol) in the reaction mix followed by electrophoresis of 1–2 μl of the reaction product in a sequencing gel and autoradiography.

End-labeling of Reverse Transcriptase Primer

For sequencing the transcribed RNA, end-labeled oligonucleotides, having sequences internal to the fragment to be sequenced, are used. Oligonucleotides (100 ng) are end-labeled in a 13-μl reaction mixture containing 50 mM Tris–HCl (pH 7.4), 10 mM MgCl$_2$, 5 mM DTT, 0.1 mM spermidine, 100 μCi of [^{32}P]ATP (5000 Ci/mmol), and 7 U of polynucleotide kinase. After incubation at 37°C for 30 min, the reaction mixture is heated at 65°C for 5 min followed by the addition of water so that 5 ng of oligonucleotide is present per microliter of the final reaction mix.

Sequencing of Amplified hsp60 Fragment

The transcribed RNA is then sequenced using reverse transcriptase and the end-labeled oligonucleotide as follows: 2 μl of the transcription reaction mixture and 1 μl of ^{32}P end-labeled reverse transcriptase primer are added to 10 μl of annealing buffer (250 mM KCl, 10 mM Tris–HCl, pH 8.3). The samples are heated at 80°C for 3 min and annealed for 45 min at 45°C. Then 3.3 μl of reverse transcriptase buffer containing 24 mM Tris–HCl, pH 8.3, 16 mM MgCl$_2$, 8 mM DTT, 0.8 mM dATP, 0.4 mM dCTP, 0.8 mM dGTP, 1.2 mM dTTP, and 1.5 U of reverse transcriptase is added to each of the G, A, T, C tubes. A total of 1 μl of the appropriate dideoxynucleotide (1 mM ddATP, 0.125 mM ddCTP, 1 mM ddGTP, or 1 mM ddTTP) is added to each tube followed by 2 μl of primer RNA template. The sample is incubated at 55°C for 45 min and the reaction is stopped by adding 2.5 μl of 100% formamide with 0.3% bromophenol blue and xylene cyanol FF. Samples are boiled for 3 min and 2 μl is loaded onto the sequencing gel and separated by electrophoresis; subsequently autoradiography is done. During the sequencing of each template multiple-nested oligonucleotides are used to encompass the whole template in overlapping sequencing reactions—each reaction covers about 200 nucleotides.

Results and Discussion

The mutant mna2 belongs to a class of temperature-sensitive pet mutants that lose mitochondrial RNA at restrictive temperature. It has two alleles, mna2-1 and mna2-2 (2), and can be complemented by the wild-type hsp60 gene (3). To determine the nature of the mutation in the hsp60 gene present in mna2-1 and mna2-2, we employed the polymerase chain reaction since it

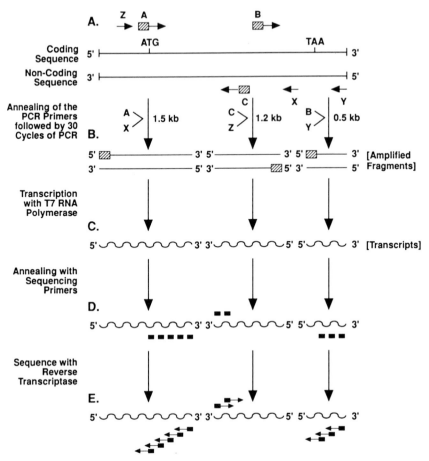

FIG. 1   Schematic representing the strategy employed in sequencing the hsp60 gene from mna2 mutants using GAWTS. (A) The coding and noncoding strands of the hsp60 gene with their 5' to 3' orientation. Three partially overlapping fragments 1.5 kb, 0.5 kb (for sequencing the noncoding strand), and 1.2 kb (for sequencing the coding strand) of this gene are amplified by PCR using oligonucleotides A and X, B and Y, and C and Z, respectively. The sequences of the oligonucleotides are given below:

A: 5' **TAATACGACTCACTATAGGGAGA**GTTTTCAAAATGTTGAG 3'
X: 5' ACCCTTGGCAAAATCATC 3'
B: 5' **TAATACGACTCACTATAGGGAGA**AGAGCTGCAGTTGAGGA 3'
Y: 5' ATTTACAAGATAATAAAATTATTACC 3'
C: 5' **TAATACGACTCACTATAGGGAGA**AGAGCTTCACCGTCAAC 3'
Z: 5' GGAATTCTGATCAAGTAGAACGCCA 3'

The oligonucleotides A, B, and C contain the T7 promoter sequence indicated by the bold letters. These primers are shaded to indicate the presence of the promoter.

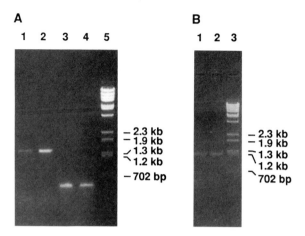

FIG. 2   Agarose gel electrophoresis of the PCR products. Agarose gel electrophoresis was done with PCR products amplified from the genomic DNA of mna2-1 and mna2-2. (A) Amplification of 1.5-kb fragment (lane 1, mna2-1; lane 2, mna2-2) 500-bp fragment (lane 3, mna2-1; lane 4, mna2-2). (B) Amplification of 1.2 kb fragment (lane 1, mna2-1; lane 2, mna2-2). λDNA digested with BstEII was used as marker [lane 5 in (A) and lane 3 in (B)].

represents a kind of *in vitro* cloning that can amplify DNA fragments of defined length and sequence. Specifically we have employed the method of GAWTS (7), since this method has several advantages. (i) It avoids purification and cloning of the PCR isolated fragments; (ii) it provides two steps of amplification of the sequence at the PCR level and at the transcription level; and (iii) a nested oligonucleotide sequencing primer provides additional specificity to generate unambiguous sequence data. The strategy applied to the yeast hsp60 gene is outlined in Fig. 1. Yeast genes are simpler than those

The PCR primers are annealed to sites just outside the sequence to be amplified. (B) Three amplified fragments with their 5′ to 3′ orientation. They are generated by 30 cycles of PCR which consists of denaturation of the DNA and annealing with primers followed by DNA polymerization. Each fragment contains the T7 promoter sequence at one end indicated by the shaded square. (C) Three RNA transcripts with their 5′ to 3′ orientation. They result from the transcription by T7 RNA polymerase from the T7 promoter sequence. These single-stranded nucleic acids are used as templates for dideoxy sequencing. (D) Nested oligonucleotides distributed along the length of the template are used as sequencing primers and are annealed to the single-stranded templates. (E) Sequencing is done by chain termination with dideoxynucleotides using reverse transcriptase.

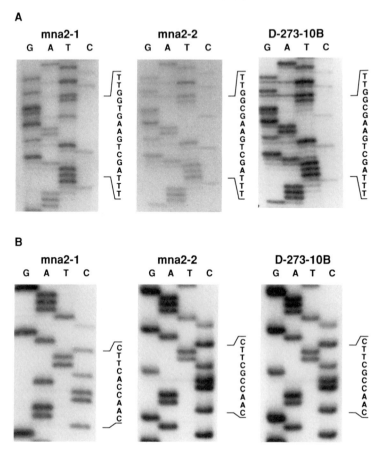

FIG. 3   Partial sequence of hsp60 gene showing mutation in mna2-1. PCR-amplified DNA fragments (illustrated in Fig. 1) isolated from strains mna2-1, mna2-2, and D-273-10B were sequenced as described under Experimental Methods. (A) Coding strand. (B) Noncoding strand. (Taken from Ref. 3.)

in higher eukaryotes in that they have few if any introns interrupting the coding sequence. The yeast hsp60 transcript is 1.9 kb long (8). We have analyzed the whole coding region of the hsp60 gene of the two mutants (mna2-1 and mna2-2). From each gene a 1.5 kb, a 500 bp, and a 1.2 kb fragment were separately generated by PCR. The strategy for generating these fragments is given in Fig. 1. Figure 2 illustrates that indeed these three fragments have been isolated. The 500 bp and the 1.5 kb fragments span the whole coding region of the hsp60 gene and were used to sequence the non-coding strand. The T7 phage promoter was included in the 5′ primer in each case so that the amplified fragment could be transcribed by T7 RNA polymerase. The resulting transcript was used as a template for sequencing with reverse transcriptase employing the chain termination method. A set of different oligonucleotides homologous to selected regions of the non-coding strand was used for internal priming for this sequencing. Each of these sequencing steps covers about 200 nucleotides of overlapping sequences. We have determined the entire hsp60 sequence of mna2-1, mna2-2, and the wild-type D-273-10B alongside of one another and the results for the altered regions are presented in Figs. 3 and 4. In the case of mna2-1 an A

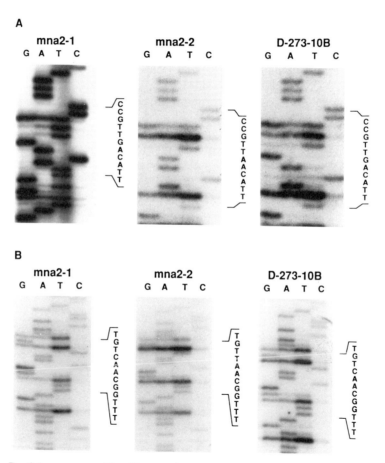

FIG. 4   Partial sequence of hsp60 gene showing mutation in mna2-2. PCR-amplified DNA fragments (as illustrated in Fig. 1) isolated from strains mna2-1, mna2-2, and D-273-10B were sequenced as described under Experimental Methods. (A) Coding strand. (B) Noncoding strand. (Taken from Ref. 3.)

instead of G was found at nucleotide 140 (Fig. 3B). Both mna2-2 and
D-273-10B contained the G at this position. In the case of mna2-2 a T rather
than a C was found at nucleotide 229. The C is observed at this position in
both mna2-1 and D-273-10B (Fig. 4B). These mutations were then confirmed
by sequencing the 1.2-kb fragment which includes 823 nucleotides downstream of ATG of the coding strand of hsp60 gene and spans the region of
mutations derived from both mna2-1 and mna2-2. The same reverse transcriptase strategy was employed for this sequencing. The results confirm a
T at position 140 in case of mna2-1 (Fig. 3A) and an A at position 229 in
case of mna2-2 (Fig. 4A). These changes result in the substitution of a valine
for alanine at amino acid 47 in the case of mna2-1 and isoleucine for valine
at amino acid 77 in the case of mna2-2 (Table I). During the course of this
sequencing we observed two differences from the previously published wild-
type hsp60 sequence (8). D-273-10B, mna2-1, and mna2-2 all have a C rather
than G at nucleotide position +1666, specifying arginine rather than alanine.
We have also found in all three sequences a G 29 nucleotides downstream
of TAA (translation termination codon) which is absent from the published sequence.

hsp60 is involved in the assembly (or refolding) of proteins imported into
mitochondria (4). A protein with similar function is present in *Escherichia
coli* as well as in chloroplasts. The bacterial counterpart is called GroEL
and that of chloroplast is called Rubisco (ribulose-bisphosphate carboxylase)-
binding protein (RBP). These three proteins share about 58% homology all
belonging to a chaperonin family (8, 9). The amino acid comparison of these

TABLE I Amino Acid Comparison of Yeast Mitochondrial hsp60 Protein
with *E. coli* GroEL and Wheat RBP at the Site of Mutation[a]

	Amino acid			
Protein	No. 47	Nucleotide No.	No. 77	Nucleotide No.
hsp60		$+140$		$+229$
		↓		↓
D-273-10B	Ala	GCG	Val	GTT
mna2-1	Val	GTG	Val	GTT
mna2-2	Ala	GCG	Ileu	ATT
GroEL	Ala		Val	
RBP	Ala		Ile	

[a] This comparison is based on the alignment of the predicted amino acid sequences of hsp60,
GroEL and RBP proteins by Reading *et al.* (8). The numbering of the amino acid is based on
the initiating methionine of the hsp60 gene. The nucleotide position is determined with the A
of initiating ATG of the hsp60 as position 1. (Taken from Ref. 3.)

three proteins at the site of the hsp60 mutations reported here is given in Table I. It is found that Ala at position 47 is conserved among GroEL, yeast hsp60, and RBP, while the mna2-1 has Val at that position. The change in Ala to Val is very conservative. A comparison of the homologous members of the hsp60 gene family in a large number of organisms (over 50) reveals Ala at position 47 for the vast majority of them suggesting a high dependence of function on this particular amino acid at this position (3). The amino acid Val at position 77 is conserved between GroEL and hsp60. The RBP has Ile at that position. The mna2-2 also contains Ile at the same position indicating another very conservative change. In contrast to the situation described at position 47, the amino acids found in the family of hsp60 gene homologues among the wide variety of organisms are more variable at position 77, consistent with the presence of Ile at this position in the normal copy of RBP (Table I). This is consistent with the observation that the functional impairment of mna2-2 is less profound than that of mna2-1 (3).

A PCR strategy similar to that outlined above has been employed to begin the characterization of spontaneous revertants of mna2-1 and mna2-2 mutants. It is clear that among about 16 such revertants none is a direct back mutation at the affected site of the hsp60 gene. These revertants are being further studied.

References

1. L. A. Grievell, *Eur. J. Biochem.* **182,** 447 (1989).
2. D. M. Mueller, T. K. Biswas, J. Baker, J. C. Edwards, M. Rabinowitz, and G. S. Getz, *Curr. Genet.* **11,** 359 (1987).
3. A. Sanyal, A. Harington, C. J. Herbert, O. Groudinsky, P. P. Slonimski, B. Tung, and G. S. Getz, *Mol. Gen. Genet.* In Press.
4. M. Y. Cheng, F.-U. Hartl, J. Martin, R. A. Pollock, F. Kalousek, W. Neupert, E. M. Hallberg, R. L. Hallberg, and A. L. Horwich, *Nature* (*London*) **337,** 620 (1989).
5. N. Arnheim and H. Erlich, *Annu. Rev. Biochem.* **61,** 131 (1992).
6. D. R. Cryer, R. Eccleshall, and J. Marmur, *Methods Cell Biol.* **12,** 39 (1975).
7. E. S. Stoflet, D. D. Koebberl, G. Sarkar, and S. S. Sommer, *Science* **239,** 491 (1988).
8. D. S. Reading, R. L. Hallberg, and A. M. Myers, *Nature* (*London*) **337,** 655 (1989).
9. S. M. Hemmingsen, C. Woolford, S. M. Van der Vies, K. Tilly, D. T. Dennis, C. P. Georgopoulos, R. W. Hendrix, and R. J. Ellis, *Nature* (*London*) **333,** 330 (1988).

[13] Comparison of the Sensitivity of Single-Strand Conformational Polymorphism and Heteroduplex Methods

Damjan Glavač and Michael Dean

Introduction

The detection of sequence variation in DNA is critical for the identification of disease-causing mutations in gene sequences and for the detection of DNA polymorphisms. Single-base alterations are the most common type of mutation and various techniques have been developed to detect these substitutions. The most commonly used techniques include RNase A cleavage, denaturing gradient gel electrophoresis (DGGE), chemical cleavage, single-strand conformational polymorphism (SSCP) and heteroduplex analysis (HA) methods.

In the ribonuclease (RNase) A mismatch cleavage method (1), the enzyme cleaves a labeled RNA probe at positions where mismatches have formed with a target DNA or RNA sequence. The fragments are separated according to their sizes so that information on the position of the mutation is also obtained. This method has been successfully used for the detection of mutations in some human cancer genes (2, 3) including familial adenomatosis polyposis (4). The efficiency of detection is not the same for all possible types of single-base mismatches and therefore the overall efficiency of this method is reported to be only 60–70% (1).

The mutation resolving capacity of DGGE (5, 6) is based on the observation that heteroduplexes between mutant and wild-type DNA fragments can be distinguished from homoduplexes because they migrate differently in a gel with an increasing gradient of denaturant (urea and/or formamide or temperature). This is a result of the instability caused by the disruption of the helix at the position of the mismatch. As the DNA migrates into the gel, the strands dissociate in discrete sequence-dependent domains when the denaturing stringency reaches the critical point. This partial melting of the dsDNA leads to an abrupt decrease of mobility. By this method about 50% of all possible single-base substitutions in DNA fragments of 50 to 1000 base pairs (bp) can be detected (5). However, the sensitivity of the method can be increased to more than 90% by attachment of a 30- to 50-bp high melting temperature GC-rich sequence to one PCR primer (6, 7). Denaturing gradient

Methods in Neurosciences, Volume 26

gel electrophoresis or GC-clamp DGGE has been used to detect point muta-tions in the β-globin gene in β-thalassemia (5, 6), rhodopsin gene (8), the p53 gene in human cancers (9–11), and in the CF gene (12). An advantage of DGGE is that detection is usually carried out by nonradioactive means. The denaturing gradient can also be generated by temperature and this approach (TGGE) has been used for the detection of mutation in the cattle β-lactoglobu-lin gene (13, 14).

In the chemical mismatch cleavage (CMC) method (15) heteroduplexes are formed between DNA probes and target DNA or RNA. Residues at the point of mutations are first modified with osmium tetroxide for T and C mismatches or with hydroxylamine for C mismatches, and then incubated with piperidine. Cleavage of the DNA occurs at the modified bases as in the Maxam and Gilbert sequencing method. A special advantage of this technique is that all mismatches react at approximately the same rate. The precise localization of the sequence alteration and the nature of the change is indi-cated by the size of the cleavage products and the cleaving reagent. The method is very sensitive and has been used for detecting point mutations in Tay-Sachs disease (16), phenylketonuria (17), and cystic fibrosis (18). An even more sensitive variation of the method has been used for the detection of mutations in collagen genes (19). Chemical modification of the mismatched base(s) is carried out with carbodiimide to modify unpaired G and T residues. The DNA is then used as a template for primer extension with *Taq* DNA polymerase and radiolabeled oligonucleotide. Extension is terminated at modified bases and the shortened extension product detected by autoradiog-raphy.

Since neither of above-described methods precisely defines the exact posi-tion and nature of the change in a fragment, DNA sequencing must be employed as a final step for all screening methods. This can be achieved by direct nucleotide sequencing of asymmetric PCR products (20), by the purification of biotin-labeled PCR product via avidin-coated magnetic beads (21), or by cycle sequencing (22). As direct sequencing becomes more effi-cient through the use of automation and new fluorescence detection technol-ogy (23), it is likely to become the primary method of mutation detection. However, at present, the determination of the nucleotide sequences of an entire gene is quite laborious and therefore inappropriate for a large number of samples.

In 1989 Orita *et al.* (24, 25) reported a new technique capable of detecting small genetic alterations, in particular point mutations, in DNA amplified by PCR. The method was based on the observation that single-stranded DNA fragments which differ only in a single-base substitution have different elec-trophoretic mobilities in nondenaturing polyacrylamide gels. They assumed that the difference in mobility was due to an altered conformation of the single-stranded DNA and named the method "single-strand conformation polymorphism" (SSCP). Another recently developed method, heteroduplex analysis (HA), involves the generation of DNA heteroduplexes between PCR products of mutant and wild-type DNA (26–28). These heteroduplexes can be detected on polyacrylamide gels because they migrate slower than their corresponding homoduplexes.

Principle of Polymerase Chain Reaction Single-Strand Conformation Polymorphism and Heteroduplex Analysis

The SSCP technique is based on the principle that single-stranded DNA molecules take on specific sequence-based secondary structures (conformers). Molecules differing by a single base substitution in up to a 1000-bp-long DNA fragment may form different conformers and migrate differently in polyacrylamide gels. The combined use of the PCR and SSCP analysis provides a simple and sensitive method for screening large groups of samples (23, 27–29). In Fig. 1 an example of PCR-SSCP detection of a point mutation in genomic DNA is shown schematically. For the PCR, either a set of two 5' ^{32}P-labeled primers (10 pmol) or a ^{32}P-labeled deoxynucleotide triphosphate (0.1 μl, 3000 Cu/mmol) as one of four deoxynucleotide substrates can be used. The low primer concentration and low deoxynucleotide concentration increase both the specificity of annealing and the proportion of incorporated labeled deoxynucleotide. The PCR reaction (9 μl) is performed in the presence of 0.1 μg of genomic DNA and 0.25 U of *Taq* polymerase for 30 to 35 cycles at 94, 55, and 72°C for 0.5, 0.5, and 1 min, respectively. A 2-μl aliquot of each PCR reaction to be analyzed is diluted prior to electrophoresis with 10 μl of sequencing stop buffer (95% formamide (v/v), 10 mM NaOH, 0.05% xylene cyanol, and 0.05% bromophenol blue). For denaturation, samples are heated to 94°C and immediately placed on ice. Electrophoresis is performed either in a cold room at 4°C (4 to 8 hr) at 50 W or at room temperature at 10 W (12 to 16 hr). The gel is dried on filter paper and exposed to X-ray film. The mobility shifts of one or both of the two complementary strands indicate the presence of a sequence variation in one of the alleles.

Figure 2 shows the principle of heteroduplex analysis. Heteroduplexes are formed by mixing equal amounts of the wild-type and mutant DNA PCR products, denaturing, and reannealing. In practice, 5 μl of each PCR amplification to be analyzed is mixed with wild-type DNA, heated to 95°C for 5 min, and cooled to room temperature slowly. Heteroduplexes do form during standard PCR cycles; however, additional incubation to 95°C for a few minutes drives this process to completion. Four distinct species are generated by this reassortment: wild-type homoduplex, mutant homoduplex, and two

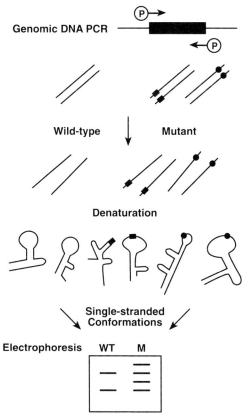

FIG. 1   The principle of PCR-SSCP analysis. Labeled double-stranded PCR products are generated for both wild-type and mutant samples. Following denaturation the single strands refold to form specific secondary structures. Mutant molecules will have a different structure than the wild-type molecules. On electrophoresis the two different wild-type strands migrate differently on the gel, as do the two mutant strands.

different heteroduplexes. All four of these DNA species are resolvable on gels with increasing concentration of denaturant. However, it has been shown that in most cases such heteroduplexes are also resolvable on pure polyacrylamide gels or polyacrylamide gels with 1 to 10% glycerol (26). Because such gels are also used for SSCP analysis, both methods can complement each other. Alternatively the same PCR product can be easily prepared for both types of electrophoretic systems.

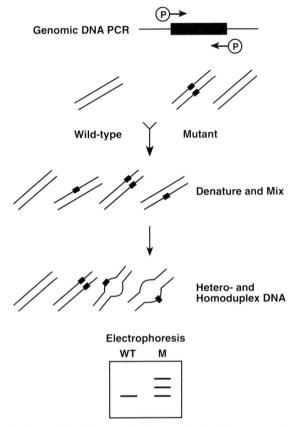

FIG. 2   The principle of PCR-heteroduplex analysis. The procedure to generate heteroduplexes is identical to the SSCP procedure (Fig. 1). Following amplification the samples are subjected to a denaturation and reannealing step. Samples are then loaded directly on a nondenaturing gel. Wild-type samples produce a single homoduplex band, whereas heterozygotes display one or more heteroduplexes that migrate slower on the gel.

Sensitivity and Variables Affecting Sensitivity

The most fundamental question of any method used for genetic analysis is its sensitivity. Because PCR-SSCP and heteroduplex analysis are relatively new techniques, only limited data are available for comparison with other methods (29–40). For SSCP there is no adequate theoretical model for predicting the three-dimensional structure and/or mobility shift of single-stranded DNA under a given set of conditions, as there is for DGGE analysis.

Furthermore there is a lack of large representative panels with many different types of mutations that could be used in sensitivity studies. Therefore at present, it is not possible to correlate electrophoretic mobility of single strands with the type of base change. However, on the basis of reports from several groups that have used SSCP in their studies, an estimation of the overall sensitivity is possible (Table I).

Conformational changes of a single-stranded molecule which are induced by a mutation are very sensitive to environmental changes such as temperature, composition of the gel, ionic strength, and additives. In fact these parameters can be used to optimize the sensitivity of SSCP for a given fragment. Because there is no theoretical basis for predicting the mobility shift, this must be done empirically. Mobility μ is defined as $\mu = d/Et$ where d is the distance migrated in millimeters, E is the potential gradient in volts/ millimeter, and t is the time in hours (41). For samples on the same gel, Et is constant and thus the migrated distance is proportional to the mobility of the single-stranded DNA fragments.

Temperature and Ionic Strength

Most SSCP analyses have been done at room temperature, at room temperature with a cooling fan, or in the cold room. A temperature change during electrophoresis is especially deleterious to the sensitivity and/or reproducibility (24, 42). This can be avoided if the temperature is controlled with a device that precisely maintains the gel temperature during electrophoresis by providing feedback control to the power supply (e.g., StrataTherm, Stratagene, La Jolla, CA). By placing the entire gel electrophoresis apparatus in a cold room, electrophoresis can be carried out at any temperature between 4 and 30°C. Higher power (up to 50 W) is also useful in shortening the electrophoresis time and improving the resolution. In addition, most single-stranded conformations are likely to be more stable at a lower temperature. We have tested the effect of temperature on 86 β-globin mutants (38). On 8% (2.6%C (w/v)) acrylamide gels run in a 4°C cold room at 50 W, all of the mutations migated differently than the wild-type sample. The sensitivity decreased to 80% if the gel was run at 10 W at room temperature and dropped to only 20% if the gel was run at more than 20 W at room temperature. However, in many cases good resolution was obtained on gels with 5 to 10% glycerol run at room temperature (25, 32, 36).

Since the formation of higher-order structures and their stability depends on ionic strength, the type and concentration of buffer in the gel and in the buffer chamber is also important. Orita et al. (25) originally used 1× TBE (90 mM Tris, 92 mM boric acid, 2.5 mM EDTA) buffer. Less concentrated buffer mixtures (0.8× TBE or 0.5× TBE) have also been used for SSCP

TABLE I   Sensitivity of SSCP on Known Mutations

Gene	Sensitivity (detected/examined)	Length (bp)	Electrophoretic conditions Concentration, cross-linking, temperature (°C)	Ref.
Ras	10/10	100–200	5%(2%C), 1.0× TBE, 4	32
	9/10	100–200	5%(2%C), 1.0× TBE, room temperature + 10% glycerol	33
Ornitine γ-amino-transferase	4/4	100–200	5%(3.3%C), 4	
	4/4	100–200	5%(3.3%C), 4, + 10% glycerol	
	4/4	100–200	5%(3.3%C), room temperature	
	5/6	300–350	6%(5%C), 4	
	4/6	300–350	6%(5%C), 4, + 10% glycerol	
	4/5	300–350	6%(5%C), room temperature	
Factor IX	11/12	183	5.6%, 0.5× TBE, 10 + 10% glycerol	35
	14/22	307	5.6%, 0.5× TBE, 10 + 10% glycerol	
p53	18/20	134–285	4.5%, 1.0× TBE, 4	35
	10/20	134–285	4.5%, 0.5× TBE, 4	
	11/20	134–285	4.5%, 0.5× TBE, 4 + 5% glycerol	
Rhodopsin	5/8	300	6%(1.3%C), 0.5× TBE, room temperature + 5% glycerol	36
β-Globin	86/86	193	7.5%(2.6%C), 0.8× TBE, 4	38
Cystic fibrosis	135/135	200–570	8%(1.3%C), 0.8× TBE, 4	38, 39
			10%(1.3%C), 0.8× TBE, 4 + 10% glycerol	
			10%(1.3%C), 0.8× TBE, 4 + 10% sucrose	

analysis with equal or better resolution (35, 37, 38). Less concentrated buffer solutions also shorten electrophoretic time and improve the sharpness of the bands. In nonradioactive SSCP analysis run on small 20% acrylamide gels, 1.5× TBE has been used (43).

Gel Concentration and Median Pore Size

The properties of the gel can be altered significantly by changing the percentage of acrylamide and bisacrylamide in the gel (41). Two parameters can be varied; the concentration of acrylamide in the gel (%T) and the percentage of cross-linking (%C). Low cross-linking (1–3%C) produces "long fiber gels" with an increased pore size. Many early SSCP analyses were done at a cross-linker concentration (5%) that is not optimal for the detection of conformational differences. In some cases good separation on gels with lower percent of cross-linker was obtained (33, 37) while in others the percent of cross-linker was varied with no improvement in resolution of single strands (34, 35). We empirically determined the influence of gel concentration and percent cross-linking on the separation efficiency on 86 β-globin mutants and 135 CF mutations (38, 39). A series of gels were run with acrylamide concentration ranging from 3 to 15% and with a variable ratio of acrylamide : bisacrylamide (9:1, 19:1, 29:1, 37.5:1, and 75:1 (w/w)). Gels with higher acrylamide concentration and low cross-linking were optimal for separation.

The gel concentration and cross-linking can also be adjusted to the fragment size to increase the sensitivity. For example, PCR fragments from 80 to 150 bp can be analyzed on gels with 10 to 14% acrylamide at 1.3 to 2.6% cross-linking while fragments up to 600 bp are best run on 6 to 10% acrylamide gels (39). The influence of acrylamide concentration and cross-linking is shown in Fig. 3 for 45 β-globin point mutations on three different acrylamide gels.

Additives

It has been empirically determined that the presence of 1–10% glycerol in the gel quite often improves the sensitivity (24, 25). However, it is not clear how the addition of glycerol to the gel influences the separation of single strands. Hayashi (42) proposed that glycerol might act as a weak denaturant and partially open the folded structure of the single-stranded DNA. We tested the resolution of 86 β-globin point mutations on acrylamide gels with 2 to 15% glycerol relative to other "OH-rich" additives such as butanol, glucose, or sucrose. In addition additives that denature single-stranded DNA such as

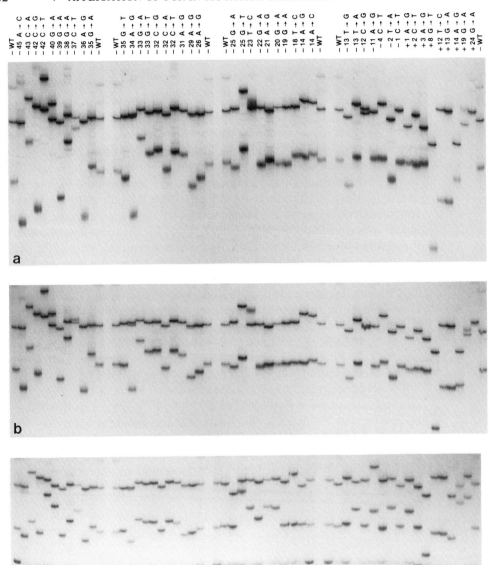

FIG. 3   PCR-SSCP analysis of 45 single base substitutions in a 193-bp β-globin fragment on three different acrylamide gels. (a) 10% acrylamide with 1.3% cross-linking, (b) 8% acrylamide with 2.6% cross-linking, and (c) 5% acrylamide with 2.6% cross-linking. All three gels were run in the cold room at 50 W in 0.8× TBE.

urea, formamide, and dimethyl sulfoxide were also tested (38). We found a significant similarity in the separation pattern of mutants on gels with glycerol and on gels with OH-rich additives. However, gels with denaturing additives also revealed a similar separation pattern for the same set of mutations. This indicates that interactions between the —OH groups of glycerol and the DNA, as well as intermolecular hydrogen bond formation, are responsible for the changes in conformation and mobility shift observed in glycerol gels. We also found that low concentrations of urea (2 to 5%) or 10 to 15% sucrose improved the separation of the β-globin mutants and many CF mutations. An added benefit of these gels is a sharp heteroduplex resolution especially when mutations with small deletions are analyzed (39, data not shown).

Fragment Size

The effect of the size of the DNA fragment on the sensitivity of SSCP is perhaps the best understood of all variables. Most studies report a decrease in sensitivity with increasing size of the fragment (34, 35, 37). In general for most DNA fragments shorter than 200 nucleotides, a sensitivity of greater than 90% can be achieved if a combination of two or three different sets of conditions is used. As the size of the PCR fragment increases from 300 to 500 bp, a drop in sensitivity of 10 to 20% should be expected (32). In practice there is rarely a need to screen longer fragments since most exons are within this size range.

Alternatively a larger PCR product can be digested with an appropriate restriction enzyme before running the sample on the SSCP gel. Optimal fragment size is also a function of base composition and may vary from one DNA fragment to another. As there is an upper limit to the size of DNA fragments for optimal SSCP sensitivity it is likely that there is also a lower limit. A high sensitivity of detection for DNA fragments as small as 100 bp has been reported (37). We observed differences in mobility shifts for β-globin fragments as short as 50 bp (38).

Type of Base Change and Base Composition

Other important parameters that play a role in the sensitivity of SSCP include the nature of the base substitution and the sequence composition of the DNA fragment. It has been shown that the base sequence around a point mutation has a greater effect on the mobility shift of single strands than the nature of the base substitution (35, 38). We have used an asymmetric PCR-SSCP technique to follow the relative position of the purine and pyrimidine-rich single strands for individual mutations and correlated the mobility shift with the nature and/or position of the base change. We found that the most dramatic shifts occur in the purine-rich strand, which appears to be much more sensitive to changes in the gel than the pyrimidine-rich strand. In contrast, on gels with glycerol the pyrimidine-rich strand appears to be more informative. We have also studied the influence of the neighboring sequence for 25 G→A and 18 A→G mutations in the β-globin fragment. On glycerol gels most A→G substitutions in "GC-rich" regions result in an increase in the mobility of the purine-rich strand. In contrast most G→A mutations decrease the mobility of the purine strand relative to the wild type (38).

These observations can be used to predict the sensitivity of detecting fragments of different base composition. For example it is more likely that for DNA fragments with a high AT content (more than 60%) detection will be best on glycerol gels. This approach is useful when predominantly AT-rich or GC-rich DNA fragments are to be analyzed. However, more SSCP data on fragments with diverse base composition are needed to confirm this observation. Since HA is not as widely used as SSCP, there are much less data available for estimating its sensitivity. Heteroduplex analysis has been used to detect individual mutations in cystic fibrosis (26), as well as the antithrombin (44) and rhodopsin genes (45). The sensitivity of heteroduplex analysis can be increased by two approaches. Heteroduplexes can be formed between samples and a 1- to 3-bp deletion mutant which is used instead of wild type (46). Alternatively the sample can be mixed first with wild-type sample and then with one more mutant control sample to increase the possibility for additional heteroduplex formation (47).

Nonisotopic Protocols

The development of nonisotopic SSCP detection methods is of great importance for clinical laboratories. Several approaches have been developed using silver staining, ethidium bromide staining, or fluorescence labeling. Nonisotopic SSCP detection has been used for the diagnosis of Tay-Sachs disease (48), phenylketonuria (49), the detection of p53 mutations in breast cancer cells (50), and the identification of novel mutations in the CFTR gene (51). Nonradioactive SSCP is usually performed on shorter gels with a higher concentration of loaded DNA. These conditions reduce the sensitivity of the method. This problem can potentially be overcome with the use of 4 to 20% gradient polyacrylamide gels together with a precise temperature-controlled system (43). An alternative is to employ fluorescence-labeled primers and perform the analysis on an automated DNA sequencer (52, 53).

Applications of Polymerase Chain Reaction Single-Strand Conformation Polymorphism and Heteroduplex Analysis

Soon after the SSCP and HA methods were described they were used for the identification of mutations in genes involved in human hereditary diseases and in human cancers. One of the first genes that has been extensively studied with SSCP is the cystic fibrosis transmembrane conductance regulator (CFTR) gene (Fig. 4) (54, 55). Subsequently SSCP has been used to identify sequence variations in the neurofibromatosis type 1 (NF1) gene (56), the B1 variant of Tay-Sachs disease (48), hemophilia B (57), Alzheimer's disease (58, 59), and in dystrophin gene in Duchenne muscular dystrophy (60).

In cancer research the PCR-SSCP technique has been employed for the detection of mutations in the p53 gene in surgical samples of several human

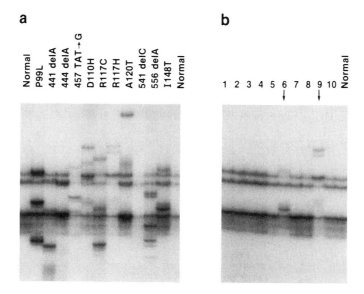

FIG. 4 Optimization of PCR-SSCP analysis on samples of known mutations in exon 4 of the CFTR gene. (a) The best separation of mutants was obtained on a 10% (1.3%C) acrylamide gel with the addition of 10% sucrose. The gel was run in a cold room at 50 W in 0.8× TBE. (b) It is often desirable to circumvent sequencing simply by deciding whether a gene alteration is one of previously established mutations. Since each mutation of exon 4 is characterized by a characteristic "fingerprint" on the gel (a) this provides an indication of the identity of the mutation. This comparison can be performed by comparing the "fingerprints" to patterns of CF samples under investigation. From this analysis it was established that sample 6 carries the I148T mutation and sample 9 the R117H mutation.

cancers (61–63). SSCP has also been used successfully to identify new tumor-suppressor genes, including the gene responsible for familial adenomatus polyposis coli (APC) (64, 65), the Wilm's tumor suppressor gene (WT1) (66), and the von Hippel-Lindau disease tumor suppressor gene (67).

Based on the principle of SSCP, some other interesting techniques have been developed such as RNA-SSCP (35, 68, 69) dideoxy fingerprinting, a combination of SSCP and direct sequencing (70), and amplification refractory mutation system (ARMS-SSCP) (71). Although these methods have been used successfully in individual applications, they are too labor intensive for screening large groups of samples.

Conclusions

Because of the simplicity and high sensitivity of the PCR-SSCP and/or HA techniques, they have been applied in a wide range of applications in molecular biology and medicine. Both methods can detect insertions, deletions, or single-base substitutions in PCR products. The efficiency of each method is high if parameters that affect the separation are carefully optimized for a particular DNA fragment. In many cases more than one electrophoretic condition must be employed to achieve high sensitivity. With the further development of nonradioisotopic detection, these methods will be used increasingly in routine clinical diagnostic testing for hereditary diseases or human cancers.

Acknowledgments

We thank Mary Carrington and Bernard Gerrard for comments on the manuscript. The content of this publication does not necessarily reflect the views or policies of the Department of Health and Human Services, nor does mention of trade names, commercial products, or organizations imply endorsement by the U.S. Government.

References

1. R. M. Myers, Z. Larin, and T. Maniatis, *Science* **230,** 1242 (1985).
2. D. Shibata, C. Almoguera, K. Forrester, J. Martin, N. Arnheim, and N. Perucho, *Cell* (*Cambridge, Mass.*) **53,** 549 (1988).
3. K. Forrester, C. Almoguera, K. Han, W. E. Grizzle, and M. Perucho, *Nature* (*London*) **327,** 298 (1988).
4. I. Nishishio, Y. Nakamura, Y. Miyoshi, Y. Miki, H. Ando, A. Horii, K. Koyama, J. Utsunomiya, S. Baba, P. Hedge, A. Markham, A. J. Krush, G. Petrersen,

S. R. Hamilton, M. C. Nilbert, D. B. Levy, T. M. Bryan, A. C. Preisinger, K. J. Smith, L.-K. Su, K. W. Kinzler, and B. Vogelstein, *Science* **253,** 665 (1991).

5. R. H. Myers, N. Lumelsky, L. S. Lerman, and T. Maniatis, *Nature (London)* **313,** 495 (1985).

6. V. C. Shefield, D. R. Cox, L. S. Lerman and R. M. Myers, *Proc. Natl. Acad. Sci. U.S.A.* **86,** 232 (1989).

7. R. M. Myers, S. G. Fisher, L. S. Lerman, and T. Maniatis, *Nucleic Acids Res.* **13,** 3131 (1985).

8. V. C. Sheffield, G. A. Fishman, J. S. Beck, A. E. Kimura, and E. M. Stone, *Am. J. Hum. Genet.* **49,** 699 (1991).

9. J. E. Finkelstein, C. A. Francomano, S. W. Brusilow, and M. D. Traystman, *Genomics* **7,** 167 (1990).

10. R. Ridnap and K. Husgafvel-Pursianinen, *Hum. Mol. Genet.* **2,** 639 (1993).

11. G. A. Rouleau, P. Merel, M. Lutchman, M. Sanson, J. Zucman, C. Marineau, K. Hoang-Xuan, K. Hoang-Xuan, S. Demczuk, C. Desmaze, B. Plougastel, S. M. Pulst, G. Lenoir, E. Bijlsma, R. Fashold, J. Dummanski, P. de Jong, D. Parry, R. Eldrige, A. Aurias, O. Delattre, and G. Thomas, *Nature (London)* **363,** 515 (1993).

12. P. Fanen, N. Ghanem, M. Vidaud, C. Besmond, J. Martin, B. Costes, F. Plassa, and M. Goossens, *Genomics,* **13,** 770 (1992).

13. R. M. Wartell, S. H. Hosseini, and C. P. Moran, *Nucleic Acids Res.* **18,** 2699 (1990).

14. M. K. Tee, C. Moran, and F. W. Nicholas, *Anim. Genet.* **23,** 431 (1991).

15. R. G. H. Cotton, N. R. Rodrigues, and D. R. Campbell, *Proc. Natl. Acad. Sci. U.S.A.* **85,** 4397 (1988).

16. S. Akli, J. Chelly, J.-M. Lacorte, L. Poenaru, and A. Kahn, *Genomics* **11,** 124 (1991).

17. S. M. Forrest, H. H. Dahl, D. W. Howells, I. Dianzani, and R. G. Cotton, *Am. J. Hum. Genet.* **49,** 175 (1991).

18. C. T. Jones, I. McIntosh, M. Keston, A. Ferguson, and D. J. H. Brock, *Hum. Mol. Genet.* **1**(1), 11 (1992).

19. A. Ganguly and D. J. Prockop, *Nucleic Acids Res.* **18,** 3933 (1990).

20. U. B. Gyllensten and H. A. Erlich, *Proc. Natl. Acad. Sci. U.S.A.* **85,** 7652 (1990).

21. G. Ruano and K. K. Kidd, *Proc. Natl. Acad. Sci. U.S.A.* **88,** 2815 (1991).

22. T. Hultman, S. Stahl, E. Hornes, and M. Uhlen, *Nucleic Acids Res.* **17,** 4937 (1989).

23. A. Rosenthal and J. D. S. Charnock, *DNA Seq.* **3,** 61 (1992).

24. M. Orita, H. Iwahana, H. Kanazawa, and T. Sekiya, *Proc. Natl. Acad. Sci. U.S.A.* **86,** 2766 (1989).

25. M. Orita, Y. Suzuki, T. Sekiya, and K. Hayashi, *Genomics* **5,** 874 (1989).

26. M. B. White, M. Carvalho, D. Derse, S. J. O'Brien, and M. Dean, *Genomics* **12,** 301 (1992).

27. R. Sorrentino, C. Iannicola, S. Costanzi, A. Chersi, and T. Roberto, *Immunogenetics* **33,** 118 (1991).

28. M. Carrington, M. B. White, M. Dean, D. Mann, and F. E. Ward, *Hum. Immunol.* **33,** 114 (1992).

29. M. Orita, T. Sekiya, and K. Hayashi, *Genomics* **8,** 271 (1990).
30. S. E. Poduslo, M. Dean, U. Kolch, and S. J. O'Brien, *Am. J. Hum. Genet.* **49,** 106 (1991).
31. M. Iizuka, S. Mashiyama, M. Oshimura, T. Sekiya, and K. Hayashi, *Genomics* **12,** 139 (1991).
32. K. Hayashi and D. W. Yandel, *Hum. Mutat.* **2,** 338 (1993).
33. Y. Suzuki, M. Orita, M. Shiraishi, K. Hayashi, and T. Sekiya, *Oncogene* **5,** 1037 (1990).
34. J. Michaud, L. C. Brody, G. Steel, G. Fontaine, L. S. Martin, D. Valle, and G. Mitchell, *Genomics* **13,** 389 (1992).
35. G. Sarkar G, H. S. Yoon, and S. S. Sommer, *Nucleic Acids Res.* **20,** 871 (1992).
36. A. Condie, R. Eeles, A. L. Borresen, C. Coles, C. Cooper, and J. Prosser, *Hum. Mutat.* **2,** 58 (1993).
37. V. C. Sheffield, J. S. Beck, A. E. Kwitek, D. W. Sandstrom, and E. M. Stone, *Genomics* **16,** 325 (1993).
38. D. Glavac and M. Dean, *Hum. Mutat.* **2,** 404 (1993).
39. M. Ravnik-Glavac, D. Glavac, M. Chernick, P. diSant'Agnese, and M. Dean, *Hum. Mutat.* **3,** 231 (1994).
40. M. Ravnik-Glavac, D. Glavac, and M. Dean, *Hum. Mol. Genet.* **3,** 801 (1994).
41. .A. Chrambach and D. Rodbard, *Science* **172,** 440 (1970).
42. K. Hayashi, *PCR Methods Appl.* **1,** 34 (1992).
43. T. Hongyo, G. S. Buzard, R. J. Calvert, and C. M. Weghorst, *Nucleic Acids Res.* **21,** 3637 (1993).
44. R. J. Olds, D. A. Lane, C. H. Beresford, U. Abildgaard, P. M. Hughes, and S. L. Thein, *Genomics* **16,** 298 (1993).
45. J. Keen, D. Lester, C. Inglehearn, A. Curtis, and S. Bhattacharya, *Trends Genet.* **7,** 5 (1991).
46. E. van den Akker, J. E. F. Braun, G. Pals, M. V. M. Lafleur, and J. Retel, *Nucleic Acids Res.* **20,** 6745 (1992).
47. P. Guldberg and F. Guettler, *Nucleic Acids Res.* **21,** 2261 (1993).
48. P. J. Ainsworth, L. C. Surth, and M. B. Couler, *Nucleic Acids Res.* **19,** 405 (1991).
49. B. Dockhorn-Dworniczak, B. Dworniczak, L. Broemmelkamp, J. Buelles, J. Horst, and W. W. Boecker, *Nucleic Acids Res.* **19,** 2500 (1991).
50. E. P. H. Yap and J. O'D. McGee, *Nucleic Acids Res.* **20,** 145 (1992).
51. J. Reiss, U. Lenz, F. Rininsland, P. Ballhausen, D. Drews, and H.-G. Posselt, *Hum. Genet.* **90,** 303 (1992).
52. R. Makino, H. Yayzu, Y. Kishimoto, T. Sekya, and K. Hayashi, *PCR Methods Appl.* **2,** 10 (1992).
53. J. Ellison, M. Dean, and D. Goldman, *BioTechniques* **15,** 684 (1993).
54. M. Dean, M. D. White, J. Amos, B. Gerrard, C. Stewart, K. T. Khaw, and M. Leppert, *Cell (Cambridge, Mass.)* **61,** 863 (1990).
55. M. Ravnik-Glavac, D. Glavac, R. Komel, and M. Dean, *Hum. Mutat.* **2**(4), 286 (1993).
56. M. Claustres, M. Laussel, M. Desgeorges, M. Giansily, J.-F. Culard, G. Razakatsara, and J. Demaille, *Hum. Mol. Genet.* **2**(8), 1209 (1993).

57. R. M. Cawthon, R. Weiss, G. Xu, D. Wiskochil, M. Culver, J. Stevens, M. Robertson, D. Dunn, R. Gesteland, P. O.'Connell, and R. White, *Cell (Cambridge, Mass.)* **62,** 193 (1990).

58. D. B. Demers, S. J. Odelberg, and L. M. Fisher, *Nucleic Acids Res.* **18,** 5575 (1990).

59. M.-C. Chartier-Harlin, F. Crawford, H. Houlden, A. Warren, D. Hughes, L. Fidani, A. Goate, M. Rossor, P. Roques, J. Hardy, and M. Mullan, *Nature (London)* **353,** 844 (1991).

60. O. Takamiya, G. Kemball-Cook, D. M. A. Martin, D. N. Cooper, A. von Felten, E. Meili, I. Hann, D. R. Prangnell, H. Lumley, E. G. D. Tuddenham, and J. H. McVey, *Hum. Mol. Genet.* **2,** 1359 (1993).

61. E. Zietkiewicz, L. R. Simard, S. B. Melancon, M. Vanasse, and D. Labuda, *Lancet* **339,** 134 (1992).

62. S. Mashiyama, Y. Murakami, T. Yoshimoto, T. Sekiya, and K. Hayashi, *Oncogene* **6,** 1313 (1991).

63. R. Mazars, P. Pujol, T. Maudelonde, P. Jeanteur, and C. Theillet, *Oncogene* **6,** 1685 (1991).

64. C. H. Hensel, R. H. Xiang, A. Y. Sakaguchi, and S. L. Naylor, *Oncogene* **6,** 1067 (1991).

65. J. Groden, A. Thliveris, W. Samowitz, M. Carlson, L. Gelbert, H. Albertsen, G. Joslyn, J. Stevens, L. Spirio, M. Robertson, L. Sargeant, K. Krapcho, E. Wolff, R. Burt, J. P. Hughes, J. Warrington, J. McPherson, J. Wasmuth, D. Le Paslier, H. Abderrahim, D. Cohen, M. Leppert, and R. White, *Cell (Cambridge, Mass.)* **66,** 589 (1991).

66. D. R. Rosen, T. Siddique, D. Patterson, D. A. Figlewicz, P. Sapp, A. Hentati, D. Donaldson, J. Goto, J. P. O'Regan, H.-X. Deng, Z. Rahmani, A. Krizus, D. McKenna-Yasek, A. Cayabyab, S. M. Gaston, R. Berger, R. E. Tanzi, J. J. Halperin, B. Herzfeldt, R. Van den Bergh, W.-Y. Hung, T. Bird, G. Deng, D. W. Mulder, C. Smyth, N. G. Laing, E. Soriano, M. A. Pericak-Vance, J. Haines, G. A. Rouleau, J. S. Gusella, H. R. Horvitz, and R. H. Brown, Jr., *Nature (London)* **362,** 59 (1993).

67. J. Pelletier, W. Bruening, C. E. Kashtan, S. E. Mauer, J. C. Manivel, J. E. Striegel, D. C. Houghton, C. Junien, R. Habib, L. Fouser, R. N. Fine, B. L. Silverman, D. A. Haber, and D. Housman, *Cell (Cambridge, Mass.)* **67,** 437 (1991).

68. F. Latif, K. Tory, J. Gnarra, M. Yao, F.-M. Duh, M. L. Orcutt, T. Stackhouse, I. Kuzmin, W. Modi, L. Geil, L. Schmidt, F. Zhou, H. Li, M. H. Wei, F. Chen, G. Glenn, P. Choyke, M. M. Walhter, Y. Weng, D.-S. R. Duan, M. Dean, D. Glavac, F. M. Richards, P. A. Crossey, M. A. Ferguson-Smith, D. L. Paslier, I. Chumakov, D. Cohen, A. C. Chinault, E. R. Maher, W. M. Linehan, B. Zbar, and M. I. Lerman, *Science* **260,** 1317 (1993).

69. P. V. Danenberg, T. M. Horikoshi, M. Volkenandt, K. Danenberg, H. J. Lenz, C. C. L. Shea, A. P. Dicker, A. Simoneau, P. A. Jones, and J. R. Bertino, *Nucleic Acids Res.* **20,** 573 (1992).

70. G. Sarkar, H. S. Yoon, and S. S. Sommer, *Genomics* **13,** 441 (1992).

71. Y. M. D. Lo, P. Patel, W. Z. Mehal, K. A. Fleming, J. I. Bell, and J. S. Wainscoat, *Nucleic Acids Res.* **20,** 1005 (1992).

[14] Analysis of p53 Mutations in Human Gliomas by RNA Single-Strand Conformational Polymorphism

Theresa M. Cheng, Vinod Ganju, Steve R. Ritland, Gobinda Sarkar, and Robert B. Jenkins

Introduction

Determination of the genetic cause(s) and pathway(s) of oncogenesis for human cancers is important so that effective diagnosis and treatment modalities may be developed. These pathways are thought to vary from one tumor type to another, although the components are often the same negatively and positively acting gene product cell-cycle regulators. An important negative regulator of tumorigenesis (and the normal cell cycle) is the p53 protein. Inactivation of the gene by mutation or of the p53 protein itself by oncogene products of tumor viruses is important in several (if not most) tumors (1–4). Germline p53 mutations in patients from pedigree affected with Li-Fraumeni syndrome (as well as other families not known to have the Li-Fraumeni syndrome) have also been shown to predispose carriers to a higher incidence of initial primary and second primary cancers, such as brain tumors, sarcomas, leukemias, breast carcinomas, and other neoplasms (5–9). Thus, detection of somatic or germline mutations are important influences in the treatment and prognosis of these patients.

We sought to examine the leukocytes and tumor tissue of patients with brain tumors for p53 mutations. Because most mutations which occur in the p53 gene are single base pair mutations, we developed a technique sensitive for the detection of such alteration using RNA single-strand conformational polymorphisms (rSSCP).

Principle of Method

A 53 kDa protein p53 is composed of 393 amino acids encoded by 2510 base pairs, dispersed among 11 exons. The gene itself is composed of a total of 19,786 base pairs including intron and exon coding sequences. Because of the size of the p53 gene, detection of single base pair mutations which occur most frequently in cancers is often difficult using standard molecular biology

Methods in Neurosciences, Volume 26

techniques. Several methods exist which can be used to determine single base pair mutations; however, these are time-consuming, reproduce poorly, have high false-negative rates, and require complicated instrumentation (10–13). DNA single-strand conformational polymorphism (DNA–SSCP) has become popular because of its simplicity and potential for high output (14, 15). However, informativeness of DNA-SSCP is influenced by DNA sequence length and composition, electrophoresis temperature, acrylamide gel concentration, electrophoresis buffer concentration, and electrophoresis running time (16). Single-stranded RNA (ssRNA) molecules should have a larger repertoire of secondary structure than single-stranded DNA (ssDNA) molecules. For example, stable duplexes can be formed in ssRNA by shorter hairpin loops than in ssDNA and the 2'-hydroxyl group in RNA is available for sugar–base and sugar–sugar hydrogen bonds. Based on these observations, a novel technique based on rSSCP was developed by Sarkar *et al.* (16) involving the separation of single strands of RNA on a nondenaturing polyacrylamide gel. In an examination of a total of 2.6 kb of factor IX genomic sequence in nine regions ranging from 180 to 497 nucleotides, rSSCP was much more sensitive than DNA-SSCP (70% versus 35% overall rate) in detecting sequence changes at 20 different sites. For 307 bp segments, DNA-SSCP and rSSCP detected mutations in 59 and 95% of the cases, respectively. This improved to 92–100% for rSSCP (different rates for T7 and Sp6 polymerases) and 75–83% for DNA-SSCP depending on the electrophoresis conditions. The false-negative rates for rSSCP and DNA-SSCP were 0 and 1%, respectively.

Based on the results of this study, we developed a novel approach for the detection of single base pair mutations in the p53 gene by rSSCP. Since smaller fragments were shown to be more informative than larger ones, we designed our primers to divide the gene into the 11 exon coding sequences containing partial intron flanking sequences on both sides (size of fragments ranged from 145–252 bp). We also constructed the primers to contain both T7 and Sp6 phage promoter sequences, one upstream and one downstream, so rSSCP could be performed on both of the strands in case there were ambiguities. In addition, instead of using ^{32}P as our radiolabel, we incorporated ^{35}S because of its longer half-life and better band resolution of ^{35}S.

Specific oligonucleotide primers were designed by using the computer program OLIGO (National Biosciences, Plymouth, MN). Sites for the first round of PCR amplification (i.e., primers 1–12 in Fig. 1) were chosen to lie outside a group of exon coding sequences, generating a larger DNA fragment (size of fragment ranged from 231 to 895 bp). A second round of PCR is then performed using the PCR product from the first round as the DNA template (nested PCR). Primers for the nested PCR (i.e., primers 13–27) are designed to lie outside of the individual exon coding sequences but within the sites

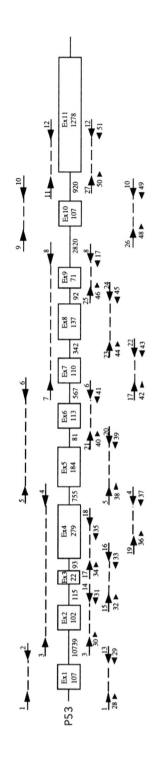

used for the first round of PCR reactions. For example, nested PCR using primers 15 and 16 uses the product from the first round of PCR (which used primers 3 and 4) as the DNA template. This nested PCR produces a product which includes the entire exon coding sequence (170–273 bp including the phage promoter sequences). Because of the size of exon 4, it had to be divided into two overlapping segments. The purpose of the nested PCR amplification is to produce a "clean" PCR product specific for the individual exon coding sequences. Also, T7 and Sp6 phage promoters were incorporated into each primer to enable abundant RNA transcription of the sense and antisense strands from the PCR-amplified DNA segments. Including both of these steps in the technique prevents the need for purification steps at any point in the procedure. Upstream and downstream sequence primers (primers 28–51) are synthesized to lie within the sites used for the nested PCR amplifications, but does not include T7 or Sp6 polymerase sequences at the end of primer. A schematic diagram of the p53 gene indicating intron and exon sequences, PCR primer locations, and sequencing primers is shown in Fig. 1. The sequences of all of the primers are described in Table I. Further detailed explanation of the procedures is described under PCR Amplification Procedure in the Methods section.

Reagents

DNA Extraction

Red blood cell (RBC) lysis buffer 1: 0.2% (w/v) NaCl. Autoclave; store at room temperature. Red blood cell lysis buffer 2: 1.5% (w/v) NaCl. Autoclave; store at room temperature. 2× nucleic acid purification grade lysis buffer (Applied Biosystems, Inc., Foster, CA). Tris–NaCl–CDTA buffer: 50 mM Tris–Cl, pH 7.6, 100 mM NaCl, 10 mM diaminocyclohexane tetraacetic acid (CDTA). Autoclave and store at room temperature. Tris–EDTA (TE) buffer: 10 mM Tris–Cl, pH 7.6, 1 mM EDTA, pH 8.0. Adjust pH to 8.0 with concentrated HCl, autoclave, and store at room temperature. Phenol/chloroform/water (Applied Biosystems Inc., Foster, CA): 68% phenol : 14% chloro-

FIG. 1 Primer map for p. 53. ➡ Denotes a PCR oligonucleotide primer containing Sp6 or T7 phage promotor sequences incorporated into the primer; ▶ denotes a sequencing oligonucleotide primer; *n*, oligonucleotide primer number whose sequence is noted in Table I. T7, phage promotor sequence: taa tac gac tca cta tag gga ga; Sp6, phage promotor sequence: cat aca cat acg att tag gtg aca cta tag aat ac.

TABLE I   p53 Oligonucleotide Primer Sequences

Primer	Sequence location	Phage promotor[a]	Primer sequence (5' to 3')
1	In-1 770-51D	Sp6	ggg gtt gat ggg att g
2	In-1 1080-41U	T7	cca ctc acc ccc aaa ctc
3	In-1 11582-52D	Sp6	gtc tca gac act ggc at
4	In-4 12399-39U	T7	aag ggt gaa gag gaa t
5	In-4 12982-50D	Sp6	tgc cgt gtt cca gtt
6	In-6 13529-39U	T7	ata agc agc agg aga a
7	In-6 13937-53D	Sp6	cct gct tgc cac agg tct
8	In-9 14850-41U	T7	tgc ccc aat tgc agg taa
9	In-9 17468-53D	Sp6	tgt tgc ttt tga tcc gtc
10	In-10 17768-39U	T7	acc atg aag gca gga t
11	In-10 18503-52D	Sp6	agc ctt agg ccc ttc aa
12	Ex-11 18792-39U	T7	ttc tga cgc aca cct a
13	In-1 1016-41U	T7	ctg aaa ata cac gga gcc
14	In-2 11861-39U	T7	cca cag gtc tct gct a
15	In-2 11841-49D	Sp6	ccc cct agc aga ga
16	In-3 12011-35U	T7	ggt gaa aag agc
17	In 3 11947-51D	Sp6	tgg gac ctg gag ggc t
18	Ex-4 12192-37U	T7	agg ggg ctg gtg ca
19	Ex-4 12110-49D	Sp6	agc tcc cag aat gc
20	In-5 13266-39U	T7	tgt cgt ctc tcc agc c
21	In-5 13264-49D	Sp6	aca ggg ctg gtt gc
22	In-7 14138-39U	T7	agt gtg cag ggt ggc a
23	In-7 14412-51D	Sp6	tcc tta ctg cct ctt g
24	In-8 14649-41U	T7	tga atc tga ggc ata act
25	In-8 14638-51D	Sp6	gcc tca gat tca ctt t
26	In-9 17521-52D	Sp6	aac tca ggt act gtg aa
27	In-10 18533-51D	Sp6	gaa aag ggg cac aga c
28	In-1 804-13D		tgc tca aga ctg g
29	In-1 998-14U		5' gag agc ccg tga ct 3'
30	In-1 11662-15D		gct gga tcc cca ctt
31	In-2 11854-16U		tct ctg cta ggg ggc t
32	In-2 11857-16D		tgt ggg aag cga aaa t
33	In-3 11985-13U		gtc ctc agc ccc c
34	In-3 11973-13D		ggg ggc tga gga c
35	Ex-4 12169-17U		ggt gta gga gct gct gg
36	Ex-4 12153-17D		cca gca gct cct aca cc
37	In-4 12352-14U		gat acg gcc agg ca
38	In-4 13010-15D		act tgt gcc ctg act
39	In-5 13243-12U		ctc acc atc gct
40	In-5 13290-12D		ggc ctc tga ttc
41	In-6 13487-16U		cca ctg aca acc acc c
42	In-6 13965-15D		cac tgg cct cat ctt
43	In-7 14123-14U		aag tgg ctc ctg ac
44	In-7 14429-16D		5' ttc tct ttt cct atc c 3'

(*continued*)

TABLE I   *(continued)*

Primer	Sequence location	Phage promotor[a]	Primer sequence (5' to 3')
45	In-8 14606-16U		ctt gtc ctg ctt gct t
46	In-8 14661-16D		ttt cct tgc ctc ttt c
47	In-9 14764-16U		gat aag agg tcc caa g
48	In-9 17547-18D		ttc tcc ccc tcc tct gtt
49	In-10 17753-16U		tga gaa tgg aat cct a
50	In-10 18574-14D		tcc tcc ctg ctt ct
51	Ex-11 18781-14U		acc tat tgc aag ca

[a] Sp6 phage promotor sequence: cat aca cat acg att tag gtg aca cta tag aat ac., T7 phage promotor sequence: taa tac gac tca cta tag gga ga.

form : 18% water. *Chloroform* (Baxter Scientific, McGaw, IL)/isoamyl alcohol (Sigma Chemical, St. Louis, MO): 24:1 mixture. Store at room temperature in amber bottle.

Synthesis of Oligonucleotide Primers

(See Fig. 1 for Map and Table I for Specific Primer Sequences).

All oligonucleotide primers are synthesized with a Model 394 Applied Biosystems, Inc., automated DNA synthesizer and stored at −20°C until purification. The primers are stabilized with ammonium chloride salt which needs to be removed by passing it over a NAP-10 Sephadex G-25 DNA grade column from Pharmacia LKB Biotechnology (Milwaukee, WI) pre-equilibrated with diethyl pyrocarbonate (DEPC)-treated water. The primers are eluted with approximately 3 ml of DEPC-treated water to achieve a final concentration of 20 μM.

PCR Amplification of Genomic DNA

5× PCR buffer: 250 m*M* KCl, 50 m*M* Tris–Cl (pH 8.3), 7.5 m*M* MgCl$_2$. Autoclave, aliquot into 1- to 2-ml tubes, and store at −70°C. *AmpliTaq mix:* Immediately prior to thermocycling, mix 1.0 U of AmpliTaq (Perkin–Elmer, Norwalk, CT) with 1 μl of DEPC-treated water, and 0.8 μl of 5× PCR Buffer. Store on ice until use. This gives a final concentration of 0.5 U AmpliTaq/ μl. *Ethidium bromide:* 10 mg/ml in water. Store at 4°C in light-tight container. *6× sample buffer:* 0.25% (w/v) bromophenol blue, 15% (w/v) Ficoll 400, 9 m*M* Tris-base, 9 m*M* boric acid, 0.4 m*M* EDTA, pH 8.0. *2% NuSieve agarose*

3:1 gels (FMC BioProducts, Rockland, ME): Mix 2 g of agarose in 100 ml of 0.5× TBE (see below) in a 500-ml Erlenmeyer flask. Dissolve agarose by heating the slurry in a microwave. Add 10 μl of ethidium bromide.

RNA Single-Strand Conformational Polymorphism Reactions

5× transcription reaction buffer (Promega, Madison, WI) or 200 mM Tris–Cl, pH 7.5, 30 mM MgCl$_2$, 10 mM spermidine, 50 mM NaCl. Sterilize and store at −70°C. [α-^{35}S]UTP (DuPont NEN, NEG-039H, Wilmington, DE): 1500 Ci/mmol in 0.08 ml of 10 mM Tricine/1 mM dithiothreitol (DTT). All electrophoresis reagents are molecular biology grade quality. *40% polyacrylamide : bisacrylamide* (19 : 1) in nanopure water. Filter with 45-μm pore-size filter paper (otherwise dark spots will occur on the autoradiograph). Store in an amber bottle at 4°C. *5× Tris–borate–EDTA (TBE) buffer:* 0.45 M Trisbase, 0.45 M boric acid, 40 mM EDTA, pH 8.0. Store at room temperature. *rSSCP gels* (5.6% nondenaturing polyacrylamide electrophoresis gels containing 10% glycerol): 8.25 ml of 19 : 1 40% polyacrylamide : bisacrylamide, 5.5 ml of 5× TBE, 5.5 ml glycerol, 550 μl of 10% ammonium persulfate dissolved in water, 12 μl of TEMED. Fill to 55 ml with nanopure water.

Sequencing Reactions

10× primer end-labeling buffer: 10× T$_4$ polynucleotide kinase buffer (Promega) or 500 mM Tris, pH 7.4, 100 mM MgCl$_2$, 50 mM DTT, 1 mM spermidine. Sterilize and store at −70°C. [γ-^{32}P]ATP (DuPont NEN, NEG-002Z): 10 mCi/ml, >5000 Ci/mmole. *Annealing buffer:* 250 mM KCl, 10 mM Tris, pH 8.3. Sterilize; store at −70°C. *Reverse transcriptase buffer:* Add 120 μl of 1 M Tris–Cl, pH 8.3, 80 μl of 1 M MgCl$_2$, 400 μl of 100 mM DTT, 40 μl of 100 mM dATP, 20 μl of 100 mM dCTP, 40 μl of 100 mM dGTP, 60 μl of 100 mM dTTP, 500 μl of 1 mg/ml of actinomycin D, and 2790 ml of water. Aliquot and store in amber tubes at −70°C (actinomycin is light-sensitive). All solutions except dNTPs and actinomycin D should be autoclaved prior to mixture. Final concentrations of buffer and dNTPs after combination into reverse transcription reaction are 24 mM Tris, pH 8.3 (26), 16 mM MgCl$_2$ (17.3), 8 mM DTT (8.6), 0.86 mM dATP, 0.86 mM dGTP, 1.3 mM dTTP, 0.43 mM dCTP, 108 μg/μl actinomycin D. *Sequencing stop buffer:* 85% formamide (deionized), 25 mM EDTA, 0.1% bromophenol blue, 0.1% xylene cyanol. Sterilize; store at −70°C. *Sequencing gels* (5.6% denaturing polyacrylamide electrophoresis gels containing 7 M urea): Dissolve 23.1 g of electrophoresis grade urea in 5 ml of water and 5.5 ml of 5× TBE by gently swirling in a 65°C water bath for approximately 10–15 min. Add 8.25 ml of cold 19 : 1 40% polyacrylamide : bisacrylamide, 550 μl of 10% ammonium persulfate dissolved in water, and 12 μl of TEMED. Fill to 55 ml with nanopure water. Gently mix.

Materials and Enzymes

7-ml Venoject/vacutainer blood collection tubes containing 15% EDTA solution (Turumo Medical Corp, Elkton, MD). *Proteinase K* (Sigma Chemical, St. Louis, MO): 20 mg/ml in sterile water. Store at −20°C. *AmpliTaq* (Perkin–Elmer Cetus, Norwalk, CT): 5 U/μl. *dNTPs*, lithium salt (Boehringer-Mannheim, Indiana, IN): 100 mM stock. *ddNTPs* (Boehringher-Mannheim): Dilute stock dideoxynucleotides (ddNTP) (100 mM) with DEPC-treated water to a final concentration of 1 mM for ddGTP, ddATP, ddTTP, and 0.25 mM for ddCTP. Aliquot into sterile 0.5-ml microcentrifuge tubes and store at −70°C until ready to use in sequencing reactions. *rNTPs* (Promega, Madison, WI): Mix together rATP, rUTP, rGTP, and rCTP from a stock of 10 mM in a 1:1:1:1 ratio. Aliquot small amounts into sterile 0.5-ml microcentrifuge tubes and store at −70°C until ready to use in sequencing reactions. It is best to avoid repeated freezing and thawing to maintain stability of the nucleotides. *T7 RNA polymerase* (Promega): 20 U/μl. *Sp6 RNA polymerase* (*Promega*): 20 U/μl. *RNasin ribonuclease inhibitor* (Promega): 40 U/μl. *T$_4$ polynucleotide kinase* (Promega): 8 U/μl. *Avian myeloblastosis virus* (*AMV*) *reverse transcriptase* (Promega): 7.5–10 U/μl. *Model H3 horizontal slab gel electrophoresis apparatus* and *Model 250 power supply* (GIBCO BRL Life Technologies, Inc., Gaithersburg, MD). *Model S2 sequencing gel electrophoresis apparatus* and *Model 4000 power supply* (GIBCO BRL Life Technologies, Inc., Gaithersburg, MD). *33 × 45-cm and 22 × 40-cm glass plates* for electrophoresis. *49 well sharks tooth electrophoresis comb* for 0.4-mm spacers (5.7 mm point-to-point spacing) and 0.4-mm spacers (GIBCO BRL Life Technologies, Inc.). *Slab gel dryer and vacuum pump. Kodak* (Rochester, NY) *X-OMAT AR X-ray film:* 35 × 43 cm and X-ray cassette holders. *Sorvall GLC-2 centrifuge* (DuPont Instruments, Newton, CT). *Adjustable water baths. 480 Automatic DNA thermocycler* (Perkin–Elmer Cetus, Norwalk, CT). *Biofuge microcentrifuge* (Baxter Scientifics, McGaw, IL). *Savant vacuum dryer* (Savant, Farmingdale, NY).

Methods

Blood Collection and Leukocyte Preparation

Use protective clothing, eyewear, face mask, and gloves when handling the specimens. Whole blood is collected in three EDTA Venoject tubes. The leukocytes are spun down into a buffy coat layer by centrifuging the tubes at 3000 rpm for 30 min at 15°C on the Sorvall centrifuge. Remove the buffy coat layer with a sterile glass Pasteur pipette and place into a sterile 50-ml Falcon clear polypropylene conical bottom tube with a screw cap and graduated markings (Becton–Dickinson, Lincoln Park, NJ). Add 20 ml of red blood cell (RBC) lysis buffer 1 to the tube and mix well for 1–2 min at room temperature. Add 20 ml of RBC lysis buffer 2 to the mixture and again mix for 1–2 min at room temperature. Centrifuge at 2300 rpm for 10 min at 15°C to pellet the white blood cells (WBC). Discard the supernatant. Resuspend the WBC pellet with 1.0 ml of Tris–NaCl–CDTA buffer. Transfer equal amounts of the resuspended WBC pellet into two sterile 2.0-ml Sarstedt tubes (Sarstedt, Inc., Newton, NC). Store the WBC resuspension at −70°C until nucleic acid extraction.

Tissue Collection

Fresh tissue from brain tumors are collected from the patients intraoperatively, divided into approximately 0.5-cm^3 pieces, and immediately frozen in liquid nitrogen. Tissue is stored in 2-ml Sarstedt tubes at −70°C until nucleic acid extraction.

In an environmentally controlled room set up for handling PCR, DNA, and RNA, perform the following procedures using protective clothing, eyewear, and gloves at all times. All supplies and reagents should be sterile and filter pipette tips should be used in the appropriate situations.

DNA Extraction

Frozen tissue is sliced into 10-μm-thick sections using a cryostat with a temperature setting of −20°C. Sections are carefully and quickly placed into a sterile 50-ml centrifuge tube, which has been prechilled on dry ice. Great care should be taken not to thaw the sections at this point because the tissue may undergo autolysis and the DNA may degrade. Tissue sections are stored on dry ice until DNA extraction. Representative sections of the tumor tissue can be mounted on a slide and stained with hematoxylin–eosin for analysis. Thaw one Sarstedt tube containing the Tris–NaCl–CDTA resuspended WBC pellet on ice (the other tube may be saved for future RNA or DNA extractions). Transfer to a sterile 50-ml tube when liquified. Quickly add an additional 1.5 ml Tris–NaCl–CDTA to each 50-ml tube containing leukocytes and 3.0-ml Tris–NaCl–CDTA to each 50-ml tube containing tissue sections. Add 3.0 ml of cold 2× nucleic acid lysis buffer to each tube. Add 100 μl of proteinase K to each tube and mix well. Incubate the mixture at 55°C on a shaker for at least 6 hr to digest the cells. Add an equal volume of cold phenol/chloroform/water mixture to the lysed cells and mix thoroughly. Centrifuge at 3500 rpm for 10 min at 4°C. Carefully remove the upper aqueous layer and transfer to a new sterile 10-ml centrifuge tube. Repeat phenol/chloroform/water extraction step, again transferring the upper aqueous layer to a new sterile 10-ml tube. To the aqueous layer, add an equal volume of chloroform/isoamyl alcohol and mix well. Centrifuge at 3500 rpm for 10 min at 4°C. Carefully remove aqueous supernatant and transfer to a sterile 10-ml centrifuge tube. Add 2× volume of cold 100% ethanol and 1/50 (final volume) of sterile 5 M NaCl. Mix thoroughly. Store overnight at −20°C or for 4 hr at −70°C. Centrifuge at 10,000 rpm for 30 min at 4°C. Carefully discard supernatant. Wash the DNA pellet by resuspending the DNA in 70% ethanol and transfer to a sterile 2-ml Sarstedt tube. Microcentrifuge the mixture at 10,000 rpm for 10 min (in a cold room if possible) to pellet the DNA. Carefully discard the supernatant. Dry the pellet in a Savant vacuum for approximately 10 min or until the pellet is slightly moist. If the pellet is dried too much, the DNA will be difficult to resuspend in TE. Resuspend the DNA pellet in 200 μl of TE. Incubate at 37°C for 30 min. Rotate overnight at room temperature to dissolve the DNA. Determine the DNA concentration by spectrophotometry and dilute the DNA further as needed to achieve a concentration of approximately 2 μg/μl. Human genomic DNA extracted above from both the leukocytes and brain tumor of each patient is diluted 1:10 with DEPC:water and stored at 4°C for PCR amplification reactions. The undiluted DNA can be stored at 4°C for several months or at −20 to −70°C for long-term storage.

PCR Amplification Procedure

Mix the following reagents to a 0.5-ml sterile microcentrifuge PCR tube in an ice–water bath: 5 μl 5× PCR buffer, 14.8 μl DEPC-treated water, 0.05 μl 100 mM stock of each dNTP (total of 0.2 μl for all 4 dNTPs for a final concentration of 200 μM per dNTP), 1 μl primer 1, 1 μl primer 2, 1 μl DNA template, 2 μl AmpliTaq Mix. Add a thin layer of mineral oil to the top of the PCR mixture. Place tube in the automated DNA thermocycler at the following settings: denaturation at 94°C for 1 min, annealing at 55°C for 2 min, elongation at 72°C for 1 min. Repeat the above for a total of 35 cycles, then place at a final extension of 72°C for 10 min, followed by cooling at 4°C. Store first-round PCR products at −70°C until further use. Repeat steps 1–3 for primer sets 1 and 2, 3 and 4, 5 and 6, 7 and 8, 11 and 12. For primer set 9 and 10, follow the same procedure above except use an annealing temperature of 52°C. Perform nested PCR amplication of the first-round PCR

products as shown in Fig. 1 and described under Principle of Method. Store
nested PCR products at −70°C until further use. To test the quality and
quantity of PCR product for each primer set, samples are run on a 2%
NuSieve agarose gel in 0.5× TBE for 1.5 hr at 145 W in room temperature.
A 123- or 100-kb ladder should be used for determining the molecular weight
of the product. A photograph is taken for future reference.

RNA Single-Strand Conformational Polymorphism

Transcription reactions are done with both T7 and Sp6 polymerases in separate reactions by mixing the following together in a sterile 0.5-ml microcentrifuge tube in an ice–water bath: 2 μl 5× transcription buffer, 1 μl 100 mM DTT,
2.25 μl DEPC-treated water, 2 μl rNTP mixture, 0.25 μl RNase inhibitor, 0.5
μl RNA polymerase, 0.5 μl [α-^{35}S]UTP, 1.5 μl DNA template. Incubate the
transcription reaction mixture at 37°C for 2 hr. The reaction is stopped by
freezing the samples. Prior to running the ^{35}S-labeled transcribed RNA on
a rSSCP gel, add 5 μl of sequencing stop buffer to each tube. The mixture
is heated in boiling water for 4 min, followed by quick chilling in ice–water
for 10 min. One microliter of the mixture is loaded onto a 5.6% nondenaturing
polyacrylamide gel containing 10% glycerol. Electrophoresis is carried out
at 5 W for 15–17 hr (overnight) or until green dye front is 3–4 cm from the
bottom of the glass plates. After electrophoresis, dry the gel and subject it
to autoradiography for 6–24 hr at room temperature without an intensifying
screen. Note that the intensity of the rSSCP signal can be increased by
decreasing the amount of 95% formamide dye solution 10-fold.

Sequencing Procedure

PCR fragments showing shifts with rSSCP are sequenced following the procedure described in Stoflet et al. (17), except that the reactions are stopped
by freezing the samples. The nucleotide sequences of the respective exons
can be read and compared to the published sequences, which can be obtained
in the computer program GOPHER (University of Minnesota, Minneapolis,
MN). The mutations in any of the exons of the p53 gene which had migrational
shifts by rSSCP can be readily detected and confirmed by this method. To
further confirm the presence of the sequence mutation, we sequenced the
opposite PCR DNA strand by using the sequencing oligonucleotide primer
facing the opposite direction as that was end-labeled previously. In addition,
to ensure that the mutation is not an artifact of the procedure, the original

DNA extracted from the tumor/blood should be used to reamplify only the respective PCR fragment and confirm the sequence abnormality.

Results and Discussion

Examples of the gel migration patterns for p53 are shown in Fig. 2. The single base pair mutation was confirmed by direct sequencing as shown in Fig. 3. Potential pitfalls and helpful hints of this technique have been described under Methods. Since the p53 gene is large, we have found rSSCP useful as a screening technique to determine which of the 11 exons we should sequence for mutations. We use a conservative approach in our interpretation of rSSCP data. Any questionable gel migration anomaly is subjected to direct DNA sequencing since we do not want to miss a mutation. This conservative approach will give a higher false-positive rate (i.e., an apparent rSSCP gel migration shift without demonstrable mutation on DNA sequencing. How-

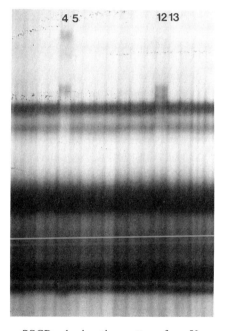

FIG. 2   Example of an rSSCP gel migration pattern for p53 on a 5.6% nondenaturing polyacrylamide gel containing 10% glycerol. Conformational changes in the structure of RNA of the tumor (lanes 4 and 12) as compared to the leukocytes of the patient (lanes 5 and 13) can be seen as migrational differences of the various strands of RNA.

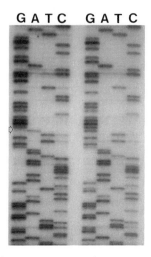

FIG. 3   The single base pair sequence mutation corresponding to the rSSCP migrational shift for the tumor depicted in Fig. 2.

ever, there may also be rare situations where rSSCP may detect a mutation not detected by direct sequencing. For example, the percentage of tumor cells may be too low to result in a DNA-sequencing anomaly but high enough to result in an rSSCP gel migration shift. We are currently comparing rSSCP/ sequencing data with immunostaining results. We have sequenced all 11 exons from 80 specimens which had negative rSSCP results. No mutations were observed. The low false-negative rate of 0% ensures that most, if not all, DNA mutations can be detected by sequencing only those exons which have an rSSCP gel migration anomaly. We have used this technique on several different types of brain tumors including astrocytomas, oligodendrogliomas, ependymomas, meningiomas, mixed oligodendroglioma–astrocytomas, pilocytic astrocytomas, gangliogliomas, metastatic tumors, hemangioblastomas, central neurocytomas, plasmacytomas, subependymomas, neurofibromas, and hamartomas. We did not have any problems with any of the different tumor tissue types.

One of the drawbacks in studying tumor tissue is the heterogeneity of the tumor with normal tissue interposed between tumor tissue as well as different clonal populations of cells within various areas of the tumor. Minimizing the surrounding and interposed areas of normal tissue will help decrease this problem. Also, the abundance of transcript generated by first-round PCR, nested PCR, and rSSCP can compensate for low copy numbers of various mutations. In addition, because of the multiple additional conformational polymorphic bands created by rSSCP, the chances of detecting heterogeneic band migration abnormalities are much higher than those with other techniques since the mutation may change the migration of one band and not another.

Another advantage of rSSCP is that there does not seem to be variation in informativeness with different electrophoresis conditions except that running the gel as long as possible simplifies the interpretation of the autoradiographic band separation. In addition, since T7 and Sp6 phage promoter sequences were incorporated into the primers, and nested PCR reactions were performed, no purification step is needed at any stage. Even though no technique to date is able to detect all mutations with certainty, the probability of finding the single base pair mutation is much higher with rSSCP and reproducibility is excellent. The simplicity and ease of execution renders rSSCP an attractive method for detection of mutations as other members of our laboratory have been able to readily use this technique for the analysis of p53 mutations in ovarian tumors without any problems. In addition, we are certain that one can apply rSSCP to detect a variety of p53 and other gene mutations in many different types of tumor systems as well.

Acknowledgments

We thank the following for their assistance: Paul Stalboerger for preparation of the tissue, Michael Strausbauch and Kevin Battaile for sequencing advice, and Dr. Gerard Vockley's laboratory for their generosity in allowing us the use of equipment. This work was supported by National Institutes of Health Grant CA 50905.

References

1. A. J. Levine, J. Momand, and C. A. Finlay, *Nature* (*London*) **351**, 453 (1991).
2. M. Hollstein, D. Sidransky, B. Vogelstein, and C. C. Harris, *Science* **253**, 49 (1991).
3. D. P. Lane, *Nature* (*London*) **358**, 15 (1992).
4. B. Vogelstein, *Nature* (*London*) **348**, 681 (1990).
5. S. Srivastara, Z. Zhiqiang, K. Pirollo, W. Blattner, and E. H. Chang, *Nature* (*London*) **348**, 747 (1990).
6. D. Malkin, K. Jolly, N. Barbier, A. T. Look, S. H. Friend, M. C. Gebhardt, T. I. Andersen, A. Borresen, F. P. Li, J. Garber, and L. C. Strong, *N. Engl. J. Med.* **326**, 1309 (1992).
7. D. Malkin, F. P. Li, L. C. Strong, J. F. Fraumeni, Jr., C. E. Nelson, D. H. Kim, J. Kassel, M. A. Gryka, F. Z. Bischoff, M. A. Tainsky, and S. H. Friend, *Science* **250**, 1233 (1990).
8. J. Toguchida, T. Yamaguchi, S. H. Dayton, R. L. Beauchamp, G. E. Herrera,

K. Ishizaki, T. Yamamuro, P. A. Meyers, J. B. Little, M. S. Sasaki, R. R. Weichselbaum, and D. W. Yandell, *N. Engl. J. Med.* **326,** 1301 (1992).

9. T. Frebourg, J. Kassel, K. T. Lam, M. A. Gryka, N. Barbier, T. I. Andersen, A. Borresen, and S. H. Friend, *Proc. Natl. Acad. Sci. U.S.A.* **89,** 6413 (1992).

10. S. G. Fischer and L. S. Lerman, *Proc. Natl. Acad. Sci. U.S.A.* **80,** 1579 (1983).

11. A. Ganguly, J. E. Rooney, S. Hosomi, A. R. Ziegler, and D. J. Prockop, *Genomics* **4,** 530 (1989).

12. A. Ganguly and D. J. Prockop, *Nucleic Acids Res.* **18,** 3933 (1990).

13. R. M. Myers, N. Lumelski, L. S. Lerman, and T. Maniatis, *Nature (London)* **313,** 495 (1985).

14. M. Orita, Y. Suzuki, T. Sekiya, and K. Hayashi, *Genomics* **5,** 874 (1989).

15. R. K. Saiki, D. H. Gelfand, S. Stoffel, S. J. Scharf, R. Higuchi, G. T. Horn, K. B. Mullis, and H. A. Erlich, *Science* **239,** 487 (1988).

16. G. Sarkar, H.-S. Yoon, and S. S. Sommer, *Nucleic Acids Res.* **20,** 871 (1992).

17. E. S. Stoflet, D. D. Koeberl, G. Sarkar, and S. S. Sommer, *Science* **239,** 491 (1988).

Section VI

Generation of Probes by PCR

[15] PCR and Generation of Antisense RNA Probes for Use in RNase Protection Assays

Honghao Yang and Peter W. Melera

Introduction

The RNase protection assay has been widely utilized to study the structure of RNA molecules and particularly for the mapping of 5' transcription initiation sites (1), exon–intron boundaries (2), and 3' polyadenylation sites (3). The assay has also been used to detect mutations in DNA molecules (4). Moreover, due to its great sensitivity (5), the RNase protection assay is also useful in identification and quantitation of RNA species that are expressed at extremely low levels (5, 6).

Utilization of the RNase protection assay was initially reported by Zinn *et al.* (7) and later described in detail by Melton *et al.* (5). The principle of the assay is based on the use of a sequence-specific antisense radiolabeled RNA probe, which, after hybridizing to cellular RNA or DNA, protects the complementary sequence region from single-strand-specific RNase digestion. To prepare such an RNA probe, by standard procedures (Fig. 1A), a DNA fragment that contains an appropriate sequence is cloned into a vector in reverse orientation downstream of a bacteriophage RNA polymerase promoter. By doing so, an antisense RNA probe can later be synthesized from this cloned DNA template via *in vitro* transcription that initiates from the promoter. While in many cases, this cloning step is relatively simple and straightforward, it can become technically difficult and time-consuming particularly if there are no convenient restriction sites available at appropriate positions that can be used either for the initial construction of the vector or for linearization of the DNA template before synthesizing the RNA probe (Fig. 1A). Since the size and sequence of the RNA probe is dependent on the DNA template, the cloning process which requires that restriction sites be available for vector construction substantially limits the freedom to routinely modify the probe. In fact, it can be shown that such modification is critical if optimal results are to be obtained from the RNase protection assay (Figs. 4 and 5).

S1 nuclease protection is another method that has been frequently used to analyze the structure of RNA molecules. S1 nuclease is a single-strand-specific endonuclease that digests both single-stranded RNA and DNA to nucleotides (8). However, the requirement for low temperature and high

Methods in Neurosciences, Volume 26

227

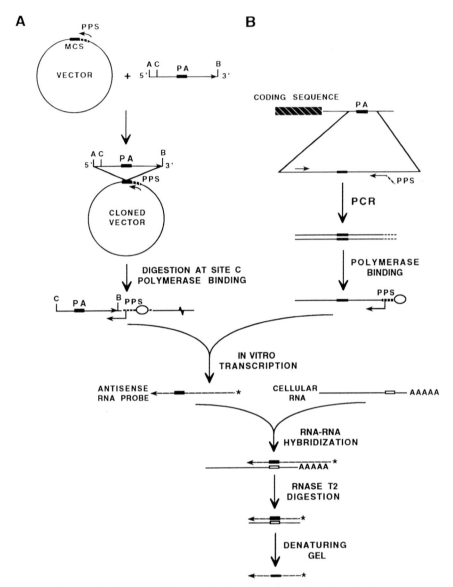

FIG. 1   Schematic diagram of the standard and PCR-mediated methods to generate probes for RNase protection assays. Mapping of a 3′ polyadenylation site in mRNA is used here as an example. (A) The standard method. A DNA template containing the appropriate sequence is cloned into an expression vector in a reverse orientation downstream of a bacteriophage RNA polymerase promoter (PPS). After the DNA template is linearized by digestion at restriction site "C," an *in vitro* transcription

salt concentration (>200 mM) for preferential digestion of single-stranded molecules over double-stranded duplexes (9) can cause technical problems during protection studies. In addition, the nonspecificity of S1 nuclease at AT-rich sequences and its inherent exonuclease activity (10) can result in undesirable experimental errors. However, despite being more sensitive, more accurate, and less problematic than the S1 nuclease protection assay (5, 10), RNase protection experiments are not problem free. One commonly encountered difficulty is high nonspecific background. This is believed to result partially from the relatively high potential for cellular RNA or the radiolabeled RNA probe to form secondary structures and is, therefore, difficult to avoid. Many adjustments to the conditions under which the assay is performed have been suggested in an attempt to limit the degree of nonspecific background (11). Generally, they involve changing the hybridization stringency, or modifying the conditions for ribonuclease digestion. While these adjustments are sometimes helpful, often they are not (12). In these circumstances, modification of the RNA probe itself by changing its length and sequence has been shown to be very useful and thus represents an extremely valuable approach to this problem.

Using a pair of oligonucleotide primers, the polymerase chain reaction (PCR) can amplify specific DNA sequences from various templates, such as homogeneous plasmid DNAs, heterogeneous genomic DNAs, and cellular RNAs, (13). PCR can also be used to produce large amounts of RNA from DNA templates (14, 15). This can be accomplished by attaching an RNA

---

reaction from this linearized template would produce a radiolabeled (noted as *) runoff antisense RNA probe. MCS, multiple cloning site of the vector. (A) and (B) Two restriction sites used for cloning. PA, polyadenylation signal sequence. (B) The PCR-based method. A RNA probe similar to that as generated by the standard procedure shown in A can also be synthesized by a PCR-mediated procedure. To accomplish this, a pair of PCR primers were designed to hybridize to the sequences flanking the putative polyadenylation site (PA). A SP6, T7, or T3 RNA polymerase promoter sequence (PPS) was attached to the 5' end of the antisense primer. After PCR amplification, a linear DNA template was generated with a PPS (noted as dashed lines) attached to its 5' end. Transcription initiated from the RNA polymerase promoter can thus produce a radiolabeled RNA probe. In the diagram, the short arrows → and ← represent the sense and antisense primers used for PCR amplification. *, Radiolabeled RNA probe. The RNA probe generated by either procedure shown in (A) or (B) can then be used for hybridization to cellular RNA. The single-stranded unannealed RNA fragments are removed by T2 RNase digestion and the size of the remaining double-stranded protected RNA fragment is eventually identified on a denaturing polyacrylamide gel.

polymerase promoter sequence to one of the primers. The subsequent PCR amplification generates a linear DNA product that contains a promoter sequence at one end and can be subsequently used for the synthesis of RNA transcripts. Hence, both sense and antisense RNA transcripts can be generated from any piece of DNA whose sequence is known. In this chapter, we present a detailed experimental procedure for a modified RNase protection assay in which the PCR technique is adapted to generate RNA probes. We also provide evidence showing that the efficiency and quality of the protection assay can be substantially improved by this PCR-mediated approach.

Design and Synthesis of PCR Primers

For PCR amplification, a pair of oligonucleotide primers are designed to complement the sequences flanking the mapping site of interest (Fig. 1B). The primer sequence is designed such that nonspecific hybridization during PCR amplification is prevented. The frequency with which the four bases G, A, T, and C occur in the sequence should be randomized as much as possible, and long stretches of identical residues in the sequence avoided. Computer-aided primer searching programs (16) can be helpful in determining the specificity of the primer sequence. It is also helpful to utilize more G and C rather than A and T residues in the probe sequence in order to increase the stability of the primer–DNA template hybrids. Moreover, it is important to place GC residues at the ends (especially at the 5′ end) of the primer sequence. Stable annealing at the ends of the hybrids formed between the RNA probe and cellular RNA is critical for the prevention of "breathing" of the hybrids during ribonuclease digestion (Fig. 5).

The antisense PCR primer sequence is specifically designed to later generate an antisense RNA probe. The 5′ end of the complementary sequence of the antisense primer is extended by attaching a bacteriophage RNA polymerase promoter sequence (either SP6 or T3 or T7) (Fig. 1B) (5, 17–19). The subsequent PCR amplification incorporates this promoter sequence into the 5′ end of DNA product which in turn can be used as a template for *in vitro* transcription to synthesize an RNA probe. The SP6, T3, and T7 promoter sequences are shown in Table I. To demonstrate that the incorporation of the promoter sequence into the linear DNA template can be accomplished by PCR, we compared the electrophoretic mobility of two PCR products, one of which was generated with the RNA polymerase promoter sequence already attached to the antisense primer and another that was generated using the same primers but without the attached promoter sequence. As is shown in Fig. 2, the PCR-amplified DNA with the attached promoter sequence (lane 2) moved slower in the 6% polyacrylamide gel than did the

TABLE I   Bacteriophage RNA Polymerase
              Promoter Sequences[a]

Phage	Sequence
SP6	5' GGATTTAGGTGACACTATAGAATAC 3'
T3	5' AATTAACCCTCACTAAAGGG 3'
T7	5' TAATACGACTCACTATAGGGCGA 3'

[a] The sequences of the three bacteriophage RNA polymerase promoters are referenced from the catalogs of Promega Corp. and Boehringer-Mannheim Biochemicals.

amplified DNA without the attached promoter sequence (lane 1). The size difference between these two PCR products predicted from the gel is about the length of the attached promoter sequence (24 nucleotides). This suggests that indeed the promoter sequence was successfully incorporated into the DNA template through PCR amplification.

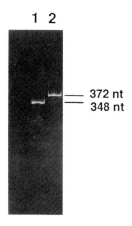

FIG. 2   Comparison of the electrophoretic mobility of two PCR-amplified DNA templates. The PCR products from two DNA templates, one containing an RNA polymerase promoter and the other one not, were electrophoresed through a 6% polyacrylamide/7 M urea denaturing gel and detected by ethidium bromide staining. The PCR product with an attached promoter sequence (372 nucleotides) is about 24 nucleotides longer than the one without (348 nucleotides). Lane 1, PCR product amplified by priming with a pair of primers neither of which contains RNA polymerase promoter sequence. Lane 2, PCR product amplified with a pair of primers one of which contains the SP6 RNA polymerase promoter sequence. Reproduced with permission from BioTechniques (20). © 1992 by Eaton publishing.

Detailed designs for the sequences of both sense and antisense PCR primers utilized during our studies mapping the 3' polyadenylation site of Chinese hamster dihydrofolate reductase (DHFR) mRNA are shown in Table II (20). As depicted in Table II, five additional nonspecific nucleotides (in this case, GAATT) are attached to the 5' end of the promoter sequence to facilitate polymerase binding. In addition, six nucleotides (i.e., gaatac for SP6 promoter, gggcga for T7 promoter, and gggacc for T3 promoter) were placed downstream of the transcriptional initiation site but upstream of the complementary sequence of the antisense primer. Thus, transcription initiated from the attached promoter would read through these six nucleotides and make the undigested RNA probe six nucleotides longer than the largest possible fragment protected by the probe. This difference in the size makes them easily distinguishable by polyacrylamide gel electrophoresis.

Two parameters, i.e., hybridization specificity and stability, need to be considered when deciding on the length of PCR primers. The major issue is whether the length of the primer is long enough to provide sufficient specificity and stability to the primer–DNA template hybrids. For the sense primer, a length of 15 to 20 nucleotides is generally appropriate. For the antisense primer, the length of the complementary sequence should be extended considering the fact that a noncomplementary promoter sequence is attached to its 5' end. The attachment of such a noncomplementary fragment tends to destabilize the hybridization between the primer and DNA template (21). However, extension of the complementary sequence to 25 to 30 nucleotides has been found to be adequate for most PCR applications, including amplification from purified plasmid DNA templates and amplification directly from genomic DNA templates. In fact, direct genomic PCR amplification generates products with qualities similar to those formed from purified plasmid DNA templates as shown in Fig. 3. The lack of background in the PCR signal in the gel reflects the specificity with which such amplification can be carried out.

All oligonucleotide primers discussed here were synthesized by the phosphoramidite method (22), using an Applied Biosystems synthesizer Model 391, and purified using the Oligonucleotide Purification Cartridges (OPC) supplied by Applied Biosystems, Inc., Foster City, CA.

Preparation of DNA Template by PCR

PCR is performed in a 0.5-ml microcentrifuge tube using a Perkin–Elmer Cetus (Norwalk, CT) GeneAmp PCR reagent kit. Either 1–10 ng of plasmid DNA or 100 ng of genomic DNA is suspended in a 100-μl reaction mixture containing buffer [50 mM KCl + 10 mM Tris–HCl, pH 8.3 + 1.5 mM MgCl$_2$ + 0.01% (w/v) gelatin], 1.0 μM of each primer, and 200 μM each of

TABLE II Sequences of the Three Pairs of PCR Primers Used for Mapping of the Three Poly(A) Sites of DHFR Gene

Sense primers		Antisense primers	
Name	Sequence	Name	Sequence[a]
PA1-5′	5′ GCCACTCCCAAAGTCATGC 3′	PA1-3′	5′ GAATTGGATTTAGGTGACACTATA̲gaatacCT GCTGGGGAGCCACTTGAGGCCGCATGGG 3′
PA2-5′	5′ GGATATTGCTTGAAATG 3′	PA2-3′	5′ GAATTAATACGACTCACTATA̲gggcga GGGAGGGGGATTTGGATCTACATATATG 3′
PA3-5′	5′ CTCTTCCCTATCCTTCAGGC 3′	PA3-3′	5′ GAATTGGATTTAGGTGACACTATA̲gaatac GCTGTGGACAGCAGTCAGCATGGAG 3′

[a] The SP6 promoter sequence in PA1-3′ and PA3-3′ and the T7 promoter sequence in PA2-3′ are underlined. ⌐→ indicates the initiation site and orientation of the *in vitro* transcription.

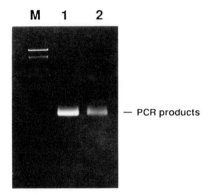

FIG. 3   PCR amplification from a purified plasmid DNA template and a genomic DNA template with one of the PCR primers attached to a SP6 RNA polymerase promoter. Both PCR-amplified products were electrophoresized through a 1% agarose gel and stained by ethidium bromide. Lane M, λ/HindIII DNA size marker. Lane 1, PCR product amplified from the pMQ8-2.1 plasmid DNA template. Lane 2, PCR product amplified directly from the genome of DC-3F/A3 cells. Reproduced with permission from BioTechniques (20). © 1992 by Eaton Publishing.

dATP, dCTP, dTTP, and dGTP. Before adding *Taq* polymerase, the tube is preheated at 95°C for 3 min to denature the DNA template. This preheating step also promotes the inactivation of potentially contaminating DNase and other protein factors. Before the temperature of the tube drops below the hybridization temperature, i.e., about 50–60°C, 2.5 units of Perkin–Elmer Cetus AmpliTaq DNA polymerase is added and the tube vortexed to ensure mixing. The tube is then overlaid with 50 μl of mineral oil and subjected to 30 or 40 cycles of denaturation at 94°C for 1 min, annealing at 50 or 54°C for 2 min, and extension at 72°C for 3 min, in a thermal cycler.

After the appropriate number of cycles are complete, the reaction mixture is extracted once with an equal volume of chloroform to separate the aqueous phase from the organic mineral oil. The top aqueous phase which contains DNA product is carefully removed and then filtrated through a Sephadex G-50 spin column (Boehringer-Mannheim Biochemicals, Indianapolis, IN) (23) to purify the DNA product away from unincorporated free primers and other reagents. The diluted DNA solution is then concentrated by ethanol precipitation and the resulting precipitate resolubilized to a final concentration range of 0.5–1 μg/μl.

In Vitro Transcription

Between 0.2 and 1 μg of the PCR-amplified DNA template is applied to each *in vitro* transcription reaction. In addition to the DNA template, the reaction

mixture also contains 40 mM Tris–HCl (pH 7.5); 6 mM MgCl$_2$; 2 mM spermidine; 10 mM NaCl; 10 mM dithiothreitol (DTT); 1 unit/μl of RNasin; 500
μM of each rATP, rUTP, rGTP; and 12 μM rCTP, as well as 50 μCi radiolabeled [α-^{32}P]rCTP (New England Nuclear Corp., Boston, MA). Depending
on the specific promoter utilized, the reaction is initiated by adding 5–10
units of SP6, T3, or T7 RNA polymerase (Promega Corp., Madison, WI and
Boehringer-Mannheim Biochemicals, Indianapolis, IN), followed by incubation at 37 or 40°C for 1 hr. Ten units of RNase-free DNase I (GIBCO
BRL, Gaithersburg, MD) is then added to remove the DNA template. After
digestion for 15 min at 37°C, approximately 120 μl of diethyl pyrocarbonate
(DEPC)-treated distilled H$_2$O is added to increase the volume to 150 μl. The
newly synthesized RNA probe is then extracted by phenol, followed by three
rounds of ethanol precipitation (75% ethanol and 0.5 M sodium acetate),
which removes 98–99% of unincorporated free radioisotopes (11). The vacuum-dried RNA pellet is then dissolved in 50–100 μl of hybridization buffer.
Repeated pipetting and heating of RNA solution at 65°C for 10–15 min helps
to ensure that the probe is completely dissolved. One-microliter aliquot is
then removed to determine its specific radioactivity.

Incorporation of an RNA promoter sequence into a DNA template as
described above places the promoter at the very 5' end of the resulting DNA
molecules. This location conceivably could interfere with the binding of RNA
polymerase to the DNA template and thus affect the efficiency and quality
of *in vitro* transcription. To prevent this, we have further extended the 5' end
of the attached promoter sequence by five nucleotides therefore providing a
short flanking sequence outside the promoter to enhance polymerase binding
(Table II). As a result, *in vitro* transcription initiated from these specially
designed constructs has been shown to be very efficient at generating RNA
probes with specific radioactivities of 10^8 to 10^{9}cpm/μg (12). This level of
specific radioactivity is directly comparable to those achieved by standard
procedures in which linearized plasmid DNA templates are used (11, 12).
Since the sensitivity of RNase protection assays relies largely on the specific
radioactivity of the probe, the PCR-based assay described here should provide a level of sensitivity similar to that of the standard procedure.

In general, the quality of the RNA probes prepared by this method is
satisfactory and they can be used directly for RNase protection assays. If,
however, one finds a high abundance of prematurely terminated transcripts,
a careful reexamination of each step of the procedure, particularly the conditions used for transcription, can often eliminate the problem. If not, then
gel purification of full-length probes must be considered.

The size of the RNA probe is, in fact, a critical parameter that can affect
the success of this assay. Short RNA probes (e.g., those less than 80–100
nucleotides) increase the nonspecific background of the assay (5) and also
increase the potential for poor yields during the ethanol precipitation steps

(12). Longer probes (e.g., greater than 300 nucleotides), on the other hand, tend to give rise to prematurely terminated RNA molecules during *in vitro* transcription (11). Furthermore, the mapping results obtained using long RNA probes can be less precise than those using shorter probes (Fig. 5). In conventional RNase protection assays, the choice of the size of the RNA probe is largely limited by the availability and the location of the restriction sites used to linearize the DNA template prior to *in vitro* transcription (Fig. 1A). The use of PCR to generate these probes, however, provides the opportunity to generate probes of any size as desired. For most of our studies, 150–250 nucleotides have been found to be adequate.

RNA–RNA Hybridization

Total cellular RNA is extracted from washed cell pellets either by the guanidinium isothiocyanate/cesium chloride gradient procedure (24) or by the RNasol method (25). Purified RNA samples can be stored in ethanol and kept at −20 or −70°C for long periods. For use in RNase protection experiments, small aliquots of RNA sample can be taken from the ethanol stock solution, pelleted, dried, and dissolved in RNase-free distilled H_2O.

The amount of RNA sample applied for each protection assay depends on the level of RNA of interest expressed in the cells. If the expression level is reasonably high, using 1 to 5 μg of the total RNA is enough. However, if the expression is extremely low, about 30 to 50 μg of total RNA or 0.5–1 μg of poly(A)$^+$ mRNA would be required. Approximately 2–5 × 10^5 cpm of the antisense RNA probe should be used for hybridization to ensure that the probe is in excess (10, 11). Both the probe and cellular RNA are mixed in 30 μl of hybridization buffer containing 80% deionized formamide, 0.4 M NaCl, 40 mM PIPES (PH 6.4), and 1 mM EDTA. The probe–RNA mixture is then heated at 85–90°C for 5 min, to ensure denaturation of the RNA, and then allowed to slowly cool to the desired hybridization temperature. Hybridization should be continued for a minimum of 3 to 4 hr with longer times of up to 12 hr, i.e., overnight, often employed.

Preliminary experiments should be performed to establish an optimal hybridization temperature. For our studies, 30–35°C hybridization temperature provided the best results. The percentage of formamide used and the salt concentration in the hybridization solution can also be adjusted if the preliminary experiments are not satisfactory. Theoretically, the stringency of hybridization should be low enough to prevent the loss of specifically hybridized probe–RNA duplex, but high enough to avoid nonspecific annealing.

RNase Digestion

The use of a combination of RNase A and T1 or RNase T2 alone is the most popular way to conduct RNA–RNA hybridization digestion. RNase One commercially available from Promega has also been found to be suitable for RNase protection studies. The choice as to which RNase to use is largely a matter of personal preference and convenience. However, on a case by case basis, it may be found that one enzyme or set of enzymes is better than another. For our studies, RNase T2 has been found to provide the most consistent digestion patterns (12). For each protection study, the amount of RNase should be optimized. The ideal concentration of RNase should provide complete digestion of unhybridized probe and minimal, if any, digestion of RNA–RNA hybrid. The amount of RNase T2 used in our experiments is in the range of 30–35 units/ml, and the digestion is carried out at 30°C for 1 hr in 350 μl of digestion buffer which contains 50 mM sodium acetate and 2 mM EDTA. After incubation with 2.5 μl of proteinase K (20 mg/ml) and 10 μl of 20% sodium dodecyl sulfate (SDS) at 37°C for 5 min to inactive the ribonuclease, the protected RNA–RNA hybrids are phenol-extracted, ethanol-precipitated, and dried under vacuum. The RNA pellet is subsequently suspended in 6–10 μl of loading buffer which contains 80% (vol/vol) deionized formamide, 1 mM EDTA, 0.1% bromphenol blue, and 0.1% xylene cyanol, which provides sufficient sample for duplicate electrophoretic analyses on 6 or 8% polyacrylamide/7 M urea denaturing gels.

Improvements Afforded to RNase Protection Assay by Use of PCR

The use of PCR to generate antisense RNA probes for use in RNase protection assays greatly simplifies the overall procedure, primarily because there is no need to subclone the DNA templates required for probe synthesis. As a result, the efficiency of the assay is dramatically increased. Using PCR to replace the cloning step also substantially increases the flexibility of the assay, since prior to mapping studies, sequence information is generally available. Hence, it should be possible to readily generate antisense RNA probes of various lengths and different sequences, simply by choosing different pairs of PCR primers. This flexibility also offers a facile approach for reducing the nonspecific background problems frequently associated with RNase protection assays, to the extent that they can be overcome by using alternative probes.

To demonstrate this, we show the result of RNase protection studies which were performed to map the second poly(A) site of the Chinese hamster

DHFR gene (26). The sequences around the second poly(A) site are very AT-rich, and the initial RNase protection results were poor and difficult to interpret because of the nonspecific background constantly present in the gels (Fig. 4A). When adjustment of hybridization stringency and ribonuclease digestion conditions failed to solve the problem, the RNA probe was shortened to prevent its complementary sequences from overlapping with the AT-rich region. This was accomplished simply by designing a pair of primers (PA2-5′ and PA2-3′ in Table II) that allowed amplification of a shorter DNA

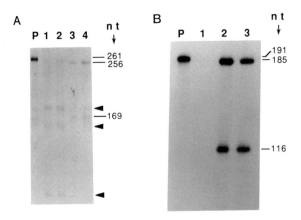

FIG. 4   Mapping of the second poly(A) site of the Chinese hamster DHFR gene. (A) A 261-nt long antisense RNA probe generated from a PCR-generated DNA template was initially hybridized to 10 μg of total RNA from Chinese hamster cell lines DC-3F (lane 2), DC-3F/A3 (lane 3), and DC-3F/MQ19 (lane 4), as well as 10 μg of yeast tRNA (lane 1). Based on the results from multiple experiments, the 169-nt fragment was considered to be the specific protected fragment representing the DHFR RNA polyadenylated at the second poly(A) site. The 256-nt protected fragment represents the readthrough (RT) DHFR transcript which is polyadenylated at a downstream poly(A) site. The arrowheads indicate the nonspecific protected fragments. (B) A smaller RNA probe, 191 nt in length, was hybridized to 10 μg of total RNA from DC-3F/A3 (lane 2) and DC-3F/MQ19 (lane 3), as well as 10 μg of yeast tRNA (lane 1). The 116-nt protected fragment represents the RNA polyadenylated at the second poly(A) site. The 185-nt fragment which is 6 nt shorter than the probe, represents the RT DHFR RNA that is polyadenylated at a downstream poly(A) site. Lane P is an undigested RNA probe. For the experiments illustrated here and in Fig. 5, the cell lines DC-3F/A3 and DC-3F/MQ19 were used as the source of DHFR mRNA. It should be noted, first, that DC-3F cells contain two polymorphic DHFR alleles that differ in their polyadenylation profiles and, second, that DC-3F/MQ19 amplifies one of these two alleles, while DC-3F/A3 amplifies the other. DC-3F/MQ19 cells do not utilize the third poly(A) site as well as DC-3F/A3 cells (see Fig. 5), but both utilize the second site with similar efficiency.

template. The result of this modification is shown in Fig. 4B. As noted in Fig. 4, two RNA fragments, 185 and 116 nt in length, were protected by this modified RNA probe. The shorter one represents the DHFR transcript polyadenylated at the first poly(A) site, whereas the longer one represents the readthrough DHFR transcript that is processed at a downstream poly(A) site. The fact that only two distinct protected fragments are seen in the gel shows that the nonspecific background has been successfully eliminated.

The ability to freely adjust the length and sequence of the probe indirectly by PCR not only can help to solve the background problem, but also can allow more detailed mapping studies to be conducted. One typical example is provided by mapping the first poly(A) site of the DHFR gene (Fig. 5). Initially, a relatively long RNA probe (277 nt) was used for the assay (Fig. 5A). As a result, a 142-nt protected fragment was seen in the gel, representing the DHFR transcript polyadenylated at the first poly(A) site. However, the 142-nt band was broad and heterogeneous and it was not clear whether it represented a single fragment or multiple fragments. In order to clarify this problem, the length of probe was shortened to 158 nt. As can be seen in Fig. 5B, use of this probe produced multiple protected fragments clustered together as ladders with the most predominant fragment, 92 nt, located in the middle. Although the basis for these multiple fragments was not clear, we speculated that they may result from "breathing" at the ends of the probe–RNA hybrids during ribonuclease digestion. To prevent this, the 158-nt RNA probe was extended by use of primer PA1-3' (Table II) at its 5' end to include additional GC residues. The length of the resulting probe was 171 nt. As shown in Fig. 5C, four distinct groups of fragments were protected by this probe, locating the 3' ends of the DHFR transcripts at four different positions clustered within a 13-nucleotide region. Among these fragments, the most predominant one is 105 nt in length which maps the 3' end of DHFR transcript at the same position as demonstrated by sequencing of a DHFR cDNA clone (26). Genomic DNA sequence analysis indicates that three potential poly(A) signals coexist in close proximity upstream of the polyadenylation cleavage sites defined by the RNase protection analyses (26). The first two of these, ATTAAA and AATATA, overlap each other by 2 nucleotides, while the third, AAGAAA, lies 9 nucleotides downstream of the first. All of these are known to be functional poly(A) signals, although the efficiency with which they each direct polyadenylation is different (27). The close proximity of these three functional poly(A) signals in the DHFR gene, therefore, most likely explains why multiple bands, i.e., cleavage sites, are present at this specific poly(A) site (Fig. 5C, lanes 2 and 3). To have prepared the three probes utilized for this study by standard cloning procedures would have been extremely difficult and laborious.

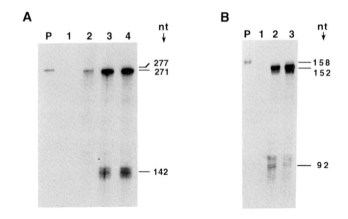

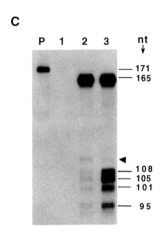

FIG. 5   Mapping of the first poly(A) site of the Chinese hamster DHFR gene by using different length RNA probes. Radiolabeled RNA probe (5×10^5 cpm) and 10 μg of total RNA were used for these studies. (A) A 277-nt RNA probe was hybridized to total cellular RNA extracted from DC-3F (lane 2), DC-3F/A3 (lane 3), and DC-3F/MQ19 (lane 4), as well as 10 μg of yeast tRNA (lane 1). The 271-nt fragment corresponds to the RT transcript, while the 142-nt band corresponds to transcript polyadenylated at the first poly(A) site. Lane P represents an undigested probe. (B) A smaller probe, 158 nt in length, was then used for hybridization. Lane P, undigested probe; 1, yeast tRNA; 2, DC-3F/MQ19 RNA; and 3, DC-3F/A3 RNA. The 152-nt fragment represents the RT transcript, while the fragments around 92 nt represent the transcript polyadenylated at the first site. (C) A 171-nt probe was used. Lane P, undigested probe; 1, yeast tRNA; 2, DC-3F/A3 RNA; 3, DC-3F/MQ19 RNA. The 165-nt fragment again corresponds to the RT transcript. A cluster of four distinct bands as noted (i.e., 95, 101, 105, and 108 nt) represent DHFR transcripts polyadenylated at

Additional Concern Associated with PCR-Mediated RNase Protection Assay

One unique problem that may complicate the use of PCR for RNase protection analyses is the relatively high frequency with which *Taq* polymerase incorporates the wrong nucleotides during PCR amplification. This error rate has been reported to be approximately 1 in 5000 nucleotides (28). In general, the short size of the probes used in the protection assays should reduce the probability of sequence errors in the PCR-amplified DNA templates. However, to ensure that these potential errors do not compromise final results, multiple experiments should be performed using probes generated from independent PCR amplifications. Any experimental errors caused by the incorrect sequence of one probe would not be expected to be reproduced in other independent experiments. In practice, we have not found this to be a major source of detectable error in our attempts to map the 3′ ends of the DHFR transcripts in Chinese hamster lung cells.

References

1. M. Trudel, J. Magram, L. Brudckner, and F. Costantini, *Mol. Cell. Biol.* **7,** 4024 (1987).
2. T. Shimada, K. Inokuchi, and A. W. Nienhuis, *Mol. Cell. Biol.* **7,** 2830 (1987).
3. D. Solnick and S. T. Lee, *Mol. Cell. Biol.* **7,** 3194 (1987).
4. R. M. Myers, Z. Larin, and T. Maniatis, *Science* **230,** 1242 (1985).
5. D. A. Melton, P. A. Krieg, M. R. Rebagliati, T. Maniatis, K. Zinn, and M. R. Green, *Nucleic Acids Res.* **12,** 7035 (1984).
6. R. P. Hart, M. A. Mcdevitt, H. Ali, and J. R. Nevins, *Mol. Cell. Biol.* **5,** 2975 (1985).
7. K. Zinn, D. DiMaio, and T. Maniatis, *Cell (Cambridge, Mass.)* **34,** 865 (1983).
8. J. M. Greene and K. Struhl, *in* Current Protocols in Molecular Biology'' (F. M.

the first poly(A) site. The size difference of these four fragments indicated that the first poly(A) site was located at four slightly different positions. The difference in intensity of these four bands between lanes 2 and 3 reflects the different amount of DHFR transcript polyadenylated at the first site in DC-3F/A3 and DC-3F/MQ19 cells, respectively. The band indicated by the arrowhead results from an RNase cleavage at a nucleotide mismatch (C vs T) between the RNA probe from one allele and cellular RNA from the other located six bases downstream of the most 3′ proximate polyadenylation cleavage site (26).

Ausubel, R. Brent, R. Kingston, D. D. Moore, J. G. Seidman, and K. Struhl, eds.), Vol. 1, p. 4.6.1. Wiley, New York, 1987.

9. R. Lehman, *in* The Enzymes'' (P. D. Boyer, ed.), Vol. 14A, p. 198. Academic Press, Orlando, FL, 1982.

10. RPA II™ Ribonuclease Protection Assay Kit Instruction Manual, Ambion, Inc. (1990).

11. M. Gilman, *in* Current Protocols in Molecular Biology'' (F. M. Ausubel, R. Brent, R. Kingston, D. D. Moore, J. G. Seidman, and K. Struhl, eds.), Vol. 1, p. 4.7.1. Wiley, New York, 1987.

12. H. Yang and P. W. Melera, unpublished observations (1992).

13. M. A. Innis, D. H. Gelfand, J. J. Sninsky, and T. J. White, eds., "PCR Protocols: A Guide to Methods and Applications." Academic Press, San Diego, 1990.

14. D. Y. Kwoh, G. R. Davis, K. W. Whitfield, H. L. Chappelle, L. J. DiMichele, and T. R. Gingeras, *Proc. Natl. Acad. Sci. U.S.A.* **86,** 1173 (1989).

15. E. S. Stoflet, D. D. Koeberl, G. Sarkar, and S. S. Sommer, *Science* **239,** 491 (1988).

16. L. J. Korn and C. Queen, *DNA* **3,** 421 (1984).

17. M. J. Chamberlin and T. Ryan, *in* "The Enzymes" (P. D. Boyer, ed.), Vol. 15B, p. 87. Academic Press, New York, 1982.

18. C. E. Morris, J. F. Klement, and W. T. McAllister, *Gene* **41,** 193 (1986).

19. S. Tabor and C. C. Richardson, *Proc. Natl. Acad. Sci. U.S.A.* **82,** 1074 (1985).

20. H. Yang and P. W. Melera, *BioTechniques* **13,** 922 (1992).

21. S. M. Freier, R. Kierzek, J. A. Jaeger, N. Sugimoto, M. H. Caruthers, T. Neilson, and D. H. Turner, *Proc. Natl. Acad. Sci. U.S.A.* **83,** 9373 (1986).

22. M. H. Caruthers, *in* Methods of DNA and RNA Sequencing'' (S. M. Weisman, ed.), p. 1. Praeger, New York, 1983.

23. T. Maniatis, A. Jeffrey, and D. G. Kleid, *Proc. Natl. Acad. Sci. U.S.A.* **72,** 1184 (1975).

24. J. M. Chirgwin, A. E. Przybila, R. J. MacDonald, and W. J. Rutter, *Biochemistry* **18,** 5294 (1979).

25. P. Chomczynski and N. Sacchi, *Anal. Biochem.* **162,** 156 (1987).

26. K. W. Scotto, H. Yang, J. P. Davide, and P. W. Melera, *Nucleic Acids Res.* **20,** 6597 (1992).

27. M. Wickens, *Trends Biochem. Sci.* **15,** 277 (1990).

28. P. Kartovsky, *Trends Biochem. Sci.* **15,** 419 (1990).

[16] *In Vitro* Transcription of cRNA from PCR-Generated DNA Fragments

Sherry Leonard

The use of cRNA probes has become widely accepted for many hybridization studies. Not only is cRNA single-stranded and, therefore, a more efficient probe, but hybrids of DNA–RNA and RNA–RNA are more stable under stringent washing conditions than are DNA–DNA hybrids. Generation of these probes by RNA polymerases requires the presence of the specific polymerase promoter and is usually accomplished by the linearization of a plasmid containing both promoter sequence and the gene of interest. In many cases, however, the cloned cDNA is not available, is not cloned in a vector suitable for *in vitro* transcription, or restriction enzyme sites are not present which will give the desired cRNA product length. The method presented here provides a simple approach for synthesis of a DNA template containing RNA polymerase promoter sites, using the polymerase chain reaction (PCR). A general schemata for the synthesis of a template with promoters at each end is shown in Fig. 1. We have found that several RNA polymerases will transcribe from these DNA fragments, yielding cRNA probes of high quality. It is thus possible to generate a cRNA probe for any gene for which the sequence is known.

Primers for DNA Template Synthesis

Primer sequences for PCR are designed from the gene of interest. As examples here, we have used murine acidic fibroblast growth factor (aFGF; Genbank Accession Number M30641) and human nerve growth factor (β-NGF; EMBL Accession Number X52599). The forward and reverse primers should be matched according to melting temperature, as well as possible, and pretested in a PCR reaction to be sure they amplify the desired fragment. The PCR product can be verified by hybridization of a Southern blot with an internal oligonucleotide, complementary to the desired sequence. For primer selection, we used OLIGO primer analysis software (National Biosciences, Hamel, MN). Care in choosing the region of the gene to be used for the cRNA probe is important, since considerable homology exists within gene families. It is best to compare both the PCR primers and the PCR product with known sequences in a sequence databank, such as GenBank (1) or

Methods in Neurosciences, Volume 26

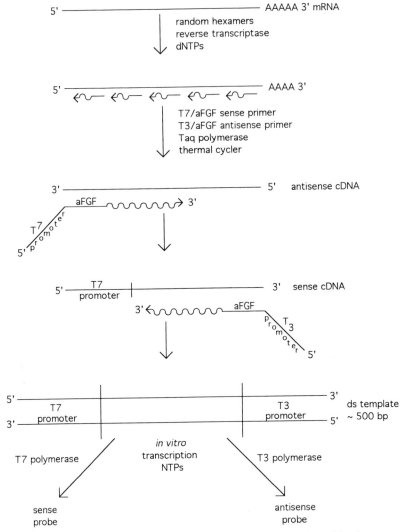

FIG. 1 Generation of DNA fragments for *in vitro* transcription of both sense and antisense cRNA probes. Primers are designed to amplify a PCR product containing RNA polymerase promoters at each end. The DNA fragment is then used in a standard *in vitro* transcription reaction to synthesize cRNA.

EMBL (2), and to determine whether there could be a problem with cross-reactivity under the probe hybridization conditions to be used. If considerable homology with other mRNAs is found, a different region of the gene should be selected for probe construction.

Once, the gene specific primer sequences have been selected, new primers are prepared containing both the specific primer sequences and RNA polymerase promoter sequences. We have evaluated the efficacy of various RNA polymerases for this application (3). Both T7 and T3 RNA polymerases transcribe efficiently from their specific promoters in DNA fragments. The SP6 RNA polymerase, however, appears to require additional DNA sequence or perhaps secondary structure and, therefore, should be not be used for this application.

There is no cross talk between either T7 or T3 and, thus, the promoters can be included in the same DNA fragment, enabling the synthesis of both sense and antisense cRNA probes from the same DNA fragment. Although both polymerases transcribe from a minimal promoter sequence (T7, 5' TAA-TACGACTCACTATAGGGAGA 3';T3, 5' AATTAACCCTCACTAAAGG-GAGA 3'), we have found that the transcription efficiency increased if an additional 9–10 nucleotides 5' of the essential promoter sequence were included. Additionally, for these polymerases there is a preference for a G nucleotide at the start of transcription (+1 position). If G is not the first nucleotide in the specific gene primer sequence, one should be included. Here we include the G, as well as 5 additional nucleotides of promoter sequence, 3' of the start site.

Primers for generating DNA templates containing single-promoter sites (aFGF) or dual-promoter sites (β-NGF) are shown in Table I, as well as the PCR fragment sizes. The single-promoter templates are designed to generate either sense (T7) or antisense (T3) aFGF cRNA probes from separate PCR products. The composite primers for human NGF contain both T7 and T3 RNA promoter sequences. All promoters include nine nucleotides 5' of the required sequence for transcription and five nucleotides of promoter sequence 3' of the G start position. Our primers are synthesized on an Applied Biosystems PCR-Mate Oligonucleotide Synthesizer (Applied Biosystems, Foster City, CA).

Generation of DNA Template

Total RNA is used for generation of the DNA templates and is prepared from whole mouse brain by the method of Chomczynski and Sacchi (4). We also routinely add an RNase-free DNase digestion followed by two phenol/chloroform extractions prior to the final ethanol precipitation to avoid PCR

TABLE I Primer Sequences for PCR-Generated Minigenes[a]

Primer set	Template	Upstream primer	Downstream primer	PCR product size (bp)
1	**T7**/aFGF	5′ CCAAGCTTC**TAATA CGACTCACTATAGG GAGA**/TGAAGGGGA GATCACAACC 3′	aFGF 5′ GAAACAAGATGGC TTTCTGGC 3′	469
2	**T3**/aFGF	5′ CAGAGATGCAA**TTA ACCCTCACTAAAGG GAGA**/ **GAAACAAGA TGGCTTTCTGGC** 3′	aFGF 5′ TGAAGGGGGAGATC ACAACC 3′	469
3	**T3**/β-NGF	5′ CAGAGATGCAA**TTA ACCCTCACTAAAGG GAGA**/ACAGTTTTA CCAAGGGAGC 3′	**T7**/β-NGF 5′ CCAAGCTTCT**AAT ACGACTCACTATA GGGAGA**/AAGATG GG ATGGGGATGATG AC 3′	503

[a] Consensus promoter sequences are in boldface type and delineated from the gene-specific sequence by a slash (/).

products generated from contaminating DNA. The DNA template is then synthesized in a 0.5-μl microfuge tube, using the reverse transcriptase polymerase chain reaction (RT-PCR) (5). The RT step reaction of 40 μl contains 1 mM deoxyribonucleoside triphosphates (dNTPs), 0.5 U/μl placental RNase inhibitor, 0.01 M dithiothreitol (DTT), 2.5 U/μl Moloney murine leukemia virus (M-MLV) reverse transcriptase, 1× RT buffer, 300 pmol random hexamers, and 200 ng mouse total RNA. Although we use buffer included with the M-MLV from GIBCO BRL/Life Technologies (Gaithersburg, MD), a standard reverse transcriptase buffer of 20 mM Tris (pH 8.4 at room temperature), 50 mM KCl, 2.5 mM MgCl$_2$, 1 mM each dNTPs, 1 mM dithiothreitol, and 1 mg/ml nuclease-free bovine serum albumin (BSA) could be used as well. Random hexamers can be purchased from Pharmacia LKB Biotechnology Inc. (Piscataway, NJ). The RNA is incubated at 65°C for 5 min, quick-chilled on ice, and added to the RT reaction mixture. After 10 min at room temperature to allow annealing of the random hexamers, the reaction is incubated at 37°C for 1 hr. The reverse transcriptase is then heat-inactivated at 100°C for 5 min.

PCR reaction mix (60 μl), containing upstream and downstream primers to a final concentration of 1 μM each, MgCl$_2$ to 2 mM, 1× PCR buffer, 200 μM dNTPs, and 2.5 U *Taq* polymerase is then added to the cDNA template generated in the RT reaction. PCR buffer included with the *Taq* polymerase from Perkin–Elmer (Norwalk, CT) is used for this experiment, but a standard PCR buffer of 10 mM Tris (pH 8.4 at room temperature), 50 mM KCl, and 1.5 mM MgCl$_2$, would also be suitable. The tubes are placed in a Perkin–Elmer DNA Thermal Cycler with the following program: 1 min at 94°C, 2 min at 54°C, and 3 min at 72°C, for 4 cycles; then 1 min at 94°C, 1 min at 65°C, and 3 min at 72°C, for 36 cycles, and finishing with an extension period of 7 min at 72°C. We found that, with the composite primers, the 4 cycles at a lower annealing temperature increase the yield of the template product. The temperature for annealing is calculated using the OLIGO software and should be determined for each construct. The reaction mixture is run on a 2% agarose gel, the single band excised and electroeluted to isolate the DNA fragment.

In Vitro Transcription of Sense and Antisense cRNA Probes from PCR-Generated DNA Fragment

Sense and antisense cRNA probes are then synthesized by *in vitro* transcription of the DNA-generated templates, using either T7 or T3 polymerase. Reaction mixtures of 10 μl contain 1× transcription buffer; 0.5 U/μl placental RNase inhibitor; 10 mM dithiothreitol; 0.5 mM each ATP, CTP, and GTP;

5 μM UTP; 25 μCi [α-^{32}P]UTP; 0.5 μg of the PCR-generated DNA template; and 10 U/μl of the appropriate RNA polymerase. Manufactured kits are available (Ambion, Austin, TX) which include transcription buffer. However, a standard *in vitro* transcription buffer of 40 mM Tris (pH 8.1 at 37°C), 6 mM MgCl$_2$, 2 mM spermidine, 5 mM dithiothreitol, 5 mM NaCl, and 50 μg/ml nuclease-free bovine serum albumin can be used instead. The reaction should be assembled at room temperature; on ice, 2 mM spermidine will precipitate the DNA template.

If the cRNA probe is to be used for *in situ* hybridization, 200 μCi of [α-^{35}S]UTP may be substituted for the [α-^{32}P]UTP, with no changes in the protocol.

The reaction is begun by adding the RNA polymerase and incubating at room temperature for 30 min. We have found that incubation at room temperature results in more full-length transcript. If a large yield of cRNA is desired, the incubation temperature can be increased to 37°C, and an additional 10 U of polymerase added at the end of 30 min, followed by another 30 min incubation.

The template is then removed from the reaction by the addition of 1 μg (1 U) of RNase-free DNase I and an incubation of 15 min at 37°C. The reaction is terminated by adding 1 μl of 0.2M EDTA and diluted to 50 μl. The percentage incorporation of [α-^{32}P]UTP can be determined by dilution of a 2-μl aliquot from the final reaction to 200 μl in 1× TE (10 mM Tris, pH 7.4; 1 mM EDTA), containing 50 μg/ml of carrier tRNA. The dilution is counted directly and 100 μl of the dilution is precipitated by addition of 2 ml of cold 5% trichloroacetic acid. The precipitate is collected by vacuum filtration through GF/C glass fiber filters and counted for determination of incorporation.

The labeled cRNA probe is then separated from unincorporated nucleotides by passing through a Sephadex G-25 spin column (Boehringer-Mannheim, Indianapolis, IN). If ^{35}S is used, the elution buffer should contain 1% SDS, 10 mM Tris (pH 7.4), 1 mM EDTA, and 10 mM DTT. All solutions for cRNA synthesis should be prepared in water that has been treated with 0.1% diethyl pyrocarbonate (12 hr at 37°C; autoclave for 20 min on a liquid cycle).

The probes may be stored for 1 week at −70°C. Examples of the incorporation obtained using the above reaction conditions for single (aFGF) or double (β-NGF) polymerase promoter constructs are shown in Table II. We found no difference in yield between the single and double constructs. Incorporation at 37°C is approximately 2-fold higher, but higher yields of full-length transcripts are obtained at room temperature. Incorporation by T7 polymerase, using 0.2 μg of linearized plasmid containing β-actin (pT7/actin), is also shown. Correction for the gene copy number in the PCR-generated

TABLE II   Incorporation of [α-³⁵S]UTP for Probes Synthesized by *in Vitro*
Transcription from PCR-Generated DNA Fragments

Template	Polymerase	Assay temperature (°C)	Incorporation[a] (%)
None	T7	22	00.1
None	T3	22	00.1
T7/aFGF	T7	22	29.4
T3/aFGF	T3	22	19.6
pT7/actin	T7	22	74.6
T7/aFGF	T7	37	52.5
T3/β-NGF/T7	T7	22	38.1
T3/β-NGF/T7	T3	22	28.1

[a] Percent incorporation of [α-³²P]UTP was determined by TCA precipitation of an aliquot of the final reaction.

fragment and the T7 actin plasmid suggests that T7 polymerase transcribes about 15-fold more efficiently from the linearized plasmid. Although the efficiency of transcription from the PCR-generated DNA fragment is lower, ample transcript is generated for use of the cRNA probe in several experiments.

The size of the probe can be verified by electrophoresis of an aliquot through a 5% polyacrylamide gel. Sense and antisense transcription products, generated at room temperature, for aFGF are shown in Fig. 2, indicating that the conditions used provide a single cRNA of the expected size.

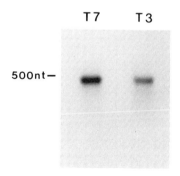

FIG. 2   cRNA products synthesized *in vitro* from PCR-generated templates. PCR-generated DNA templates for aFGF containing either T7 or T3 RNA polymerase promoter sequences were transcribed *in vitro* as described. The radioactive cRNA product was resolved on a 1.2% agarose gel which was dried and exposed to film. A size marker is shown at the left.

The results of an *in situ* hybridization experiment using sense and antisense probes for aFGF, transcribed from PCR-generated fragments with [^{35}S]UTP as label, on 12-μm sections of mouse brain are shown in Fig. 3. *In situ* hybridization as described (3).

Comments

Transcription from a PCR-generated DNA fragment has several advantages. Primers can be designed from any gene for which the sequence is known, enabling the investigator to prepare any probe of interest. There is no need to clone the fragment; both T7 and T3 polymerases transcribe efficiently from the PCR product containing specific promoter sequences. Probes of any length can be designed by varying the primer choices. We have found that cRNA probes between 200 and 500 nucleotides are optimal for *in situ* hybridization. Both sense and antisense cRNA probes can be generated from

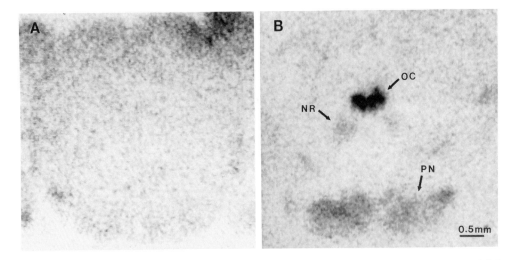

FIG. 3   *In situ* hybridization of mouse brain sections with sense and antisense aFGF cRNA probes transcribed *in vitro* from a PCR-generated template. Mouse brain was removed following decapitation and frozen in liquid nitrogen. Sections of 15 μm were thaw-mounted onto slides, fixed in paraformaldehyde, and hybridized with sense (A) and antisense (B) cRNA probes transcribed *in vitro* from a PCR-generated fragment containing sequences for aFGF. Following a stringent wash, the sections were exposed to βMAX Hyperfilm (Amersham) for 10 days. OC, oculomotor complex; NR, nucleus ruber; PN, basilar pontine nucleus.

the same construct, containing different promoter sequence at each end, by varying the RNA polymerase used for transcription.

As transcription from these constructs yields a principal product of uniform size, they are ideally suited for generation of cRNA for nuclease protection assays. Additionally, PCR fragments containing one promoter site can be used for synthesis of mRNA for *in vitro* translation into protein (6, 7). The method is also of particular use when many different gene products are to be examined.

Acknowledgments

This work was supported by the Veterans Administration Medical Research Service.

References

1. H. S. Bilofsky, C. Burks, J. W. Fickett, W. B. Goad, F. I. Lewitter, W. P. Rindone, C. D. Swindell, and C.-S. Tung, *Nucleic Acids Res.* **14**, 1 (1986).
2. G. H. Hamm and G. N. Cameron, *Nucleic Acids Res.* **14**, 5 (1986).
3. J. Logel, D. Dill, and S. Leonard, *BioTechniques* **13**, 604 (1992).
4. P. Chomczynski and N. Sacchi, *Anal. Biochem.* **162**, 156 (1987).
5. E. Kawasaki, *in* PCR Protocols: A Guide to Methods and Applications'' (M. A. Innis, D. H. Gelfand, J. J. Sninsky, and T. J. White, eds.), p. 21. Academic Press, San Diego, 1990.
6. K. S. Browning, *Amplifications* **3**, 14 (1989).
7. K. C. Kain, P. A. Orlandi, and D. E. Lanar, *BioTechniques* **10**, 366 (1991).

Section VII

PCR in the Context of Cloning and Constructing Libraries

[17]   Direct Cloning of DNA Fragments Generated by PCR

David Kovalic and Bernard Weisblum

Introduction

Cloning of amplified DNA from polymerase chain reactions has become an important task for many researchers, as the popularity of the polymerase chain reaction (PCR) has increased. Unfortunately the difficulty often encountered in cloning these fragments stands in marked contrast to their ease of production. Double-stranded DNA products obtained by primed amplification with *Thermus aquaticus* (*Taq*) DNA polymerase (and other polymerases that lack proofreading function) contain a single 3' untemplated deoxyadenosine residue gratuitously added by the polymerase to its product (1). To clone the amplified products efficiently, either the extra deoxyadenosine residues must be removed or the vector has to be modified to accommodate them. It would be desirable to use the latter method in concert with a simple vector preparation, which would save the additional time and materials consumed in modifying the PCR product.

Construction of the Vector and Rationale for Its Use

A general method is described for direct cloning of DNA fragments generated by PCR that is based on digesting the cloning vector pDK101, with *Xcm*I restriction endonuclease. This reaction yields a unit linear molecule with 3' unpaired thymidine residues at both ends and a 16-nucleotide "central stuffer." Such vectors are capable of ligation directly with products that are obtained by primed enzymatic amplification with *Taq* DNA polymerase bearing complementary 3' unpaired deoxyadenosine residues. Other methods for direct cloning of PCR products have been described which involve enzymatic tailing of a vector by addition of a single thymidylate residue with either terminal transferase and ddTTP (2) or *Taq* DNA polymerase and dTTP (3).

Two partially complementary 24-mer DNA oligonucleotides containing the *Nco*I four base overhang (shown below) were chemically synthesized,

Methods in Neurosciences, Volume 26

255

annealed, and ligated with plasmid pGEM5fZ(+) (Promega, Madison, WI) that had been prepared by digestion with *Nco*I in the multiple cloning sequence, as follows:

```
      NcoI                                          NcoI
5'-----C        CATGGATAACATGGCCAACAAAAC        CATGG------3'
3'-----GGTAC        CTATTGTACCGGTTGTTTTGGTAC        C------5'
```

The resultant construction yielded the sequence:

```
              1 2 3 4 5 6 7 8 9
    5'-----CCATGGATAACATGGCCAACAAAACCATGG-----
    3'-----GGTACCTATTGTACCGGTTGTTTTGGTACC-----
                          9 8 7 6 5 4 3 2 1
```

The numbers 1 through 9 represent the nine indifferent nucleotides in the center of the *Xcm*I recognition sequence, and on digestion with *Xcm*I, those nucleotides would be cleaved to yield a vector with the desired unpaired 3'-thymidylate residues and the central stuffer, as shown:

```
                        MscI
    5'-----CCATGGAT    AACATGGCCAACAAA    ACCATGG------
    3'-----GGTACCT    ATTGTACCGGTTGTT    TTGGTACC------
```

Note that two tandem *Xcm*I sites, [CCA---------TGG][CCA---------TGG], generate a *Msc*I site, TGGCCA. This site occurs only once in pDK101 and can therefore be used to spot-test for the presence of the *Xcm*I adaptor.

The continuity of the β-galactosidase open reading frame through the multiple cloning site of pGEM5fZ (+) is maintained after insertion of the *Xcm*I adaptor to form pDK101, as shown below, and allows for blue-white screening of transformants:

pGEM5fZ(+)

```
      I    P    R    P    W    R    P    G    A    C
GATATCCCGCGGCCATGGCGGCCGGGAGCATGC
CTATAGGGCGCCGGTACCGCCGGCCCTCGTACG
EcoRV              NcoI                      SphI
```

pDK101

```
    I   P   R   P   W   I   T   W   P   T   K   P   W   R   P   G   A   C
GATATCCCGCGGCCATGGATAACATGGCCAACAAAACCATGGCGGCCGGGAGCATGC
CTATAGGGCGCCGGTACCTATTGTACCGGTTGTTTTGGTACCGCCGGCCCTCGTACG
EcoRV           XcmI            MscI            XcmI            SphI
                NcoI                            NcoI
```

Since the overhanging 3'-deoxythymidylate residues obtained by digestion with XcmI lack self-complementarity, the probability of religation of a digested preparation to reconstitute the empty vector is markedly reduced. Transformation with this vector would therefore self-select for inclusion of an insert with overhanging 3'-deoxyadenosyl termini to reconstitute a circular plasmid molecule. The probability of inadvertently recloning the excised stuffer or of transforming with undigested plasmid is minimized by agarose gel purification of the T-tailed pDK101 linears.

Applications: General Description

1. In the most direct application of plasmid pDK101, prepared XcmI-digested vector is ligated with PCR product drawn directly from the amplification reaction, followed by transformation, selection of ampicillin-resistant colonies, screening of transformant colonies for the lac⁻ phenotype, and checking for the presence of the desired insert. RNA transcripts of the inserted DNA can be obtained by transcription with the appropriate RNA polymerase. We have used this approach successfully to clone subfragments of the 23S rRNA gene to obtain transcripts of 23S rRNA domain V for use as substrate of RNA methylating enzymes.

2. Methods have been described for cloning PCR products on the basis of restriction sites incorporated into the primers (4, 5). In the event that the PCR product cannot be subcloned directly after attempts to cleave these sites, possibly because of their proximity to the ends, the product is first cloned into pDK101 (as outlined above), following which it is excised for further constructions. Successful excision of the insert provides assurance that it contains the desired cohesive ends.

3. The construction of gene cassettes can be simplified by ligase-mediated PCR with pDK101. This requires either the use of phosphorylated primers in the initial PCR reaction or addition of kinase to the subsequent ligation reaction and avoids the initial transformation step. The use of 5' phosphorylated inserts allows direct amplification of the DNA insert by a second PCR reaction primed by the β-galactosidase forward and reverse

sequencing primers which bracket the multiple cloning site. Cleavage at restriction sites incorporated into the initial primers then can be performed efficiently and without regard to their proximity to the 5' ends. Digestion of the amplified insert to form the cassette can be monitored easily because the PCR product primed by forward and reverse sequencing primers looses ca. 240 nucleotides as a result of digestion. The increase in electrophoretic mobility resulting from digestion can be easily followed by gel electrophoresis. We have used this approach successfully to construct and express an *ermC* methylase (6) cassette bracketed by the restriction sites *Nhe*I and *Hind*III.

Solutions and Reagents

1. Plasmid pDK101 is available from the American Type Culture Collection (Rockville, MD) as ATCC 77406.

2. *Xcm*I restriction endonuclease (Cat. No. 533, New England Biolabs (NEB), Tozer, MA), and 10× *Xcm*I digestion buffer (NEBuffer 2), supplied with the enzyme.

3. T4 phage DNA ligase (Cat. No. 202, New England Biolabs) and 10× ligase buffer supplied with the enzyme.

4. T4 phage DNA polynucleotide kinase (Cat. No. 201, New England Biolabs).

5. Purification of plasmid DNA from 1.5-ml cultures, or gel slices, was performed initially by use of Magic Miniprep and Magic PCR Prep kits, respectively (Promega, Madison WI, Cat. No. A7100 and No. A7170). Subsequent experiments revealed that the commercial binding "resin" can be replaced satisfactorily with an aqueous suspension of 1.5% diatomaceous earth (Sigma Chemical Co., Cat. No. D-5384, 1.5 g/100 ml) in $7M$ guanidine hydrochloride (Sigma Cat. No. G-4505, 66.9 g/100 ml). The rationale for this method of DNA purification has been discussed (7, 8).

6. Forward sequencing primer (NEB Cat. No. 1218); reverse sequencing primer (NEB Cat. No. 1222).

7. *Escherichia coli* cells are prepared and used for electroporation as described (9).

8. PCR inserts for cloning are obtained by standard protocols optimized for the particular target sequence. In our original description (10), PCR products that were obtained with unphosphorylated primers were used; however, for reasons mentioned above, it is more desirable to use PCR products carrying 5' phosphoryl ends.

Procedures

Preparation of Vector

1. Grow *E. coli,* strain ATCC 77406, from a single colony, overnight in 10 ml LB medium containing ampicillin, 100 μg/ml.

2. Divide the overnight culture into six Eppendorf microfuge tubes and prepare six individual minipreps according to Magic Miniprep instructions. Combine and pool the six eluates. Yield: 10–15 μg plasmid DNA in 300 μl Tris–EDTA buffer (Tris hydrochloride, 10 m*M* (pH 8.0); Na$_2$EDTA, 1 m*M*).

3. Digest the pDK101 DNA sample from step 2 with 5 units *Xcm*I/μg pDK101 DNA—by addition of 39 μl NEB buffer 2 and 50 μl *Xcm*I (concentration 1 unit/μl). Incubate at 37°C for 1 hr.

4. Extract the digestion reaction twice with and equal volume of phenol/chloroform/isoamyl alcohol (25/24/1). Extract the upper (aqueous) phase once with an equal volume of chloroform.

5. Purify the extracted preparation from step 4 electrophoretically on a preparative 1% low melting point (LMP) agarose gel (NuSieve GTG, FMC Bioproducts, Rockland, ME) in Tris acetate EDTA buffer (Tris acetate, 40 m*M* (pH 8.0); Na$_2$EDTA, 1 m*M*) containing ethidium bromide (0.5 μg/ml).

6. Locate and excise the pDK101 linear band with the briefest possible exposure to ultraviolet light, and purify using Magic PCR Prep according to the manufacturer's directions.

7. Analyze *Xcm*I-digested plasmid DNA preparation by gel electrophoresis and by self-ligation plus transformation to assure purity and low background. Store prepared DNA at −20°C until needed.

Ligation of PCR-Amplified DNA Obtained Using Unphosphorylated Primers and Phosphorylation of the PCR Product

1. Mix in 10 μl total volume:

10× ligation buffer (NEB)	1 μl
*Xcm*I-digested pDK101	4 μl containing ca. 200 ng DNA
PCR-amplified DNA	4.5 μl containing ca. 200 ng DNA
Phage T4 polynucleotide kinase (10 units/μl)	0.5 μl (5 units)

Incubate for 10 min at 37°C

2. Add 0.5 μl phage T4 DNA ligase (400 units/μl)
   Incubate for 4–16 hr at 16°C
3. Heat-inactivate kinase and ligase at 65°C for 20 min.
4. Transform *E. coli* host strain directly, or perform a second round PCR using universal forward and reverse sequencing primers. The PCR reaction is performed for 30 cycles in a 100-μl reaction volume and contains 1 μl heat-inactivated ligation reaction (step 2) as template.

Other T-Vectors

The preparation of T-vectors by digestion with restriction endonucleases has utilized either *Hph*I (11) or *Xcm*I (10). Note that *Hph*I-based T-vector clones can be digested with *Hph*I to yield (reusable) T-vector linear molecules whereas *Xcm*I-based T-vector clones cannot. This is because the *Hph*I enzyme recognition site is on the plasmid side of the cutting site and is situated entirely external to the stuffer. Thus *Hph*I can be used to excise inserts and to regenerate (re)usable T-vector. In contrast, the two specific parts of the *Xcm*I recognition site (CCA and TGG) straddle the location at which this enzyme cuts, and cloning into the prepared site is very unlikely to regenerate a *Xcm*I. Thus *Xcm*I cannot be used to excise inserts in pDK101, nor can it be used to regenerate (re)useable cloning vector.

Acknowledgments

This work was supported by Research Grants AI-18283, S10-RR01684, and CA-07175 from the National Institutes of Health, DMB-8514305 from the National Science Foundation, as well as by research support from the University of Wisconsin Graduate School.

References

1. J. M. Clark, *Nucleic Acids Res.* **16,** 9677 (1988).
2. T. A. Holton and M. W. Graham, *Nucleic Acids Res.* **19,** 1156 (1991).
3. D. Marchuk, M. Drumm, A. Saulino, and F. S. Collins, *Nucleic Acids Res.* **19,** 1154 (1990).
4. V. Jung, S. B. Pestka, and S. Pestka, *Nucleic Acids Res.* **18,** 6156 (1990).
5. D. L. Kaufman and G. A. Evans, *BioTechniques* **9,** 304 (1990).
6. S. Horinouchi and B. Weisblum, *J. Bacteriol.* **150,** 804 (1982).

7. R. Boom, C. J. A. Sol, M. M. M. Salimans, C. L. Jansen, P. M. E. Wertheim-VanDillen, and J. Van Der Noordaa. *J. Clin. Microbiol.* **28,** 495 (1989).
8. M. J. Carter and I. D. Milton, *Nucleic Acids Res.* **21,** 1044 (1993).
9. J. Sambrook, E. F. Fritsch, and T. Maniatis, "Molecular Cloning: A Laboratory Manual," 2nd ed. Cold Spring Harbor Lab., Cold Spring Harbor, NY, 1989.
10. D. Kovalic, J.-H. Kwak, and B. Weisblum, *Nucleic Acids Res.* **19,** 4650 (1991).
11. D. A. Mead, N. K. Pey, C. Herrnstadt, R. A. Marcil, and L. A. Smith, *Biotechnology* **9,** 657 (1991).

[18] Subtractive cDNA Cloning Using Oligo(dT)$_{30}$–Latex and PCR

E. Hara, Y. Furuichi, and K. Oda

Subtractive cDNA libraries provide a powerful approach for identifying and isolating genes that are differentially expressed in defined tissues or cell lines. Several methods commonly referred to as "subtraction" have been developed (1–5). In most cases, the mRNA common to both types of cells has been eliminated by hydroxyapatite chromatography or the avidin–biotin system after cDNA–mRNA hybridization (6–8). To improve the subtraction system, however, several problems still remain to be solved: (i) how to increase resolution of unhybridized mRNA from the cDNA–mRNA hybrid, (ii) how to minimize the frequency of mRNA degradation, and (iii) how to isolate cDNA clones representing low-abundance mRNAs that are expressed differentially.

To construct a subtractive cDNA library, we made a latex-bound primer, oligo(dT)$_{30}$–latex, by covalently linking oligo(dC)$_{10}$-(dT)$_{30}$ at its 5' proximal region to the carboxyl residues on the surface of latex particles. The poly(A)$^+$ mRNA annealed efficiently (95%) to oligo(dT)$_{30}$–latex in a short reaction period (10 min), and the cDNA synthesis was carried out with AMV reverse transcriptase using the annealed mRNA as the template and the covalently linked oligo(dT)$_{30}$ as the primer (9, 10). This cDNA–latex particle can be easily precipitated by a brief centrifugation. Previously, we have used this cDNA–latex particle to develop a method for subtractive cDNA cloning (11). The subtractive hybridization was carried out in an Eppendorf tube between the cDNA linked to latex particles and mRNA prepared from another cell type; and unhybridized mRNA was separated by a brief centrifugation. The subtracted mRNA was subsequently amplified by PCR after conversion to cDNA.

We have revised our subtractive cDNA cloning method by using sense-strand DNA instead of mRNA for hybridization to the cDNA linked to latex particles (12), because the cDNA inserts in a library constructed by the previous method sometimes had an average length shorter than 1 kb. The sense-strand DNA was made by asymmetric PCR using only one primer. This method minimizes the frequency of mRNA degradation and makes it easy to construct the subtractive library with longer cDNA inserts sufficient to analyze the sequence in the coding region. With this improved method, we could construct a subtractive cDNA library, which effectively concentrated cDNA clones specific to senescent human diploid fibroblasts.

Methods in Neurosciences, Volume 26

Preparation of Poly(A)-Containing mRNA

Poly(A)-containing mRNAs have often been purified from total cellular RNA by traditional column chromatography using oligo(dT)-cellulose (13). Here, we introduce a new, convenient batchwise procedure with Oligotex-$(dT)_{30}$ (2) (referred to here as Oligotex-$(dT)_{30}$, oligo$(dT)_{30}$–latex, or briefly Oligotex) a fine suspension of nonpolar latex particles, homogeneous in size (0.22 mm in diameter) and carrying oligo$(dT)_{30}$-mers covalently bound to the surface (10). Because the density of oligo$(dT)_{30}$–latex is nearly equivalent to that of water (1 g/ml), it forms a stable milky suspension that still is easily precipitated to a small pellet by centrifugation with a table-top Eppendorf centrifuge (15,000 rpm, 10 min). Its small size provides a large surface area, and, thus, the rate of hybridization between Oligotex-$(dT)_{30}$ and mRNA poly(A) residues is extremely high [see Kuribayashi-Ohta et al. (10) for more details]. One cycle of mRNA affinity purification can be achieved within an hour, and because the Oligotex-$(dT)_{30}$ is stable to alkali and heat (>100°C), the beads can be sterilized, for example by autoclaving, to avoid ribonuclease contamination formidable to mRNA purification.

Total RNAs are prepared by the method described elsewhere (13). The usual method extracts RNAs with high concentrations of guanidine thiocyanate and isolates them by ultracentrifugation in cesium trifluoroacetate. Poly(A)$^+$ mRNAs are purified from the suspension of total RNAs recovered from the pellet after the ultracentrifugation.

Reagents

Oligotex-$(dT)_{30}$: available in a 5-ml sterilized suspension from Takara Co., Ltd. (4-jo Shimogyo-ku, Kyoto) or Dai-ichi Chemicals (Nihonbashi, Tokyo) in Japan, from Quiagen (Chatsworth, CA), and from Diagen (Hilden, Germany). A 50- to 100-μl suspension of Oligotex-$(dT)_{30}$ can isolate 1 μg of poly(A)$^+$ mRNA of 1200 bases in size, according to the manufacturer (Japan Synthetic Rubber Co., Ltd., Tsukiji, Tokyo, and Nippon Roche K.K., Marunouchi, Tokyo).

Elution buffer: 10 mM Tris-HCl (pH 7.5), 1 mM ethylenediaminetetraacetic acid (EDTA), 0.1% sodium dodecyl sulfate (SDS) in distilled water.

5 M NaCl: Sterilized by autoclaving.

3 M sodium acetate (pH 5.6): Sterilized by autoclaving.

Washing buffer: 10 mM Tris–HCl (pH 7.5), 1 mM EDTA, 0.1% SDS, and 0.1 M NaCl in sterilized water.

TE buffer: 10 mM Tris-HCl (pH 7.5), 1 mM EDTA.

Procedure

Total RNA (1 mg) is dissolved in 1 ml of elution buffer, Oligotex-$(dT)_{30}$ (1 ml) is then added, and the mixture is incubated at 65°C for 5 min to disrupt any internal base pairing and aggregation of the RNA molecules. After being chilled on ice for 3 min, 0.2 ml of 5 M NaCl is added, and the mixture is incubated at 37°C for 10 min. During the incubation, poly(A) residues hybridize to the oligo$(dT)_{30}$-mers by base pairing, and the mRNA molecules are caught on the Oligotex-$(dT)_{30}$ particles. The reaction mixture is centrifuged for 10 min at 15,000 rpm, and the precipitate containing the complex of poly(A)$^+$ mRNA–Oligotex-$(dT)_{30}$ is suspended by pipetting in 2.5 ml washing buffer. Note that the pellet of poly(A)$^+$ mRNA–Oligotex-$(dT)_{30}$ is tight; therefore, a thorough pipetting is needed to yield a homogeneous suspension. The suspension is left for 10 min at room temperature and centrifuged for 10 min at 15,000 rpm, and the supernatant containing the unbound RNAs, such as rRNA and tRNA, is removed. To recover the bound poly(A)$^+$ mRNA, the pellets are suspended in 1 ml TE buffer, and the suspension is incubated for 5 min at 65°C. This process breaks the hydrogen bonding between poly(A) and oligo$(dT)_{30}$ and releases mRNAs from the Oligo$(dT)_{30}$–latex particles. After centrifugation (15,000 rpm, 10 min, room temperature), the supernatant, which contains poly(A)$^+$ mRNA, is carefully isolated. Now, the pellet is not as tight as before; thus, care must be taken not to disturb the pellets. If further purification is needed, the above process can be repeated by the addition of new Oligotex-$(dT)_{30}$ (1 ml). The poly(A)$^+$ mRNA is precipitated by adding 100 μl of 3 M sodium acetate and 2 ml of cold ethanol to the supernatant and keeping the mixture at −80°C (or in dry ice) for 10–15 min. The pellet is obtained by centrifugation (15,000 rpm, 10 min, 4°C) and rinsed with cold 70% (v/v) ethanol followed by centrifugation. Finally, the resulting RNA pellet is dissolved in 50 μl TE buffer. From 1 mg of total RNA, 10–50 μg of poly(A)$^+$ mRNA is obtained, although the yields vary depending on the source.

Comments

In case the mRNA solution contains any contamination by free Oligotex-$(dT)_{30}$, a conventional phenol extraction can be used to remove the trace amount of Oligotex particles.

cDNA Synthesis on Oligotex-$(dT)_{30}$

All the procedures for constructing of a subtractive cDNA library are schematically illustrated in Fig. 1.

Reagents

All solutions must be sterilized either by autoclaving or by filtration through Millipore (Bedford, MA) filters. It is recommended that gloves and a mask be worn until the double-stranded cDNA is made.

1× TMK buffer: 50 mM Tris–HCl (pH 8.3), 100 mM KCl, 10 mM MgCl$_2$.
10× reverse transcriptase (RT) buffer: 500 mM Tris–HCl (pH 8.5), 300 mM KCl, 80 mM MgCl$_2$.
TE: 10 mM Tris–HCl (pH 7.5), 1 mM EDTA.
1 M dithiothreitol (DTT): To be freshly prepared.
100 mM dNTP: A mixture of 100 mM dGTP, dATP, dCTP, and dTTP.
Water: distilled water.
Reverse transcriptase: avian myeloblastosis virus (AMV) reverse transcriptase (Seikagaku Kogyo or Bio-Rad, Richmond, CA) RNase free.
RNase inhibitor (Takara).

Procedure

Add 50 μl each of 5% (w/v) Oligotex-(dT)$_{30}$ suspension to two Eppendorf tubes. Ten micrograms each of mRNA from cell type A (young TIG-1 cells) and cell type B (senescent TIG-1 cells) is added to each tube, and the final volume is adjusted to 100 μl with water. TIG-1 cells are normal human diploid fibroblasts with a life span of about 62 population doublings (PD) (16). The suspension is heated at 70°C for 5 min and rapidly cooled in ice-water. After addition of 100 μl of 2× TMK buffer, the suspension is incubated at 37°C for 20 min and then centrifuged at 15,000 rpm for 10 min at room temperature. The precipitate [mRNA–Oligotex-(dT)$_{30}$ complex] is suspended in 400 μl of RT buffer containing 40 μl of 10× RT buffer, 2 mM each of dNTP, 2.5 mM DTT, 100 U of reverse transcriptase, and 300 U of RNase inhibitor. An excess of reverse transcriptase is added to cover the surface of the latex particles. The reaction is carried out at 43°C for 1 hr. The reaction mixture is centrifuged at 4°C for 10 min, and the precipitate is suspended in 400 μl of TE. The suspension is heated at 92°C for 3 min and rapidly cooled in ice-water. The RNA dissociated from the cDNA–Oligotex-(dT)$_{30}$ is removed by centrifugation, and the precipitate is washed several times with 400 μl of TE by centrifugation. The precipitate (cDNA–Oligotex) is suspended in 200 μl of TE and stored at 4°C.

Comments

An excess of reverse transcriptase is required for the reaction since a majority of reverse transcriptase attaches to the latex particles. The particles should

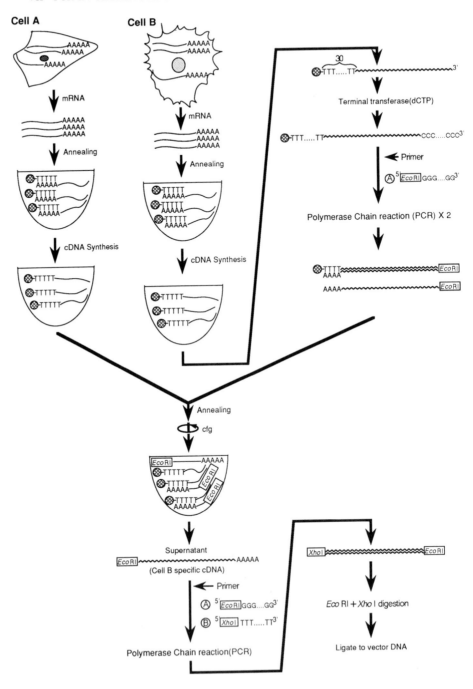

not be coated with bovine serum albumin (BSA) before the reverse transcriptase is added, because BSA usually contains a trace of RNase.

Synthesis of Sense-Strand DNA

Reagents

> 5× TT buffer: 500 mM sodium cacodylate, 10 mM $MnCl_2$, 0.5 mM DTT.
> pH is adjusted to 7.6 at room temperature.
> Terminal deoxynucleotidyltransferase from calf thymus (Takara).
> 10× PCR buffer: 100 mM Tris–HCl (pH 8.3), 50 mM KCl, 20 mM $MgCl_2$.
> Taq polymerase (Takara/Perkin–Elmer, Norwalk, CT).
> EcoRI $(dG)_{15}$ primer: 5′ CGAGGAATTC$(G)_{15}$ 3′, 2 μg/μl.

Procedure

To synthesize a sense-strand DNA having the same sequence as mRNA by asymmetric PCR, an oligo(dC) tail is added to the 3′ end of the cDNA linked to the latex particles. The cDNA–Oligotex-$(dT)_{30}$ prepared from cell type B (senescent TIG-1 cells) is washed several times with water by centrifugation. The reaction is performed in a 200-μl reaction mixture containing 40 μl of 5× TT buffer, 2 μl of 100 mM dCTP, and 200 U of terminal deoxynucleotidyltransferase at 37°C for 10 min and terminated by the addition of 20 μl of 250 mM EDTA. The mixture is centrifuged at 15,000 rpm for 10 min, and the precipitate is washed several times with water. The oligo(dC)-tailed cDNA–Oligotex is then suspended in a 100-μl reaction mixture containing 10 μl of 10× PCR buffer, 1 μl of 100 mM dNTP, 1 μl of the EcoRI $(dG)_{15}$ primer, and 10 U of Taq polymerase. Two cycles of PCR are performed at 94°C for 1.5 min, 55°C for 2 min, and 72°C for 3 min. The mixture is centrifuged at 4°C for 10 min and the supernatant (100 μl) containing the sense-strand DNA is collected and stored at −20°C. The precipitate [oligo(dC)-tailed cDNA–Oligotex] is suspended in 100 μl of TE and stored at 4°C.

FIG. 1 Schematic representation of the construction of a subtractive cDNA library using Oligotex-$(dT)_{30}$ (Oligotex). The senescent human diploid fibroblasts, TIG-1 cells (60 PDL), are represented as cell type B, and the young TIG-1 cells (35 PDL) are represented as cell type A. The Oligotex-$(dT)_{30}$ particle is shown as a shaded circle with a protruding oligo(dT).

Comments

Prior to using the sense-strand DNA, the DNA length should be checked by electrophoresing an aliquot of the DNA after amplification by PCR using both *Eco*RI $(dG)_{15}$ and *Xho*I $(dT)_{30}$ primers. If the average length of the amplified DNA is shorter than 1 kilobase (kb), the sense-strand DNA should not be used. The oligo(dC)-tailed cDNA–Oligotex can be stored without loss of the template activity for at least 3 months.

Subtractive Hybridization

Reagents

$(dA)_{30}(dG)_{10}$: 5' $(dA)_{30}(dG)_{10}$ 3'
5× hybridization buffer: 50 mM Tris–HCl (pH 7.5), 5 mM EDTA, 0.5% SDS
5 M NaCl

Procedure

The cDNA–Oligotex prepared from cell type A (young TIG-1 cells) is washed several times as described. Total cDNA–Oligotex is suspended in 100 μl of TE with 100 μg of $(dA)_{30}(dG)_{10}$ and incubated at 65°C for 5 min. Eleven microliters of 5 M NaCl is then added, and the incubation is continued at 37°C for 10 min to cover the free oligo(dT) residues on Oligotex-$(dT)_{30}$. The $(dA)_{30}(dG)_{10}$ not annealed to oligo(dT) is collected by centrifugation and stored at 4°C for reuse later. The precipitate is suspended in 100 μl of hybridization solution containing 20 μl of 5× hybridization buffer, 15 μl of 5 M NaCl, and 20 μl of sense-strand DNA. The hybridization is carried out at 55°C for 50 min. The hybridization mixture is centrifuged at room temperature for 10 min. The supernatant (the first subtractive sense-strand DNA) is collected and stored at 4°C. To dissociate the hybridized sense-strand DNA, the precipitate is suspended in 400 μl of TE, heated at 94°C for 3 min, and rapidly cooled. The suspension is centrifuged, and the supernatant is removed. The precipitate (cDNA–Oligotex) is washed several times with water to remove hybridized sense-strand DNA and suspended in the $(dA)_{30}(dG)_{10}$ supernatant previously stored. The suspension is incubated at 37°C for 10 min, and the free $(dA)_{30}(dG)_{10}$ is again collected by centrifugation. The precipitate is suspended in the first subtractive sense-strand fraction, and the second hybridization is performed at 55°C for 50 min. This subtractive hybridization step is repeated four times in total.

Comments

Latex particles cohere at NaCl concentrations higher than 1 M. In the present method, the upper limit of NaCl concentration was examined to increase the efficiency of hybridization, and the subtractive hybridization is carried out at 0.75 M NaCl for 50 min, instead of at 0.5 M for 20 min as done in the original method (11).

Amplification of Subtractive Sense-Strand DNA by PCR

Reagent

XhoI(dT)$_{30}$ primer: 5 ′ GCCA<u>CTCGAG</u>(T)$_{30}$ 3′

Procedure

Subtractive sense-strand DNA specific to cell type B (senescent TIG-1 cells) is then amplified by PCR. The subtractive sense-strand DNA in the final supernatant from the subtractive hybridization is precipitated by adding eight volumes of 75% ethanol, after the addition of 2 μg each of EcoRI (dG)$_{15}$ and XhoI (dT)$_{30}$ primers. The precipitate is suspended in 100 μl of the reaction mixture containing 10 μl of 10× PCR buffer, 1 μl of 100 mM dNTP, 4 μg each of EcoRI (dG)$_{15}$ and XhoI (dT)$_{30}$ primers, and 10 U of Taq polymerase. The reaction is performed for 35 cycles at 94°C for 1.5 min, 55°C for 2 min, and 72°C for 3 min. After 35 cycle reactions, a 5-μl aliquot is removed, and the presence of cDNA is confirmed by electrophoresis on a 1.2% agarose gel followed by staining with ethidium bromide. If cDNA is not detected, the PCR is continued for an additional 25 cycles.

Comments

It is preferable to amplify the subtractive cDNA as minimally as possible. If the subtractive cDNA is not ligated efficiently in the following step, despite the presence of sufficient cDNA, it is recommended that the PCR be repeated at an elevated annealing temperature (60°C instead of 55°C).

cDNA Cloning in Phagemid Vectors

Reagents

Sephacryl S-400 column: Sephacryl S-400 (Pharmacia, Piscataway, NJ) is washed three times with TE by decantation, and the final suspension is autoclaved. A 5-ml syringe is fixed to the inside of a 50-ml Corning tube, after the tip is packed with glasswool. Sephacryl S-400 is then packed into the syringe by successive centrifugation until an approximate column volume is obtained. Usually, a column volume is adjusted to be 10-fold that of the reaction mixture. The column is washed three times with TE by centrifugation.

10× EcoRI buffer: 1 M Tris–HCl (pH 7.5), 70 mM MgCl$_2$, 70 mM 2-mercaptoethanol, 500 mM NaCl, 10% bovine serum albumin (BSA).

10× XhoI buffer: 100 mM Tris–HCl (pH 7.5), 70 mM MgCl$_2$, 70 mM 2-mercaptoethanol, 1 M NaCl.

Phenol/chloroform: a 1 : 1 (v : v) mixture of water-saturated phenol and chloroform.

λZapII DNA (Stratagene, La Jolla, CA; Uni zap XR Vector kit).

Packaging kit (Stratagene; Gigapack II gold).

Ligation kit (Takara).

1× Ligation buffer: 100 mM Tris–HCl, pH 7.6, 5 mM MgCl$_2$.

Procedure

The amplified subtractive cDNA obtained in Amplification of Subtractive Sense-Strand DNA by PCR is precipitated with ethanol, and the precipitate is dissolved in 100 μl of water. The cDNA is digested with XhoI in 400 μl of reaction mixture containing 40 μl of 10× XhoI buffer and 100 U of XhoI and incubated at 37°C for 2 hr. The mixture is extracted twice with phenol/chloroform; the cDNA is precipitated with ethanol. The cDNA is then digested with EcoRI in 400 μl of reaction mixture containing 40 μl of 10× EcoRI buffer and 100 U of EcoRI at 37°C for 2 hr. The mixture is extracted twice with phenol/chloroform, and the supernatant obtained after centrifugation is applied on the top of the Sephacryl S-400 spin column under which an Eppendorf tube is placed. The column is then centrifuged at 1000 rpm for 3 min, and the flowthrough, which contains cDNA larger than approximately 250 bp, is collected. The cDNA is ethanol-precipitated and dissolved in 10 μl of the ligation buffer with 2 μg of λZapII DNA already cleaved with XhoI and EcoRI. The cDNA is ligated into the cloning site of the λZapII vector DNA with Takara's ligation kit. The ligation is performed at 26°C for

10 min after the addition of 10 μl of enzyme solution B. The recombinant λZapII DNA is packaged, *in vitro*, with the Gigapack II packaging extract according to the protocol of Stratagene. The subtractive cDNA library is titrated with *Escherichia coli* strain XL1-blue. The size of the library thus obtained ranges from 5×10^4 to 2×10^5, depending on the extent of cDNA amplification.

Comments

The ligation efficiency of cDNA into the cloning site of the vector DNA with Takara's ligation kit is at least fivefold higher than that of the usual method. The subtractive cDNA can be cloned into a variety of convenient vectors using an appropriate restriction enzyme recognition sequence linked to the primers.

Differential Plaque Hybridization

The cDNA clones specific to cell type B (senescent TIG-1 cells) are efficiently enriched in the present subtractive library; however, they represent only about 4% of the total clones, as stated in the following section, and a majority of clones originated from mRNA common to both cell types. To isolate the specific clones, the library is further screened by successive differential plaque hybridization (12).

Reagents

Oligo(dT)$_{12-18}$ primer (0.25 μg/μl).
Actinomycin D (10 μg/μl).
[α-^{32}P]dCTP: 3000 Ci/mmol; Amersham.
Sephadex G-50 column: Sephadex G-50 (Pharmacia) is washed three times with TE by decantation and the final suspension is autoclaved. A 1-ml column is made in a 1-ml syringe and washed with several column volumes of TE.
137 mm nylon filters (NEN Research Products).
Formamide (BRL).
Herring sperm DNA: 10 mg/ml, sonicated at 200 W for 3 to 5 min.
0.5 M NaOH
1× SSC: 0.15 M NaCl, 15 mM sodium citrate

Procedure

The poly(A)$^+$ RNAs prepared from young and senescent (60 PDL) TIG-1 cells, as described, are used as templates for synthesizing the ^{32}P-labeled cDNA probes. A typical reaction mixture contains 2 μg of poly(A)$^+$ RNA pretreated at 65°C for 3 min, 10 μl of 10× RT buffer, 2 μl of 1M DTT, 5 μl of 6.6 mM dNTP(-dCTP), 5 μl of 0.66 mM dCTP, 2 μg of oligo(dT)$_{12-18}$ primer, 5 μg of actinomycin D, 500 μCi of [α-^{32}P]dCTP, 120 U of RNase inhibitor, and 70 U of reverse transcriptase in a final 100 μl volume. The mixture is incubated at 43°C for 1.5 hr, and the reaction is terminated by the addition of 5 μl of 2 N NaOH followed by heating at 70°C for 20 min. The reaction mixture is neutralized and precipitated by ethanol. After centrifugation, the precipitate is dissolved in 100 μl of TE and applied to the Sephadex G-50 column. The flowthrough fraction is collected and used as a probe.

The subtractive cDNA library is plated at 2000 to 2500 plaques per 137 mm dish with *E. coli* strain XL1-blue, and the plaques are transferred to duplicate sets of 137-mm nylon filters. The recombinant phage DNA is denatured by dipping the filter twice in 0.5 N NaOH on Saran Wrap for 2 min. The DNA is then neutralized similarly by dipping the filter twice in 1 M Tris–HCl (pH 7.5) for 2 min. The filters are air-dried and prehybridized in 10 ml of the solution containing 50% (v/v) formamide, 1% SDS, 1 M NaCl, and 10% (w/v) dextran sulfate in a plastic bag for at least 6 hr. Hybridization is then performed at 42°C for 16 hr after the addition of 10^6 cpm/ml of ^{32}P-labeled cDNA probe prepared from either cell type A (young TIG-1 cells) or cell type B (senescent TIG-1) and 100 μg/ml of denatured herring sperm DNA. The filters are washed twice with 2× SSC containing 0.1% SDS at 65°C for 30 min and exposed to X-ray film with an intensifying screen at −80°C for 3 days. Clones that preferentially hybridized to the cDNA probe from cell type B (senescent TIG-1 cells) are isolated. These clones are subjected to the second and third screenings. The positive clones are spotted onto a bacterial lawn and incubated at 37°C for 8 to 12 hr. The plaques are transferred to duplicate sets of nylon filters, and plaque hybridization is repeated as described above. A part of the result obtained after the third hybridization is shown in Fig. 2. The clones that hybridized preferentially to the cDNA probe from senescent TIG-1 cells are finally isolated (14).

Comments

For clones selected by the second or third differential hybridization, their preferential expression in cell type B (senescent TIG-1 cells) must be confirmed by RNA dot (12) or Northern blot hybridization. The plasmid DNA,

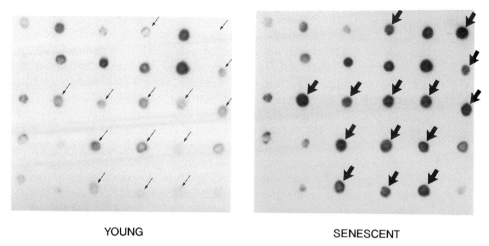

YOUNG   SENESCENT

FIG. 2   Differential plaque hybridization. The subtractive cDNA library was screened for clones preferentially expressed in senescent TIG-1 cells by successive differential plaque hybridizations. The positive clones at the second hybridization were spotted onto a bacterial lawn and incubated at 37°C for 12 hr. The phages were transferred to duplicate sets of nylon filters, and plaque hybridization was repeated with ^{32}P-labeled cDNA probes prepared from either young or senescent TIG-1 cells. The arrows indicate the clones that preferentially hybridize with the cDNA probe from the senescent cells.

pBluescript carrying the cDNA insert can be generated from a λZapII recombinant by coinfection of an *E. coli* strain, XL1-blue, with the f1 helper phage according to the manufacturer's protocol (Stratagene Uni Zap XR kit).

Characterization of Amplified Subtractive cDNA Clones

Typical results from the isolation of cDNA clones that were overexpressed in senescent human diploid fibroblasts, TIG-1, are summarized in this section. Here, senescent TIG-1 cells correspond to cell type B, and young TIG-1 cells correspond to cell type A. The total size of the subtractive cDNA library constructed by the present method was 2×10^5 plaque-forming units (pfu). Approximately 7000 plaques were screened by the first differential plaque hybridization, and 550 plaques that showed stronger intensity with the senescent TIG-1 probe were isolated. These plaques were further screened twice more by the differential hybridization, and 287 plaques that repeatedly showed preferential hybridization to the senescent TIG-1 cDNA probe were finally isolated as shown in Fig. 2. To estimate the average length of cDNA inserts, plasmid DNA was excised from each of the 287 recombinant phages by infection of *E. coli* XL1-blue with the f1 helper phage. The isolated plasmid DNAs were cleaved with *Eco*RI and *Xho*I and electrophoresed on agarose gels. The cDNA inserts ranged in length from 0.4 to about 6 kb, except for 16 clones that had very short or no cDNA inserts; the average length was estimated to be 2 kb. These results suggests that approximately 4% (271/7000 × 100) of the recombinant phages in the subtractive cDNA library contain senescent TIG-1 cell-specific cDNA inserts long enough to characterize DNA sequences in the coding region.

The 271 positive clones were classified into 28 groups by cross-hybridization. Expression levels of these genes in young and senescent TIG-1 cells were compared by the intensity of signals obtained by RNA dot hybridization. The clones in 16 groups were expressed at least three times higher in the senescent cells than in the young cells. About 400 bp of DNA sequences were determined, and a homology search was performed with the data available through the GenBank and EMBL data banks. As shown in Table I, genes encoding components of the extracellular matrix, fibronectin and procollagen, were expressed at high levels in the senescent cells, as have been reported in other senescent fibroblasts. Most of the clones originating from the low-abundance mRNAs have unknown sequences.

Comments

The present method allows for the construction of a subtractive cDNA library with large cDNAs sufficient to analyze the coding sequence with a high probability. The enrichment for cell-type-specific cDNA was effective, and several percent of the clones represented specific cDNAs. Very few clones (less than 2%) generated more than two cDNA fragments after cleavage of the plasmid DNAs with *Eco*RI and *Xho*I, indicating that the frequency of multiple cDNA insertion into a single clone is very low. Most of the false-positive cDNA clones originated from low-abundance mRNAs common to both young and senescent cells. The persistence of these common cDNAs in the library might be caused by a low efficiency of hybridization between low-abundance DNAs. It is recommended that the complete cDNA sequence be isolated from an appropriate cDNA library by using specific cDNA obtained as a probe, because PCR is often accompanied by an incorporation of wrong nucleotides at a significant frequency of approximately 10^{-5} (15).

TABLE I   Characterization of cDNA Inserts Specifically Expressed in Senescent TIG-1 Cells[a]

cDNA	Abundance	Expression level (S/Y)
Known		
Fibronectin	31	15
$\alpha1(I)$ Procollagen	20	12
$\alpha2(I)$ Procollagen	12	10
Mitochondrial cytochrome oxidase	10	7
Cytochrome P450	10	7
High homology		
Bovine cytochrome b561	6	6
Mouse nucleolin	5	5
Mouse gas3 gene	2	8
Unknown		
S-1	2	3
S-3	1	5
S-8	1	6
S-11	1	6
S-14	1	3
S-42	1	7
S-131	1	10
S-141	1	7

[a] The representative cDNA clones in 16 different groups were sequenced, and the homology with known DNA sequences was searched with the data available through the GenBank and EMBL data bank. Abundance is shown by the number of clones belonging to the same group in a total of 105 clones. The ratios of expression levels for each cDNA clone in senescent (S) and young (Y) TIG-1 cells were calculated after quantitation of the hybridization intensity obtained with the cDNA probes from senescent and young TIG-1 cells by a densitometer.

References

1. C. Timblin, J. Battey, and W. M. Kuehl, *Nucleic Acids Res.* **18,** 1587 (1990).
2. J. L. R. Rubenstein, A. E. J. Brice, R. D. Ciaranello, D. Denney, M. H. Porteus, and T. B. Usdin, *Nucleic Acids Res.* **18,** 4833 (1990).
3. A. Swaroop, J. Xu, N. Agarwal, and S. M. Weissman, *Nucleic Acids Res.* **19,** 1954 (1991).
4. M.-C. Lebeau, B. G. Alvarez, W. Wahli, and S. Catsicas, *Nucleic Acids Res.* **19,** 4778 (1991).
5. I. R. Rodriguez and G. J. Chader, *Nucleic Acids Res.* **20,** 3528 (1992).
6. T. D. Sargent and I. B. Dawid, *Science* **222,** 135 (1983).
7. M. Davis, *Proc. Natl. Acad. Sci. U.S.A.* **81,** 2129 (1984).
8. H. L. Sive and T. S. John, *Nucleic Acids Res.* **16,** 10937 (1988).

9. K. Kuribayashi, M. Hikata, O. Hiraoka, C. Miyamoto, and Y. Furuichi, *Nucleic Acids Res. Symp. Ser.* **19,** 61 (1988).

10. K. Kuribayashi-Ohta, S. Tamatsukuri, M. Hikata, C. Miyamoto, and Y. Furuichi, *Biochim. Biophys. Acta* **1156,** 204 (1993).

11. E. Hara, T. Kato, S. Nakada, S. Sekiya, and K. Oda, *Nucleic Acids Res.* **19,** 7097 (1991).

12. E. Hara, T. Yamaguchi, H. Tahara, N. Tsuyama, H. Tsurui, T. Ide, and K. Oda, *Anal. Biochem.* **214,** 58 (1993).

13. J. Sambrook, E. F. Fritch, and T. Maniatis, "Molecular Cloning: A Laboratory Manual," 2nd ed. Cold Spring Harbor Lab., Cold Spring Harbor, NY, 1989.

14. E. Hara, S. Nakada, T. Takehana, T. Nakajimna, T. Iino, and K. Oda, *Gene* **70,** 97 (1988).

15. K. A. Eckert and T. A. Kunkel, *PCR Methods Appl.* **1,** 17 (1991).

16. M. Ohashi, S. Aizawa, H. Ooka, T. Ohsawa, K. Kaji, H. Kondo, T. Kobayashi, T. Nomura, M. Matsuo, Y. Mitsui, S. Murota, K. Yamamoto, H. Ito, H. Shimada, and T. Utakoji, *Exp. Gerontol.* **15,** 121 (1980).

[19] Expression Cloning: PCR versus Episomal Vectors for Rescue of Transfected Genes

Kenton S. Miller and Mark Brudnak

Introduction

In the past few years gene cloning utilizing eukaryotic expression vectors has come of age and a plethora of genes, whose protein products are present in the cell in such vanishingly small amounts that they are difficult or impossible to purify and sequence, have now been cloned using a variety of eukaryotic expression systems. The technology for expression cloning has been refined to the point that numerous vectors, reagent kits, and manuals providing theory and "cookbook" protocols are commercially available for the novice cloner (1, 2).

The experimental rationale of eukaryotic expression cloning is straightforward. A cDNA library is constructed in an expression vector from an mRNA population known to contain an mRNA species whose translation results in a selectable or otherwise identifiable marker of interest. The cDNA library is transfected into a eukaryotic cell line which does not normally express this marker. Subsequently, those cells expressing the marker are identified in the larger population of transfected cells by an appropriate protocol. Such protocols include panning using monoclonal antibodies (MAb) (3), selection with cytotoxic genes (4), and SIB selection using assayable markers (5).

Typically eukaryotic expression cloning experiments have exploited extrachromasomally replicating vectors. Such vectors have had several distinct advantages over more traditional vectors which require integration into the host genome. First, because they replicate to high copy number in the recipient cell, such vectors usually express high levels of their respective recombinant gene products thereby facilitating the selection process (6). Second, extrachromosomally replicating vectors can be recovered after transfection and selection using the Hirt protocol for the rescue of extrachromosomally replicating virus (7).

Such vectors, however, suffer at least one major defect. They require special cell lines expressing a specific viral gene product in which to replicate. Thus, vectors based on the SV40 (simian virus 40) origin of replication require cell lines expressing the SV40 large T antigen for their replication. For example, COS cells, which are large T antigen-expressing African Green Monkey cells, have been used extensively for successful eukaryotic expres-

Methods in Neurosciences, Volume 26

sion cloning experiments (2). Several mouse (MOP and WOP) (8, 9) and hamster (CHOP and CHOP-TU) (10, 11) cell lines expressing the polyoma virus large T antigen have also been developed. These lines allow extrachromosomal replication of vectors containing the polyoma origin. Vectors expressing the EBNA-1 gene product in combination with an Epstein–Barr virus origin of replication have found extensive use in expression cloning in human cell lines (6).

Here we describe a new approach to expression cloning which exploits the power of the polymerase chain reaction (PCR) to rescue cDNAs from cell lines which have been selected for a specific gene product expressed from an integrated vector (12). We show that such a protocol can be used for several rounds of transfection and selection and that the cDNA or gene subsequently isolated remains functional. We compare and contrast the use of PCR rescue and the episomal vector systems and suggest caveats and contraindications for both. We believe the PCR rescue protocol may be of value where the use of extrachromosomally replicating vectors is obviated by the lack of an appropriate cell line.

Materials and Reagents

All materials and reagents used in cell transfection experiments should be of the highest quality available. With the exceptions noted below, all materials are purchased from Sigma (St. Louis, MO), Aldrich Chemical Co. (Milwaukee, WI), or Fluka Chemika-BioChemika, (Ronkonkoma, NY). Tissue culture flasks and apparatus are purchased from Corning or Falcon through Fisher Scientific Co. (Houston, TX).

The expression plasmids pCMV-Vec and pSGW-1 (Fig. 1) were constructed in the laboratory of KSM. The expression plasmid pcDNA I and *Escherichia coli* MC1061/P3 cells are purchased from Invitrogen (San Diego, CA). NIH/3T3 cells are from ATCC (CRL 1658) (Rockville, MD) and are maintained in Dulbecco's modified Eagle's medium (DMEM) containing 10% calf serum. Sephacryl S-1000 is purchased from Pharmacia (Piscataway, NJ).

PCR primers are purchased from Midland Certified Reagent Co. (Midland, TX). The location of each primer used is shown as large open arrowheads on the plasmid map in Fig. 1. Primer 1 (CMV Pro) is 5′ CCA CTT GGC AGT ACA TCA AGT GTA TCA TAT 3′. Primer 2 (bGH) is 5′ AAA CAC CAA GCT CTT GGT GAA GAC TCT 3′. PCR is conducted using *Taq* DNA polymerase and a DNA Thermal Cycler from Perkin–Elmer Cetus (Norwalk, CT).

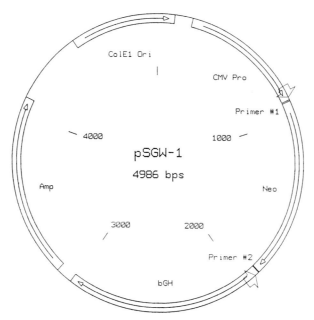

FIG. 1 Map of pSGW-1 showing PCR primer sites. ColE1 Ori, *E. coli* origin of replication; CMV Pro, human cytomegalovirus promoter; Neo, neomycin phosphotransferase II gene (G418 resistance); bGH, bovine growth hormone gene splicing and polyadenylation signals; Amp, ampicillin resistance gene. PCR primer binding sites are shown as large open arrowheads. Reproduced from ref. 12.

PCR Rescue Protocol

Library Construction

For the PCR rescue protocol, any vector capable of producing moderate to high levels of protein expression in the eukaryotic cell line of interest should be suitable for library construction. This feature renders many private and/or commercially available preconstructed libraries potentially useful. Use of an appropriate preconstructed library can save weeks to months of work. Prior to construction or purchase of such a library, the library vector should be tested in the cell line of interest by expressing a readily assayable gene product such as chloramphenicol acetyltransferase or β-galactosidase (1). Commercial sources for eukaryotic expression libraries include but are not limited to Invitrogen Co. (San Diego, CA) and Clontech Laboratories (Palo

Alto, CA). These companies will also prepare custom-made cDNA libraries from customer-supplied mRNA or tissue. In other studies, our laboratory has had good success using a CHO-K1 cDNA library constructed in the eukaryotic expression vector pCDM8 (3) and purchased from Invitrogen.

Preparation of Plasmid DNA

Plasmid DNA to be used for transfection can be prepared by any of a number of protocols which have been shown to yield transfectable DNA of high quality (1). In our laboratory, plasmid DNA is purified by the method of Birnboim (13) followed by chromatography on Sephacryl S-1000 to separate the plasmid from contaminating RNA, chromosomal DNA, and *E. coli* proteins which may be toxic to eukaryotic cells.

Transfection of Eukaryotic Cells

There are many protocols for the transfection of eukaryotic cells including electroporation (14), calcium phosphate coprecipitation (15), protoplast fusion (16), complex formation with cationic lipids (17), complex formation with Polybrene (18), and complex formation with DEAE–dextran (19). Each of these protocols has advantages and disadvantages (1); however, the DEAE–dextran protocol probably would not work with PCR rescue which requires the isolation of stably transfected clones. It is known that the DEAE–dextran protocol does not produce stable clones at high efficiency (2).

In the studies described below, NIH/3T3 cells were transfected by the calcium phosphate protocol of Chen and Okayama (15). To simulate selection of a marker from a cDNA library, the plasmid pSGW-1 was mixed at a ratio of 1 : 5000 with the plasmid pCMV-Vec. pCMV-Vec is pSGW-1 lacking the *neo* gene insert. One hundred micrograms of the simulated library was transfected into 10^5 NIH/3T3 cells in each of five 6-cm tissue culture plates. After 48 hr, the plates were trypsinized and replated into 10-cm plates for selection.

Selection for Cells Carrying Marker of Interest

Selection for cells carrying the marker of interest is the most demanding step in the design of any eukaryotic expression cloning experiment and it is critical that the parameters involved be carefully considered. For our model system we chose the neomycin phosphotransferase gene from Tn5 (*neo*)

which is easily selected using the cytotoxic agent Geneticin (G418). The *neo*/
G418 system was also chosen as a model because in actual practice we hoped
to use other cytotoxic agents for the selection process (cytotoxic lectins). In
other applications of the PCR rescue protocol, other selection methodologies
would undoubtedly be employed (see Discussion for caveats which may be
associated with various selection protocols).

The transfected NIH/3T3 cells are selected using the G418 at a concentration of 500 μg/ml. After growth for 2 weeks in the antibiotic, three clones
(Neo-1, Neo-2, and Neo-3) were isolated and expanded.

Isolation of Genomic DNA from Mammalian Tissue Culture Cells

A number of protocols for the isolation of genomic DNA suitable for PCR
are available (20). The following protocol, which is quick, has proven adequate for PCR rescue.

1. Trypsinize cells (5×10^6–10^7) and wash twice with 10 ml of phosphate-
buffered saline (PBS) by centrifugation in a 15-ml polypropylene screw-cap
tube for 5 min in a clinical centrifuge.

2. Resuspend cell pellet in the same tube in 5 ml of 10 mM Tris–HCl, pH
8.0, 100 mM NaCl, and 25 mM EDTA. Add 0.25 ml of 10% sodium dodecyl
sulfate (SDS), mix several times by gentle inversion of the tube, and incubate
5 min at room temperature.

3. Add proteinase K to a final concentration of 100 μg/ml and incubate
at 37°C for 3 hr.

4. Extract once by adding 5 ml of phenol : chloroform : isoamyl alcohol
(25 : 25 : 1) and gentle inversion of the tube followed by centrifugation.

5. Remove the organic layer (lower phase) from the tube and add DNase-
free RNase to 100 μg/ml and incubate 1 hr at 37°C.

6. Extract as in step 4 until the interface is clear. Then extract once more
with chloroform and once with water-saturated butanol. Remove the butanol
(upper phase).

7. Gently add two volumes of ethanol and mix by gentle swirling with a
plastic Pasteur pipette. The DNA will appear as a stringy mass.

8. Remove the DNA with the pipette and place in a sterile 5-ml snap-cap
tube. Lightly dry under a stream of nitrogen or in a Speed-Vac, then resuspend in 2 ml of sterile deionized water by placing on platform rocker overnight. The DNA should then be quantified by UV absorbance at 260 nm and
the A_{260}/A_{280} ratio calculated. This ratio should be greater than 1.75.

Amplification of Inserts from Plasmid DNA Integrated into the Genome

Amplification of the plasmid insert is accomplished using primers which exactly flank the cloning site of the library vector. Such primers would, of course, vary with the vector being employed. The vector used for our model system (pCMV-Vec) was constructed in our laboratory and consisted of a pBR322-based plasmid containing the *amp* gene, ColE1 origin of replication, and a cloning site with a cytomegalovirus promoter (CMV Pro) to the 5′ side and a bovine growth hormone slicing and polyadenylation site to the 3′ side. Similar plasmids are now commercially available from Invitrogen (San Diego, CA). The neomycin phosphotransferase II expression plasmid pSGW-1 (21) was derived from CMV-Vec by inserting the *neo* gene from the transposable element Tn5 into the cloning site (Fig. 1). Amplification of inserts from the stable NIH/3T3 transfectants putatively carrying this vector was accomplished using the following protocol.

To 0.5–1.0 μg of genomic DNA in PCR buffer [10 mM Tris–HCl, pH 8.3; 50 mM KCl; 20 μM of each oligonucleotide primer; 200 μM of each deoxyribonucleoside triphosphate (dNTP); 1.5 mM MgCl] add 1.5 U *Taq* polymerase for a final volume of 50 μl. The extension program employed is 5 min at 95°C then 30 cycles of 1 min, at 94°C, 1 min at 55°C; 3 min at 72°C. After 30 cycles the reactions were incubated 10 min at 72°C to complete the extensions. Longer extension times than normal (3 min at 72°C) are included to ensure completion of the longer transcripts expected from PCR rescue of a cDNA product.

Twenty-microliter aliquots of the extension reactions are analyzed by electrophoresis in a 1% agarose/Tris–acetate EDTA (TAE) gel containing 0.5 μg ethidium bromide. As shown in Fig. 2, three of three G418-resistant NIH/3T3 clones carried amplifiable inserts of the proper size. The variation in the PCR signal among the different clones may have resulted from a difference in copy number of the transfected gene between the three clones. It is known that calcium phosphate transfection product clones in which the insert occurs as tandem arrays that are highly variable in copy number (2).

Subcloning Plasmid Inserts Amplified from Genomic DNA

In order to rescue the selected gene, it is necessary to subclone the PCR amplification products asymmetrically. This is conveniently done by including different restriction site sequences in the upstream and downstream PCR primers themselves. These restriction sites should be chosen so as to minimize the likelihood that such sites will occur internally within the cDNA

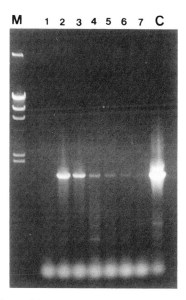

FIG. 2 PCR amplification of integrated plasmids from NIH/3T3 genomic DNA. After transfection of NIH/3T3 cells with the neomycin phosphotransferase expression plasmid pSGW-1 and selection with the antibiotic G418, genomic DNA was prepared from three separately isolated clones (Neo-1, Neo-2, and Neo-3). Plasmid inserts were then amplified by PCR from either 1 μg (lanes 1, 2, 4, and 6) or 0.5 μg (lanes 3, 5, and 7) of genomic DNA. Lane M is a λ *Hind*III digest run as marker. Lane C is 0.1 μg of pSGW-1 amplified by the same protocol. Lane 1 shows PCR products from untransfected NIH/3T3 cells. Lanes 2 and 3 show PCR products from Neo-1, lanes 4 and 5 from Neo-2, and lanes 6 and 7 from Neo-3. Reproduced from ref. 12.

being subcloned. To check for such an event, the PCR products (before and after cutting) should be run side by side in an appropriate gel. For example, a good choice of enzymes for subcloning into the vector pcDNA 3 (Invitrogen) might be 5'*Kpn* I–3'*Not* I. Alternatively, as in our model system, such sites may already exist in the original library vector.

To subclone from the vector pSGW-1 into the vector pCDNA I, three PCR reactions are run as described above. The reactions are pooled and diluted to 500 μl, and 50 μl of 10X Promega (Madison, WI) Core 1 buffer is added. Two units of *Hind*III and 4 units of *Sst*I are added and the reaction is incubated for 1 hr at 37°C. Aliquots are taken before and after to ensure the product is not degraded during digestion. The reaction is extracted once with phenol/chloroform, once with chloroform, and once with ether. Residual ether is removed under a stream of air, and the DNA is ethanol-precipitated. The pellet is resuspended in 50 μl of TAE and electrophoresed in 1%

SeaPlaque agarose containing 0.5 μg of ethidium bromide. Then, 0.5 μg of the plasmid pcDNA I is digested with *Sst*I and *Hind*III and run in an adjacent lane. After electrophoresis DNA in the gel is visualized with UV light and the appropriate bands are excised. The amount of DNA in each band is estimated by fluorescence intensity. The excised bands are weighed and melted at 60°C. An appropriate amount of DNA is removed from each tube to make a final insert to plasmid ratio of 2 : 1 (total DNA = 0.5 μg) and this is added to 2.5 volumes of NaI solution. The DNA is subsquently extracted with glass-milk as described by Volgelstein and Gilespie (22) and ethanol-precipitated. After being dried, the DNA is resuspended in 10 μl of water and an aliquot is diluted into ligation buffer, ligated at 15°C overnight, and then transformed into *E. coli* MC1061/P3 (Invitrogen).

PCR Amplification of Clones after Insert Rescue from Genomic DNA

Ten randomly selected colonies are analyzed by PCR for the occurrence of appropritely sized amplification products (Fig. 3). This is done by picking individual colonies with a sterile toothpick and transferring to 50 μl of water in a 500-μl microfuge tube. Bacteria remaining on the toothpick are transferred onto premarked LB plates for incubation.

The microfuge tubes containing the bacteria are immersed in boiling water for 10 min and centrifuged at top speed for 1 min, and then 30 μl are added to 5 μl 10X PCR buffer, 10 μl dNTP mix (2 μM each in stock), 2 μl of each primer (20 μM stock), and 0.5 μl *Taq* polymerase. The PCR reactions are conducted using the thermal cycle described above and 2 μl of the reaction is analyzed by agarose gel electrophoresis.

In our studies, 8 of the 10 transformants (Fig. 3) contained inserts and 7 were of a size appropriate to the *neo* gene. One insert seemed to have derived from a smaller fragment and was not analyzed further; however, the remaining inserts were of the correct size to have been derived from the originally transfected gene.

In order to show that the isolated inserts remained functional, one of the clones containing an appropriately sized insert (Fig. 3, lane 2) was grown in large-scale culture and the plasmid-purified. NIH/3T3 cells were transfected with this plasmid and subjected to G418 selection. After 2 weeks in culture, plates containing the cells were rinsed and stained with Giemsa to visualize the transformed colonies (Fig. 4).

No colonies were seen on plates transfected with the parental vector pcDNA I or on nontransformed plates. Thus the colonies seen on the plate transformed with rescued insert could only have resulted from the activity of the rescued *neo* gene. Subsequent PCR analysis of the secondary transfec-

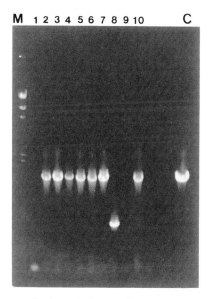

FIG. 3   PCR amplification of selected clones after insert rescue from genomic DNA. After the PCR products from NIH/3T3 clone Neo-1 were cloned into the vector pcDNA I, 10 random colonies were analyzed for inserts by PCR (lanes 1–10). Lane M contains a *Hind*III digest of λ DNA and lane C contains the PCR product of the parental plasmid pSGW-1. Reproduced from ref. 12.

tants produced products of the expected size and Southern blotting of the PCR products using a *neo* gene probe proved that these transformants carried the transfected *neo* gene.

Discussion

As demonstrated above, we have shown that PCR rescue can, in theory, be used for eukaryotic expression cloning without the need for episomally replicating vectors. However, several limitations to the actual practice must be kept in mind when designing such experiments. We encountered one such limitation when we tried to apply the PCR rescue technique to our own particular cloning application.

We originally developed the PCR rescue procedure to clone genes involved in glycoconjugate biosynthesis and its regulation. Our strategy involved transfection of an expression library followed by selection with a cytotoxic lectin. In theory, any plasmid expressing an RNA which suppresses the

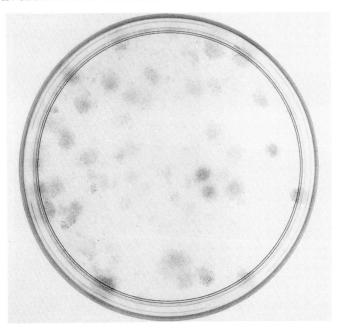

FIG. 4   Transformation of NIH/3T3 cells by a previously rescued *neo* gene. A randomly selected pcDNA I clone of the PCR products from NIH/3T3 Neo-1 (Fig. 3, lane 2) was used to transfect NIH/3T3 cells by the CaPO$_4$ procedure. After two weeks of selection, the remaining colonies were stained with Giemsa and transformation efficiency was estimated by counting. Reproduced from ref. 12.

expression of a gene required for the production of the lectin-binding site should be selectable using a cytotoxic lectin. For a number of reasons the cell lines available for use with extrachromosomally replicating vectors were unsuitable for this application.

On application of the PCR rescue protocol we found that the rate of spontaneous mutations to our lectin of choice was so high that PCR rescue did not give rise to discrete clonable bands. We believe this is due to two effects operating simultaneously. First, a high mutation frequency means that many cells survive regardless of their having taken up a plasmid or not. This generates a high background of genomic DNA, i.e., many genomes survive which do not contain integrated plasmids of any sort. Second, many of the spontaneous mutations will have taken up plasmids serendipitously, thus many surviving cells (10–20%) will carry irrelevant plasmids. This in turn would give rise to multiple bands in the PCR gel. Combined, these two effects render PCR rescue unusable as designed. Thus, any cloning experiment exploiting a cytotoxic agent for selection must ensure that the spontaneous mutation rate for resistance to that agent is sufficiently low ($\leq 10^{-6}$) to allow efficient PCR amplification from the integrated vector.

On the other hand, there are selection procedures for which PCR rescue should be particularly appropriate, e.g., in the cloning of a cDNA encoding a secreted protein such as a cytokine for which a sensitive and accurate bioassay exists. Normally, one would approach such a project using an episomally replicating vector and SIB selection (2). However, if it is important to exploit a particular cell line for such a project then PCR rescue might be ideal.

In this approach one transfects enough plates of cells with an expression library to get a statistical representation of the library in the resultant transfectants (the exact number will depend the efficiency of the transfection protocol for the particular cell line used). The library must have been constructed in a vector which simultaneously expresses an easily selected marker (i.e., *neo*). Such vectors are commercially available [pcDNA 3 (Invitrogen) is one example]. After selection and growth in G418 until colonies are visible, culture supernatant from each plate should be assayed for the presence of the desired product. Positive plates can then be replated into microtiter plates. It is not necessary to ensure clonality at this point, only to reduce the number of different transfectants per well to just a few. After a period of growth in the microtiter plate(s) each well is again assayed. Positive wells should be subcloned to produce true clones. PCR rescue can then be applied to clones assaying positive. Proof that a rescued cDNA encodes the assayed function is obtained by showing that most cells stably transfected with the subcloned cDNA also express the protein of interest. The difference between this protocol and SIB selection is that we are using pools of transfected cells rather than repeatedly transfecting subpools of plasmids.

Summary

It is clear that episomal vectors provide several advantages over PCR rescue for expression cloning in eukaryotes and should be the system of choice whenever possible. However, when it is not possible to use episomal vectors, it may be possible to clone the cDNA of interest using the PCR rescue protocol described above if the following precautions are observed: (i) The vector chosen should be capable of high expression as an integrated plasmid in the cell line to be used. This should be tested using a readily assayable marker (e.g., β-galactosidase) cloned in the vector prior to library construction. (ii) When using a cytotoxic agent for selection, it is critical that the spontaneous mutation rate be low ($\leq 10^{-6}$). (iii) When using an assay for selection, it is critical that the assay be able to reliably detect the product at low levels. The detection limits necessary can be estimated using the control plasmid constructed for point number 1. If these three conditions can be met, then an expression cloning project exploiting PCR rescue should be successful.

Acknowledgments

This work was supported by an Oklahoma Health Research Contract and the Mervin Bovard Center for Molecular Biology and Biotechnology.

References

1. J. Sambrook, E. F. Fritsch, and T. Maniatis, "Molecular Cloning: A Laboratory Manual," 2nd ed. Cold Spring Harbor Lab., Cold Spring Harbor, NY, 1989.
2. M. Kriegler, "Gene Transfer and Expression: A Laboratory Manual." Stockton Press, New York, 1990.
3. A. Aruffo and B. Seed, *Proc. Natl. Acad. Sci. U.S.A.* **84,** 8573 (1987).
4. P. Southern and P. Berg, *J. Mol. Appl. Genet.* **1,** 327 (1982).
5. G. Wong, J. S. Witek, P. A. Temple, K. M. Wilkens, A. C. Leary, D. P. Luxenberg, S. S. Jones, E. L. Brown, R. M. Kay, E. C. Orr, C. Shoemaker, D. W. Golde, R. J. Kaufman, R. M. Hewick, E. A. Wang, and S. C. Clark, *Science* **228,** 810 (1985).
6. R. F. Margolskee, P. Kavathas, and P. Berg, *Mol. Cell. Biol.* **8,** 2837 (1988).
7. B. Hirt, *J. Mol. Biol.* **26,** 365 (1967).
8. W. J. Müller, M. A. Naujokas, and J. A. Hassell, *Mol. Cell. Biol.* **4,** 2406 (1984).
9. F. G. Kern and C. Basilico, *Gene* **43,** 237 (1986).
10. M. Heffernan and J. Dennis, *Nucleic Acids Res.* **19,** 85 (1991).
11. K. S. Miller and M. Brudnak, *in preparation* (1994).
12. M. Brudnak and K. S. Miller, *BioTechniques* **14,** 66 (1993).
13. H. C. Birnboim, *in* "Methods in Enzymology (R. Wu et al., eds.), Vol. 100, p. 243. Academic Press, New York, 1983.
14. G. L. Anreason and G. A. Evans, *BioTechniques* **6,** 650 (1988).
15. C. Chen and H. Okayama, *Mol. Cell. Biol.* **7,** 2745 (1987).
16. W. Schaffner, *Proc. Natl. Acad. Sci. U.S.A.* **77,** 2163 (1980).
17. P. L. Flegner, T. R. Gadek, M. Holm, R. Roman, H. W. Chan, M. Wenz, J. P. Northrop, G. M. Ringold, and M. Danielsen, *Proc. Natl. Acad. Sci. U.S.A.* **84,** 7413 (1987).
18. W. G. Chaney, D. R. Howard, J. W. Pollard, S. Sallustio, and P. Stanley, *Somatic Cell Mol. Genet.* **12,** 237 (1986).

19. J. H. McCutchan and J. S. Pagano, *J. Natl. Cancer Inst. (U.S.)* **41,** 351 (1968).
20. M. A. Innis, D. H. Gelfand, J. J. Sninsky, and T. J. White, eds., ''PCR Protocols: A Guide to Methods and Applications.'' Academic Press, San Diego, 1990.
21. S. G. Wells and K. S. Miller, *Cell. Mol. Biol.* **38,** 159 (1992).
22. B. Volgelstein and D. Gilespie, *Proc. Natl. Acad. Sci. U.S.A.* **76,** 615 (1979).

[20] Use of PCR for Constructing Jumping Libraries

Rajendra P. Kandpal and Sherman M. Weissman

Several techniques and methodologies developed during the past few years have considerably expedited the process of gene mapping and cloning. These methods include pulsed-field gel electrophoresis (1–3), yeast artificial chromosome (YAC) cloning (4), fluorescence *in situ* hybridization (5), chromosome linking and jumping libraries (6–9), and the polymerase chain reaction (PCR) (10, 11). The advent of PCR has revolutionized many areas of biological and medical sciences. Today PCR is applied in every protocol where the amount of DNA available for experimental manipulation is very scarce. We describe in this paper the application of PCR for constructing jumping libraries.

Mapping and Cloning of Large Segments of DNA

Mapping of fairly large stretches of DNA (200–500 kb) corresponding to murine, human, and *Drosophila* genomes has been achieved by constructing clusters of overlapping cosmid clones (12–16). In these experiments, a cosmid clone containing $\approx$ 30–35 kb of genomic DNA mapping to the region of interest is isolated and unique DNA sequences from near the ends of the cosmid insert are isolated. These end pieces are used as probes to screen a cosmid library. The cosmids thus isolated will contain an additional 20–30 kb of DNA. Repeating the process of isolating the end pieces and subsequently screening a library will result in the construction of a cosmid contig. However, these genomic walks are frequently interrupted due to the presence of repetitive sequences and the presence of DNA segments in the genome which are difficult to clone. Such sequence of DNA are known to exist in the human genome (17) and are likely to hinder genome walking. In summary, genome walking by cosmid clustering is a time-consuming and labor-intensive process and suffers from the limitations described above.

To supplement cosmid cloning, alternative approaches for cloning large pieces of genomic DNA in YAC vectors (4, 18), P1 phage vector (19), and F-factor based vectors (20) were developed. Yeast artificial chromosome vectors contain yeast centromere and telomere sequences linked to selectable markers which can be ligated to large pieces (> 100 kb) of genomic DNA

Methods in Neurosciences, Volume 26

(4,18). These vectors when transformed in yeast cells can be maintained and propagated as artificial chromosomes. The YAC vectors have been extensively used by several laboratories for constructing genomic libraries (4, 18, 21–23). The average size of inserts in these libraries has varied between 200 kb and > 1 Mb. These libraries have been successfully used for constructing overlappig contigs of substantial length. In fact, some of the chromosomes such as chromosomes Y and 21 have been isolated as essentially complete YAC contigs (24–26). It is expected that more than 90% of the genome will be available as YAC contigs in the near future.

A shortcoming of the large insert YACs have been the problems of deletions, rearrangements, and chimerisms. These problems are directly proportional to the size of YACs. Rearrangement in YACs frequently contributes errors in the physical maps of the region they represent. In addition most YAC contig maps do not define the extent of the DNA sequences shared between overlapping YACs and they do not reflect the lengths of genomic DNA they span. Currently, there are no convenient ways of checking the accuracy of YAC contig-derived physical maps.

One of the ways that we have proposed to derive physical maps involves genome mapping by chromosome linking and jumping (6, 27, 28). Linking clones are defined as short clones that embed a rare cutting site and, therefore, join two fragments generated by digesting the genomic DNA with a rare cutter. Jumping clones represent the two ends of a large fragment produced with an enzyme that cuts the genomic DNA infrequently. Each jumping clone should overlap two linking clones and vice versa, so that a complete set of jumping and linking clones would assemble to give a map of genomic region. The size of the large fragments detected with linking and jumping clones would then assign physical distance to the map. In addition to providing tools for physical mapping, jumping procedures are alternative approaches for cloning over regions which are physically a considerable distance apart, usually hundreds of kilobases.

For construction of jumping libraries, large fragments of genomic DNA are produced either by partial digestion with six base recognition restriction enzymes or by complete digestion with rare cutter enzymes. These large fragments are circularized around a selectable marker such as the gene for a suppressor tRNA. After circularization, the DNA is digested completely with a six-base recognition restriction enzyme and cloned in an appropriate phage vector that requires the expression of the suppressor tRNA for growth. The ligated DNA is packaged and used to infect a suitable bacterial host that does not carry a suppressor. Such host bacteria will permit growth of the phages that have incorporated a fragment formed by the two ends of the original large fragment joined through the selectable suppressor tRNA gene. Such a clone is known as a jumping clone and represents two small fragments of DNA which were originally separated by a distance equal to the length generated by the restriction enzyme initially used to digest the genomic DNA.

The jumping protocol provides a means to exclude large stretches of intervening sequences to obtain end pieces of a given large fragment. One can perform jumps in a predetermined direction, and sometimes a jumping clone may represent DNA pieces flanking an unclonable region. Thus, jumping clones are valuable tools for physical mapping and for generating useful landmarks along the chromosome. In order to use jumping clones for constructing long-range physical maps, it is desirable to combine them with a restriction enzyme which cuts genomic DNA infrequently. One such enzyme is *Not*I, which has an eight-base pair restriction site recognition. The number of *Not*I sites in the human genome are distributed at an average of 1 in 500 kb to 1 Mb. Thus the average size of a *Not*I fragment would vary between 500 kb to 1 Mb. Despite the susceptibility of *Not*I recognition sequence for methylation, it is a desirable enzyme for constructing long-range physical maps. However, *Not*I sites are known to occur in the GC-rich regions of the genome called HTF islands (29). The CG dinucleotides in the HTF islands are less susceptible to methylation, and also the extent of methylation may vary in cultured cells. We have chosen to construct *Not*I jumping library for reasons mentioned above. Each jumping clone obtained by circularization of a *Not*I fragment will contain two ends of the *Not*I fragment and will overlap two linking clones. A *Not*I linking clone will overlap two *Not*I jumping clones in a complementary manner.

Despite such obvious advantages of linking and jumping libraries for constructing physical maps, this has not been reduced to a routine method. A major reason this method is not popular is the difficulty in constructing jumping libraries. The conventional methods for constructing jumping libraries are technically demanding and require a substantial amount of DNA for making reasonably representative libraries. We had earlier described a PCR approach for constructing jumping libraries (30). We describe here an alternative method that utilizes PCR and biotin–avidin affinity chromatography for constructing *Not*I jumping libraries (28). This method requires relatively small amounts of DNA, has versatility to yield a fairly representative jumping library, and, because of its sensitivity, can be used to construct jumping clones spanning relatively large genomic fragments.

Principle of Affinity Capture Method

A schematic flow diagram for the affinity capture method is shown in Fig. 1. The method involves digestion of genomic DNA with *Not*I. The *Not*I-

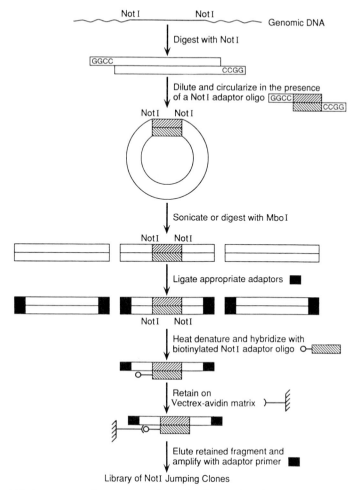

FIG. 1   Affinity capture for constructing a *Not*I jumping library. The top line represents high-molecular-weight genomic DNA containing *Not*I sites. Digestion of genomic DNA with *Not*I yields *Not*I fragments, and one such fragment containing *Not*I
overhangs is represented in the second line. The *Not*I adaptor is represented as
hatched rectangles. The adaptor-primers are shown as filled rectangles. One strand
of the adaptor-primer is used for amplification of the adaptor-ligated DNA.
The designations of the biotinylated oligonucleotide and the avidin matrix are self-
explanatory in the figure. The detailed protocol for library construction is described
in the text.

digested DNA is circularized around a *Not*I adaptor oligonucleotide at a concentration that yields principally circularization rather than concatamerization of *Not*I fragments. The circularized DNA is then cut into smaller pieces either by using a frequent cutter such as *Sau*3AI or by sonicating the DNA to yield fragments between the sizes 200 and 500 bp. The small-size DNA is then denatured by heating in a boiling water bath following by cooling in an ice-water bath. The denatured DNA is hybridized with a biotinylated affinity oligonucleotide. The affinity oligonucleotide is a biotinylated internal sequence of 25 bases represented in the *Not*I adaptor oligonucleotide. It forms a fairly stable duplex to be retained on an avidin matrix even after the matrix is washed with 150 m*M* salt at 50°C. This strategy takes advantage of avidin–biotin affinity and a hybridization protocol which allows stringent washing of the avidin matrix to reduce nonspecific retention on the matrix.

Application of PCR in Affinity Capture Protocol

As pointed out in the preceding section, construction of *Not*I jumping libraries involves circularization of *Not*I-digested DNA at a very dilute concentration. Usually, the concentration of DNA in the ligation mixture is maintained at 0.2 μg/ml or less. These conditions favor circularization of DNA and minimize concatamerization of *Not*I fragments. In order to obtain reasonable amounts of DNA for cloning after proceeding through the steps of initial ligation, digestions, extraction with phenol/chloroform, and precipitation with ethanol, it is desirable to start with 2–5 μg of *Not*I-digested DNA. This means the initial circularization will have to be carried out in 10–25 ml of ligation mixture. Manipulation of such large volumes of DNA solution for ligation, extraction, and precipitation is not very convenient.

The introduction of PCR in the affinity capture protocol circumvents some of the difficulties mentioned above and permits use of less than 1 μg of DNA for constructing jumping libraries. As shown in the scheme for *Not*I jumping library construction (Fig. 1), we have introduced PCR at two steps. After circularizing the *Not*I-digested DNA at low concentration, the circularized DNA is fragmented into smaller pieces either by digestion with a frequent cutter such as *Mbo*I or by sonication. If *Mbo*I is used for digesting the circularized DNA then it is ligated to *Mbo*I adaptor oligonucleotide. A single primer from the adaptor oligonucleotide is used to amplify the adaptor-ligated DNA. Inclusion of PCR at this step permits use of small amounts of DNA for constructing a jumping library. The adaptor-ligated DNA can be amplified to obtain desired amount of DNA for affinity capture. This DNA is denatured and hybridized to the biotinylated affinity oligonucleotide. After hybridization, the biotinylated hybrid DNA is retained onto a Vectrex–avidin (Vector

Laboratories, Burlingame, CA) matrix and specifically retained hybrids are eluted appropriately. The eluted DNA contains primer tags and can be amplified in a single primer PCR. The affinity captured DNA can then be digested with *Eco*RI and cloned in λgt10 to represent a *Not*I jumping library. Because the amount of DNA obtained after PCR amplification is not limiting, it can be processed for two or more rounds of affinity capture.

Model Systems to Test Feasibility of Affinity Capture for Constructing *Not*I Jumping Library

In order to check the suitability of affinity capture for constructing *Not*I jumping library we process a plasmid DNA (pKS) containing a *Not*I site and an anonymous cosmid DNA containing two *Not*I sites giving *Not*I fragments of 38 and 8 kb. If the affinity capture works as expected then we isolate a band corresponding to an *Mbo*I fragment of approximately 200 bp for the pKS plasmid jump and two *Mbo*I fragments representing the end pieces of the two cosmid *Not*I fragments arising after circularization of these *Not*I fragments around the *Not*I adaptor oligonucleotide. These two DNAs serve as model systems to test the affinity capture method for constructing jumping libraries.

Oligonucleotides Used

The following oligonucleotides are used for these studies.

1. *Mbo*I adaptor:
   > 5′ pGATCGGAGAATTCGCACGAGTACTAC
   > CCTCTTAAGCGTGCTCATGATGAC 5′

The lower strand is used as a PCR primer to amplify *Mbo*I digested and adaptor-ligated DNA.

2. *Not*I adaptor oligonucleotide:
   > 5′ pGGCCGGTCTTATCTGTTAATCTGTTATCTGTTATCTGACC
   > CCAGAATAGACAATAGACAATAGACAATAGACTGGCCGG 5′.

3. *Not*I affinity oligonucleotide:
   > 5′ biotin-ATAGATATGTCAGATAACAGATAACAGAT

The *Mbo*I adaptor oligonucleotide is constructed in such a way that it can only form a dimer on self-ligation. The adaptor contains an internal *Eco*RI site which facilitates cloning of the *Mbo*I fragments at *Eco*RI site after adaptor ligation and PCR amplification of the *Mbo*I fragments.

The *Not*I affinity oligonucleotide is a biotinylated oligonucleotide represented in one of the strands of the *Not*I adaptor oligonucleotide. This oligonucleotide is used to isolate the *Mbo*I fragments which contain the *Not*I adaptor oligonucleotide and which has arisen by circularization of the *Not*I DNA fragments around the *Not*I adaptor oligonucleotide.

Circularization of *Not*I-Digested pKS Plasmid and Cosmid DNA around *Not*I Adaptor

The pKS DNA (5 μg) and cosmid DNA (5 μg) are digested separately with 20 units of *Not*I in 100 μl reaction volume for 2 hr at 37°C. A total of 1 μg of the *Not*I-digested DNA is ligated to 0.5 μg of the phosphorylated *Not*I adaptor in 5 ml of ligase buffer with 8000 units of T4 DNA ligase (New England Biolabs, Beverly, MA). The ligation reaction is incubated at 4°C for 16–18 hr. After ligation, the reaction mixture is treated with 10 units of calf intestinal alkaline phosphatase (Boehringer-Mannheim, Indianapolis, IN) at 37°C for 45 min. The reaction mixture is extracted with phenol/chloroform and then concentrated by using a Centricon-30 (Amicon, Beverly, MA) device to a volume of less than 100 μl. Treatment with phosphatase renders any *Not*I fragments and adaptors which did not participate in circularization reaction incompetent for further ligation.

Amplification of Circularized DNA as *Mbo*I Fragments

The circularized and Centricon-concentrated DNA (1 μg) is diluted in a 100-μl reaction volume with 10 units of *Sau*3AI at 37°C for 1.5 hr. The reaction mixture is heated at 65°C for 20 min to inactivate the enzyme, extracted with phenol, precipitated with ethanol, and dissolved in 20 μl of Tris-EDTA (TE). The digested DNA is ligated to 2 μg of *Mbo*I adaptors in 50 μl reaction volume with 800 units of T4 DNA ligase at 16°C for 12–16 hr. The unligated adaptor and adaptor dimers are separated from the adaptor-ligated *Mbo*I fragments by electrophoresis on a 1.4% agarose gel. The DNA is extracted from the gel and concentrated by ethanol precipitation. We prefer to gel-purify the adaptor-ligated DNA. However, the adaptor-ligated DNA can be used for PCR without separating the unligated adaptors and adaptor dimers. An aliquot of the gel-purified DNA ($\approx$10 ng) is amplified by using the appropriate strand of the adaptor as primer. The amplification is carried out in a Perkin–Elmer (Norwalk, CT) PCR machine Model 9600. The template DNA (10 ng) is incubated with 10 mM Tris–Cl, pH 8.3,

50 mM KCI, 1.5 mM MgCI$_2$, 100 ng of primer and 1 unit of AmpliTaq DNA polymerase (Perkin–Elmer) in a 45-μl volume at 82°C for 2 min. Then 5 μl of 2 mM dNTPs is added to the PCR mixture and the following incubation conditions are repeated for a total of 35 cycles: 95°c, 30 sec; 55°C, 30 sec; and 72°C, 2 min. Addition of dNTPs at 82°C eliminates any nonspecific amplification of the template DNA due to false priming. We routinely use this protocol for amplification. The PCR amplification is carried out in multiple tubes to obtain a yield of 2–5 μg of the amplified DNA. The amplified DNA is pooled, and desalted and concentrated by using a Centricon-30 device. The concentrated DNA is obtained in TE. At this point, the DNA is present as *Mbo*I fragments. A small fraction of the *Mbo*I fragments will contain the *Not*I adaptor oligonucleotide. The *Not*I adaptor oligonucleotide containing *Mbo*I fragments represents the end pieces of a *Not*I fragment which has circularized around the adaptor oligonucleotide and are termed as *Not*I jumping clones. The next step in the protocol is to enrich for these *Not*I jumping clones. We have used an affinity capture method for enrichment of the jumping clones. The affinity capture protocol is described below.

Affinity Capture for Enrichment of *Not*I Jumping Clones

As mentioned above, the *Not*I jumping clones are present in the amplified DNA as *Mbo*I fragments containing the *Not*I adaptor oligonucleotide. We have synthesized a biotinylated oligonucleotide from within the *Not*I adaptor oligonucleotide sequence. If the amplified *Mbo*I fragments are denatured and hybridized to the biotinylated oligonucleotide, then the *Mbo*I fragments forming hybrids with the biotinylated oligonucleotide will represent the *Not*I jumping clones. These biotinylated hybrids can be separated from the remaining DNA by retention onto a Vectrex–avidin (Vector Laboratories) matrix.

The amplified pKS plasmid DNA (100 or 10 ng/ml) is mixed with 10 μg/ml *Mbo*I digested and PCR-amplified genomic DNA and the mixture is denatured by heating at 95°C for 5 min and cooling in an ice–water bath. The above dilution of plasmid DNA with genomic DNA is carried out to check the sensitivity of the affinity capture method to enrich for a *Not*I adaptor containing *Mbo*I fragment at an abundance of 1 in 100,000 or 1 in 10,000. Additionally, these conditions are simulated for preparing *Not*I jumping libraries corresponding to human genomic DNA. The denatured DNA is hybridized with the *Not*I affinity oligonucleotide (5 μg/ml) in 100 μl of 0.5 M sodium phosphate, pH 7.4/0.5% sodium dodecyl sulfate (SDS) at 65°C for 18–24 hr. After hybridization, the mixture is made up to 2.0 ml with 100 mM Tris, pH 7.5/150 mM NaCl (buffer A). The diluted mixture is incubated with 100 mg of Vectrex–avidin (Vector Laboratories) that has been preincubated with denatured salmon sperm DNA (100 μg/ml) for 30 min and then washed extensively with buffer A to remove unabsorbed salmon sperm DNA. After incubation with Vectrex–avidin for 30–45 min, the mixture is centrifuged at low speed (500–1000g) at room temperature for 2 min and the supernatant is removed. The matrix is successively washed three times with 5 ml of buffer A at room temperature and once at 50°C for 20 min. The DNA retained on the matrix is eluted by incubation at 65°C with 0.1 $\times$ buffer A for 20 min. The supernatant is collected after centrifuging the matrix at low speed, as above.

Amplification of the Affinity-Captured DNA

The DNA eluted from the Vectrex–avidin matrix is concentrated by using a Centricon-30 device. The Centricon-30 device concentrates the eluates and allows desalting or exchange of buffer. We exchange the sample buffer with 10 mM Tris, pH 7.5, and 0.1 mM EDTA. The sample is concentrated to a volume of 50 μl. An aliquot of 10 μl is taken from the concentrated sample and amplified by using 100 ng of MboI adaptor primer in the presence of 10 mM Tris–CI, pH 8.3, 50 mM KCI, 1.5 mM MgCI$_2$, 0.2 mM dNTPs, and 1 unit of AmpliTaq DNA polymerase. The amplification is carried out for 35 cycles by adding dNTPs at 80°C as described. An aliquot of the amplified DNA is electrophoresed on a 1.2% SeaKem GTG agarose gel. The NotI site in the pKS plasmid is contained in a 200-bp MboI fragment. After digestion of the plasmid with NotI, circularization around the NotI adaptor, digestion with MboI, ligation to the MboI adaptor, and PCR amplification with the MboI adaptor primer, the NotI adaptor is contained in a 227-bp MboI fragment. If the circularization of the NotI-digested pKS plasmid around the NotI adaptor has occurred as expected and the affinity capture protocol has been successful for enrichment of the NotI adaptor-containing MboI fragment then PCR amplification of the affinity-captured DNA should yield a DNA fragment of $\sim$ 227 bp. Indeed a DNA fragment of $\sim$ 220 bp was amplified. We detected no amplification when the affinity-captured DNA obtained from the hybridization mixture containing 10 ng pKS DNA and 10 μg genomic DNA was used for PCR. However, when a 5-μl aliquot from the first cycle PCR was reamplified for 20 cycles, a DNA band of expected size was detected on agarose gel. These results demonstrate the sensitivity and specificity of the affinity capture method. The affinity capture protocol permits enrichment of a specific NotI jumping fragment present at an abundance of 1 in 10,000. Given the size of the human genome of 3×10^9 bp, an average of one NotI site of every 10^6 bp and average size of an MboI fragment as 300 bp, it is expected that an approximate abundance of NotI jumping clones as MboI fragments will be 1 in 4000. Our results demonstrate that the affinity capture method is adequately sensitive for enrichment of such fragments to near purity.

The advantage of the affinity capture protocol is that one can process the affinity-captured DNA for a second or third round of hybridization to obtain desired purity of the jumping library. Since PCR can yield enough material from nanogram amounts of captured DNA, the amount of DNA is not limiting for performing multiple rounds of affinity hybridization. The stringency of hybridization and elution can be increased sufficiently without compromising the purity and depth of the library.

The affinity-captured DNA contains PCR primer tags, which permits its amplification by using appropriate primer. The primer sequence contains an internal *Eco*RI site. Thus, the amplified DNA can be digested with *Eco*RI and then cloned in λgt10 phage vector. The sequences flanking the *Eco*RI site of λgt10 vector can be used for amplification of the inserts cloned at this site (31). The cloned DNA can be directly amplified from the plaques. The plaques from an agar plate are picked up with a Pasteur pipette or a wide-mouth Pipetman tip, suspended in 50 μl SM buffer and an aliquot of the phage suspension is used for amplifying the cloned insert using phage sequences as primers. An aliquot of the amplified DNA can be used for sequencing by using a double-stranded cycle sequencing method (32).

Limitations of PCR in Constructing Jumping Libraries

The following are two major limitations of PCR applications.

1. Bias for amplifying small-size fragments.
2. Inefficient amplification of sequences containing a high proportion of G and C bases.

When a DNA mixture containing fragments varying in size between 100 bp and 3 kb is subjected to PCR amplification, it usually results in preferential amplification of the smaller fragments and no amplification of the largest template. The variation in amplification is not very significant if the DNA mixture contains fragments less than 1 kb. However, if the size variation in the template DNA can be reduced to a narrow range, i.e., 200–300 bp, then amplificaiton bias can be reduced significantly.

In the protocol that we have described, the amplification of *Mbo*I-digested DNA is performed. *Mbo*I digestion of genomic DNA yields fragments varying in size from less than 100 bp to greater than 1 kb, with an average size of 300 bp. Such a size variation is likely to cause a bias in amplification. In fact, some of the large fragments (>1.5 kb) may not be represented in the amplified mixture. However, the alternative that we have proposed circumvents this bias. Instead of digesting the circularized DNA, if we resort to sonication then the fragmentation can be controlled to obtain fragments of DNA ranging in size between 300 and 500 bp. Since any given *Not*I jumping fragment in the sonicated DNA may be found in a number of sonicated fragment, amplification of the sonicated DNA may be expected to contain all the jumping clones in nearly equal abundance.

The second limitation of any PCR protocol is the difficulty in amplifying certain fragments rich in G and C bases. We have previously standardized PCR conditions which result in satisfactory amplification of templates which are difficult to amplify in a conventional PCR protocol (33). Other investigators have also reported some variations in PCR conditions which permit reasonable amplification of DNA templates containing higher proportions of G and C bases (34). We have noted that not only the GC content of a template but also the particular sequences of DNA that might make the amplification difficult. In our protocol we have introduced sonication for DNA fragmentation. This would result in positioning of GC stretches in multiple configurations, some of which will have increased likelihood for amplification. The amplification of high GC stretches of genomic DNA can also be achieved by using a combination of several restriction enzymes with a four-base recognition sequence to digest the genomic DNA after circularization around the *Not*I adaptor oligonucleotide. The resulting population of DNA fragments obtained after these manipulation will contain at least a fraction of GC-rich stretches in a template form which can be amplified readily. With the modifications described above, PCR can be utilized for constructing reasonably deep *Not*I jumping libraries.

Comments on Constructing Genomic *Not*I Jumping Libraries

*Preparation of Large-Size Genomic DNA and Restriction Digestion with Not*I

We are currently using the affinity capture protocol for constructing a *Not*I jumping library from JY, a human B-lymphoblastoid cell line. To make a good jumping library, it is essential to start with undergraded high-molecular-weight DNA. We prepare genomic DNA by embedding JY cells from an actively growing culture, in low-melting agarose plugs. The cells are centrifuged at 1000g at 4°C for 15 min, washed twice with phosphate-buffered saline (PBS), and resuspended at a concentration of 10^7 cells/ml of PBS. The cells are mixed with an equal volume of 1% low-melting agarose in 125 mM EDTA. The agarose gel is maintained at 45°C after being melted in a microwave oven. The cell suspension in agarose is aliquoted out in a plug mold of 120 μl capacity. The agarose plugs are allowed to solidify on ice. The plugs are pushed out of the mold and incubated in a solution containing 0.5 M EDTA, pH 9–9.5, 1% sarcosyl, and 1mg/ml proteinase K, at 50°C for 48 hr (35). This treatment causes the cells to lyse and releases the DNA into the agarose matrix. Before digestion with any restriction enzyme, the plugs are incubated in TE containing 1 mM phenylmethylsulfonyl fluoride (PMSF) to inactivate any residual proteinase K remaining in the plugs. The incubation of plugs in TE with PMSF (usually 10 plugs in 20 ml solution) is carried out on a platform shaker at room temperature for 2–3 hr with two to three changes of solution. The plugs quenched with PMSF are finally incubated in TE to remove residual PMSF from the plugs. The DNA embedded in agarose plugs is now ready for digestion with restriction enzymes. The plug containing approximately 10 μg DNA is incubated in 250 μl of restriction enzyme buffer at 37°C for 1 hr. The plug is then transferred to a fresh tube containing 250 μl of restriction enzyme buffer, 100 μg/ml of bovine serum albumin, and 30–50 units of *Not*I (New England Biolabs). Incubation is carried out for 6–8 hr at 37°C. The digestion is stopped by adding EDTA to a final concentration of 25 mM. The plug can then be stored at 4°C until further analysis. The *Not*I-digested DNA is now ready for circularization. It can be melted and circularized at dilute conditions. Using the *Not*I digested DNA without size selection may bias the cyclization toward small-size fragments. *Not*I sites are frequently clustered in GC-rich regions of the genome, known as HTF islands. The size of *Not*I fragments in HTF islands is usually less than 100 kb. Therefore, use of *Not*I digests without size fractionation will result in a jumping library that predominantly contains jumps of smaller than 100 kb. In order to maximize the average size of *Not*I jump, we prefer to size select the DNA.

Size Selection of NotI-Digested DNA by Pulsed-Field Gel Electrophoresis

The agarose plug containing *Not*I-digested genomic DNA is electrophoresed in 0.8% low-melting agarose gel in 0.5 × TBE buffer in CHEF mapper (Bio-Rad, Richmond ,CA). The machine has a built-in autoalgorithm, which allows programming to separate DNA in a particular size range. We program the CHEF mapper to achieve separation between 10 and 200 kb. Under these conditions the DNA greater than 200 kb runs as a compressed zone. We run the DNA in multiple lanes along with a size marker which contains concatamerized λ phage containing multimers of 48.5 kb. After the run is complete, the gel is cut into two halves. One-half of the gel is stained with ethidium bromide and viewed in a UV transilluminator. The agarose block corresponding to compressed zone containing DNA of greater than 200 kb is cut out. After the gel block is cut out, the remaining gel is aligned with the unstained portion of the gel and the agarose block corresponding to compressed zone is cut out without exposing the DNA to UV radiation.

Circularization of Large-Size NotI Fragments

The agarose block corresponding to the compressed zone of NotI-digested DNA is incubated in 1–2 ml of T4 DNA ligase buffer. It has been shown that inclusion of 0.7 mM spermine and 0.3 mM spermidine with large-size genomic DNA during ligation with YAC vectors enhances the efficiency of YAC libraries toward higher average insert size (36). We, therefore, include spermine and spermidine in the ligation buffer. The agarose plug is melted at 70°C in the presence of ligase buffer containing polyamines. The volume of the melted solution is made up to achieve 0.2 μg/ml DNA concentration and 0.4 μg NotI oligonucleotide adaptor. The ligation mixture is incubated at 4°C for 4–6 hr, and T4 DNA ligase (NEB) is added to a final concentration of 1600 units/ml. At this point, extreme caution is exercised in mixing the ligation mixture. Incubation is carried out for 12–16 hr at 4°C and an additional aliquot of ligase is added. The ligation mixture is extracted with phenol and chloroform and incubated with 10 units of calf intestinal alkaline phosphatase at 37°C for 45 min. The phosphatase is inactivated by extraction with phenol and phenol/chloroform. The circularized DNA is then concentrated by using a Centricon-30 device. The concentrated DNA can be fragmented either by digesting with MboI or by sonication. If sonication is used to fragment the DNA then the recessed DNA ends would need to be repaired with T4 DNA polymerase, a large fragment of E. coli DNA polymerase, and T4 polynucleotide kinase. For MboI-digested DNA, MboI adaptor is added to the digested DNA. If sonication is performed to fragment the DNA then appropriate blunt-ended linkers are added, which can serve as primer tags.

Affinity Capture for NotI Jumping Clones

The MboI adaptor-ligated DNA is amplified in a single primer PCR as described before. The amplified DNA is hybridized with the biotinylated NotI affinity oligonucleotide. After hybridization, the biotinylated hybrids representing the MboI fragments containing the NotI adaptor oligonucleotide are retained on a Vectrex–avidin matrix and specifically eluted at appropriate stringency. The protocol is described in detail in the preceding sections.

Assessment of Affinity-Captured DNA

Various eluates from the Vectrex–avidin matrix are concentrated in a Centricon-30 device, and an aliquot from each eluate is amplified by using a single oligonucleotide as primer. The PCR-amplified DNA is electrophoresed on a 1.2% agarose gel and the gel is blotted onto a Hybond membrane. The Hybond blot is hybridized in Church and Gilbert buffer (37) with ^{32}P-phosphorylated affinity oligonucleotide. The filter is washed with 1X SSC at 50°C for 20 min and exposed to an X-ray film with intensifying screens at −80°C for autoradiography. The intensity of signal in various eluate fractions when compared to the starting material indicates the extent of enrichment. We observed that the eluate with 1X buffer A at 50°C for 20 min was maximally enriched.

Cloning and Characterization of the Jumping Library

The PCR-amplified material from the highly enriched fraction is digested with *Eco*RI and the digest is electrophoresed on a 1.4% agarose gel to separate the PCR primers removed from the amplified DNA by *Eco*RI. The agarose block corresponding to the DNA fragments of 0.2–1.0 kb is cut out and the DNA is recovered either by electroelution or by spinning the agarose gel through a Centripure-30 device (Amicon). The DNA is extracted with phenol and chloroform and precipitated with ethanol. Then 10–15 ng of the purified DNA is ligated to 0.5 μg of *Eco*RI-digested and -dephosphorylated arms of λgt10 phage (Stratagene) in 5 μl at 16°C for 12–16 hr. The ligated mixture is packaged into phage heads using packaging extracts (Strategene). An aliquot of the packaged library is used to infect C600Hfl bacterial host and plated on an agarose plate.

A representative number of plaques are picked from the plate and suspended in 50 μl of SM buffer. The plaques are incubated in the buffer for 4–6 hr at room temperature. A drop of chloroform is added to the phage suspension and stored at 4°C. An aliquot of 1 μl from the phage suspension is used for PCR amplification by using vector sequences flanking the *Eco*RI site as primer. The amplified DNA is run on an agarose gel to determine the percentage and size of inserts in the library.

An aliquot of the amplified DNA is digested with *Eag*I. If the clones in the library are genuine jumping clones, then digestion with *Eag*I will yield three fragments, one each corresponding to the two ends of the *Not*I fragment and the third fragment corresponding to the *Not*I adaptor oligonucleotide. Since the size of these fragments may be comparable they may not resolve sufficiently in an agarose gel. Therefore, the alternative method for assessing their structure is DNA sequencing.

An aliquot of the amplified DNA is used for sequencing using a double-stranded PCR cycle sequencing method (29). The clones are usually 200- to 400-bp long and hence the entire length can be sequenced in one pass. The sequence data will not only reveal the structure of these clones but it will also indicate the number of adaptor oligomers ligated to the jumping clones. The bonafide jumping clones should arise from a single *Not*I fragment. Therefore, hybridization of the jumping clones to a pulsed-field gel blot of *Not*I-digested genomic DNA will indicate the accuracy and distance of *Not*I jump.

Concluding Remarks

We have described in this paper an application of PCR for constructing *Not*I jumping library. The introduction of PCR in the protocol for *Not*I jumping library construction circumvents some of the problems encoutered with the conventional methods of library construction. It is now possible to construct jumping libraries from as little as 1 μg of high-molecular-weight DNA. Reduction in the amount of starting DNA enhances our ability to better handle the large-size DNA for circularization at a very dilute concentration without having to increase the volume of the ligation mixture for achieving desired concentration of DNA. Availability of representative jumping libraries corresponding to large-size *Not*I fragments will be extremely helpful in constructing long-range restriction maps and for generating useful landmarks along the chromosome.

Acknowledgments

This work was supported by research funds of the American Otological Society (RPK), National Institutes of Health Grant DC01682 (RPK), and an Outstanding Investigator Award of the National Cancer Institute, CA 42556 (SMW).

References

1. D. C. Schwartz and C. R. Cantor, *Cell (Cambridge, Mass.)* **37**, 67 (1984).
2. G. F. Carle, M. Frank, and M. V. Olson, *Science* **232**, 65 (1986).
3. G. Chu, D. Vollrath, and R. W. Davis, *Science* **234**, 1982 (1986).

4. D. T. Burke, G. F. Carle, and M. V. Olson, *Science* **235,** 806 (1987).
5. T. Reid, G. Landes, W. Dackowski, K. Klinger, and D. C. Ward, *Hum. Mol. Genet.* **1,** 307 (1992).
6. C. L. Smith, S. K. Lawrance, G. A. Gillespie, C. R. Cantor, S. M. Weissman, and F. S. Collins, *in* "Methods in Enzymology." (M. Gottesman, ed.), Vol. 151, p. 461. Academic Press, Orlando, FL, 1987.
7. M. R. Wallace, J. W. Fountain, A. M. Bereton, and F. S. Collins, *Nucleic Acids Res.* **17,** 1655 (1989).
8. F. S. Collins and S. M. Weissman, *Proc. Natl. Acad. Sci. U.S.A.* **81,** 6812 (1984).
9. A. M. Poustaka and H. Lehrach, *Trends Genet.* **2,** 174 (1986).
10. R. K. Saiki, D. H. Gelfand, S. Stoffel, S. J. Clark, R. Higuchi, G. T. Horn, K. B. Mullis, and H. A. Erlich, *Science* **239,** 487 (1988).
11. K. B. Mullis and F. A. Faloona, *in* "Methods in Enzymology" (R. Wu, ed.), Vol. 155, p. 335. Academic Press, Orlando, FL, 1987.
12. M. Steinmetz, D. Stephan, and K. Fisher Lindal, *Cell (Cambridge, Mass.)* **44,** 895 (1986).
13. E. H. Weiss, L. Golden, K. Fahrner, A. L. Mellor, J. J. Devlin, H. Bullman, H. Tiddns, H. Bird, and R. A. Flavell, *Nature (London)* **310,** 650 (1984).
14. F. Karch, B. Weiffenbach, M. Peifer, W. Bender, E. Duncan, S. Celniker, M. Corsby, and E. B. Lewis, *Cell (Cambridge, Mass.)* **43,** 81 (1985).
15. S. Baxendale, M. E. MacDonald, R. Mott, F. Francis, C. Lin, S. F. Kirby, M. James, G. Zehetner, H. Hummerich, J. Valdes *et al., Nat. Genet.* **4,** 181 (1993).
16. J. Buxton, P. Shelbourne, J. Davies, C. Jones, M. B. Perryman, T. Ashizawa, R. Butler, D. Brook, D. Shaw, P. DeJong *et al., Genomics* **13,** 526 (1992).
17. D. L. Mager and P. S. Henthorn, *Proc. Natl. Acad. Sci. U.S.A.* **81,** 7510 (1984).
18. R. H. Reeves, W. J. Pavan, and P. Hieter, *in* "Methods in Enzymology" (R. Wu, ed.), Vol. 216, p. 584. Academic Press, San Diego, 1992.
19. N. Stanberg, *Proc. Natl. Acad. Sci. U.S.A.* **87,** 103 (1990).
20. H. Shizuya, B. Birren, V. J. Kim, V. Mancino, T. Slepak, Y. Tachiiri, and M. Simon, *Proc. Natl. Acad. Sci. U.S.A.* **89,** 8794 (1992).
21. D. T. Moir, T. E. Dorman, A. P. Smyth, and D. R. Smith, *Gene* **125,** 229 (1993).
22. R. Anand, J. H. Riley, R. Butler, J. C. Smith, and A. F. Markham, *Nucleic Acids Res.* **18,** 1951 (1990).
23. J. Dausset, P. Ouzen, H. Abderrahim, A. Billault, J. L. Sambucy, D. Cohen, and D. LePaslier, *Beh. Inst. Mitt.* **91,** 13 (1992).
24. S. Foote, D. Vollrath, A. Hilton, and D. Page, *Science* **258,** 60 (1992).
25. C. Bellane-Chantelot, B. Lacroix, P. Ouzen, A. Billault, S. Beaufils, S. Bertrand, I. Georgges, *et al., Cell (Cambridge, Mass.)* **70,** 1059 (1992).
26. I. Chumakov, P. Rigault, S. Guillou, P. Ougen, A. Billault, G. Gausconi, P. Gervy, I. LeGall *et al., Nature (London)* **359,** 380 (1992).
27. E. R. Zabarovsky, F. Boldoz, R. Erlandsson, V. I. Kashuba, R. L. Allikmets, Z. Marcsek, L. L. Kisselev *et al., Genomics* **11,** 1030 (1991).
28. R. P. Kandpal, G. Kandpal, and S. M. Weissman, *Proc. Natl. Acad. Sci. U.S.A.* **91,** 88 (1994).
29. A. P. Bird, *Nature (London)* **321,** 209 (1986).
30. R. P. Kandpal, H. Shukla, and S. M. Weissman, *Nucleic Acids Res.* **18,** 3081 (1990).

31. S. Parimoo, S. R. Patanjali, and S. M. Weissman, *Methods Mol. Genet.* **1,** 23 (1993).
32. B. R. Krishnan, R. Blakesley, and D. Berg, *Nucleic Acids Res.* **19,** 1153 (1991).
33. R. P. Kandpal, D. C. Ward, and S. M. Weissman, *in* "Methods in Enzymology" (R. Wu, ed.), Vol. 216, p. 39. Academic Press, San Diego, 1992.
34. M. Schuchard, G. Sarkar, T. Ruesink, and T. C. Spelsberg, *BioTechniques* **14,** 390 (1993).
35. C. S. Smith, P. E. Warburton, A. Gaal, and C. R. Cantor, *Genet. Eng.* **8,** 45 (1986).
36. C. Connelly, M. K. McCormick, J. Shero, and P. Hieter, *Genomics* **10,** 10 (1991).
37. G. M. Church and W. Gilbert, *Proc. Natl. Acad. Sci. U.S.A.* **81,** 1991 (1984).

Section VIII

Site-Directed Mutagenesis by PCR

[21] Site-Directed Mutagenesis by PCR: Substitution, Insertion, Deletion, and Gene Fusion

Sailen Barik

Our ability to alter genes at specific predetermined sites has revolutionized molecular biology. Site-directed mutagenesis not only allows us to alter noncoding DNA sequences (e.g., promoter, terminator, transcription factor-binding elements) but to mutate protein-coding genes and generate mutant proteins. As a result, studies of the relationship between structure and function at either the nucleic acid or the protein level have become enormously efficient and have claimed a major area in recombinant DNA technology. Historically, such techniques owe their origin to the pioneering studies of Khorana and co-workers (1) demonstrating the replication of DNA strands *in vitro* using synthetic deoxynucleotide primers and purified DNA polymerase. As the primer, by definition, is incorporated in the product DNA, it was quickly recognized that by altering the nucleotide sequence of the primer, one can generate mutant DNA products at will.

The original method of mutagenesis designed and perfected by Smith and others (2–4) used single-stranded DNA templates such as those derived from M13 phage clones; this, however, often required the extra steps of subcloning the relevant gene from double-stranded plasmids to M13 and the converse. With the advent of the polymerase chain reaction (PCR) in the mid-1980s (5), it became possible to use plasmid clones directly in mutagenesis *in vitro*. In the years that followed, a happy marriage between PCR and primer-directed mutagenesis produced a variety of site-directed mutagenesis procedures in quick succession (6–14). It is perhaps no wonder that the two original techniques, site-directed mutagenesis and PCR, shared the 1993 Nobel Prize in chemistry (15).

High-efficiency mutagenesis procedures using modifications of PCR have been reported which would produce nucleotide substitutions as well as deletions and insertions (6–14). To the beginner, however, they often represent a bewildering variety of methodology to choose from. In this article, I attempt to compile the simplest of the available methods in a comprehensive manner. It is to be noted that all the procedures described here, except EIPCR (enzymatic inverse PCR), are variations of the basic theme of the three-primer, two-PCR mutagenesis procedure which has been named the "mega-primer" method.

Why "Megaprimer?"

The simplest possible site-directed mutagenesis scheme based on PCR is of course the one in which the mutation to be introduced is near the gene termini. Thus, one of the primers will have the desired mutation, and a straightforward PCR will produce the double-stranded mutant product (Fig. 1). The mutation could be a simple point mutation (nucleotide substitution) or a short insertion or deletion. How far into the gene one can mutate this way is in theory limited by the maximum length of the oligonucleotide primer that DNA synthesizers can make (i.e., 80–120 nucleotides), although in reality, economic considerations dictate the use of shorter primers. Moreover, the primers are often designed so as to contain restriction enzyme sites and extra nucleotides ("clamp") to facilitate subsequent restriction and cloning of the product, which further limits the distance of the mutation from the gene termini.

This, therefore, leads us to the more general situation where the desired mutation is internal to the sequence to be amplified. Thus, the "mutant" primer must be physically different from the "amplifying" primers that are terminal; hence the need for a minimum of three primers and the megaprimer method. Among the many advantages of the PCR-based mutagenesis over classical methods is the fact that the former does not depend on the availability of suitable restriction sites in the vicinity of the mutation. As a result, gene manipulations such as insertion, deletion, or gene fusion can be done precisely at any predetermined nucleotide position.

I first present an overall scheme of the individual procedures followed by general experimental considerations that are applicable to all procedures.

Nucleotide Substitution: The Basic Megaprimer Method

The basic strategy of the megaprimer method (6, 11) is best exemplified by a simple nucleotide substitution depicted in Fig. 2. Most variations of the

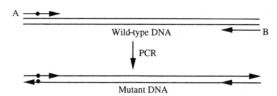

FIG. 1 Mutagenesis at gene termini by PCR. A and B represent the two PCR primers, A encoding the desired mutation. For the sake of simplicity, the double-stranded wild-type DNA template is represented by the single bold line.

PCR 1: Synthesis of mutant megaprimer

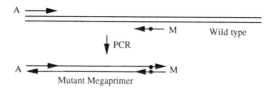

PCR 2: Use of megaprimer

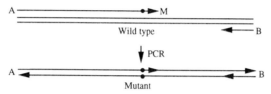

FIG. 2   The basic principle of megaprimer mutagenesis. The wild-type template and the mutant product are as indicated. A and B are primers with wild-type sequence while M represents the mutant primer. The dot in primer M represents the desired mutation which, in special cases, could be an insertion (Fig. 3) or a deletion (Fig. 4). Note that although the megaprimer is used as a double-stranded DNA, only its priming strand (AM) is incorporated in PCR 2.

megaprimer method involve two PCRs, both using wild-type DNA as template. In the first PCR, the mutant primer (M) and one of the terminal primers (A; opposite polarity of mutant primer) are used. The double-stranded product (AM), called megaprimer, is used directly in the second PCR without strand separation, along with the other terminal primer (B), to produce the full-length mutant product DNA (AB).

Application

Nucleotide substitution finds its widest application in mutating specific amino acid residues of proteins. Important examples include: (a) Alteration of phosphorylation sites (Ser, Thr, Tyr, His) to residues that cannot be phosphorylated. Ideally, the replacement residue should have an otherwise similar side chain but be devoid of the hydroxyl group; for example, Ser should be replaced by Ala, Thr by Ile, Tyr by Phe, etc. (b) In order to address the role of an acidic amino acid (e.g., in casein kinase II substrate motif), such as Asp, it may be mutated to another acidic residue (Glu), to a basic residue (Lys, Arg), or to a neutral one (Ala, Leu). (c) Mutation of specific cysteine residues into Ala or Leu may shed light on their role in disulfide linkages, zinc fingers, etc. (d) Generation of a premature termination codon in a protein reading frame will generate a truncated protein by recombinant means. Examples of site-directed mutagenesis of protein-binding sites on DNA can be equally numerous. Mutational analysis of transcription control sequences, e.g., prokaryotic promoters, TATA boxes, polyadenylation and RNA processing sequences, and transcriptional factor-binding sites, has provided seminal information on their function.

Insertion

For insertion mutagenesis, the sequence to be inserted is simply incorporated in the middle of the mutant primer (M in Fig. 3) provided that there is enough homology at either end of the primer to anneal to the template in both PCR reactions. Usually a run of 15–20 nucleotides of homology at either end of the primer is sufficient. Although the exogenous sequence is depicted as a bulge (the classical R-loop) in the annealed primer (Fig. 3), it may not necessarily exist as one. The exact structure of the annealed primer is unimportant as long as the 3' end (the "priming" end) of the primer anneals to the template comfortably. Whether the 5' end of the primer will also anneal to the template

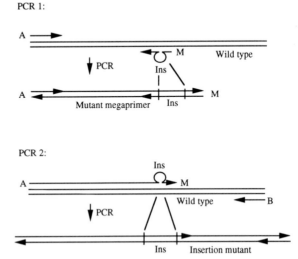

FIG. 3   Insertion mutagenesis by megaprimer PCR. The sequence to be inserted (Ins) is shown as a simplified loop in the mutant primer (M) and megaprimer (AM).

would depend on the T_m of the 5' end duplex, the annealing temperature used in the PCR, and the thermodynamic stability parameters of the bulge region, which remain largely undefined. Note that it is the complementary strand of this 5' end (of the M primer) which will become the priming end in the second PCR.

Application

The two major applications of insertional mutagenesis are (a) insertion of a stretch of amino acids within a polypeptide and (b) insertion of exogenous nucleotides to disrupt a DNA site. Although in theory the method described here will tolerate inserts of any length, in reality, very large inserts are rarely needed and unlikely to produce meaningful conclusions.

Deletion

The mutant primer (M) in deletion mutagenesis is comprised of two regions of the template with the intervening sequence (the one that is to be deleted) missing (denoted by the looped out region in the template; Fig. 4). In the

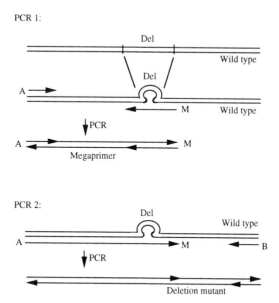

FIG. 4   Deletion mutagenesis by megaprimer PCR. The region to be deleted (Del) is shown as an unpaired loop in the template.

final product (AB), therefore, this sequence will be deleted. As in insertion mutagenesis, the 3′ end and 5′ complementary end of the mutant primer are used in priming DNA synthesis in PCR 1 and PCR 2, respectively.

Application

Deletion analyses are used wherever a specific segment of protein or DNA is to be excised to address the functional role of the sequence in question. The deleted sequence could range from a single nucleotide to a few hundred, apparantly without an upper limit of any practical concern.

Gene Fusion or Recombinant PCR

A chimeric gene can be viewed as a special case of gene insertion. The mutant primer (M; Fig. 5) in this case is a "chimeric" primer that represents the junction region of the final chimera and spans about 20 nucleotides on either side flanking the junction. While the 3′ half of the primer hybridizes

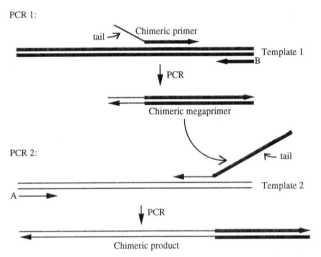

FIG. 5   Gene fusion by megaprimer PCR. The two genes to be fused are presented as templates 1 and 2 (thick and narrow lines, respectively). The chimeric primer, megaprimer, and product are shown as composite lines. See text for a better yield of the final product.

to its cognate gene template, the 5' half, derived from the other gene, would remain single-stranded during the priming reaction. This latter region is the "tail" of the primer. At present, there appears to be no significant upper limit to the length of this tail for efficient PCR amplification; primers with tails as long as 1.5–2 kb have been used with success. However, as in any primer design, it is important to ensure that the primer does not self-hybridize, i.e., the tail region does not have considerable homology with the 3' end of the primer. Clearly, the probability of self-hybridization increases with increasing length of the tail.

For gene fusion only, it is possible to combine PCRs 1 and 2 (Fig. 5) into a single PCR, since the terminal primers A and B are complementary to different templates. It is obvious from Fig. 5 that in such a situation, template 1 will undergo exponential amplification from the very beginning since both of its primers (B and chimeric primer) are available. In contrast, amplification of template 2 will begin in a linear fashion since primer A only is available to start with; once the megaprimer is made, however, amplification of template 2 will switch to the exponential mode to eventually produce large quantities of the chimeric gene. Clearly, combined PCR is not possible for those procedures (substitution, insertion, and deletion) where the same template is used in PCRs 1 and 2, since this would result in a straightforward amplification by primers A and B (to produce more of the wild-type template!) and bypass the mutant primer to a large extent.

Alternately, after a few cycles (we routinely do 10 cycles) of PCR 2 using the megaprimer and primer A, add primer B, and continue PCR2 for another 30 cycles or so (16). To add primer B, use a long round tip, stab it through the oil overlay, and mix it with the aqueous phase by pipetting back and forth a few times.

Application

The major usage of gene fusion is to produce chimera of homologous proteins from two different organisms to delineate the determinants of specificity ("domain swapping"). For example, chimeric HN (hemagglutinin) proteins derived from fusion of cytoplasmic and extracellular domains of related paramyxoviruses have provided insights into the roles of these domains. Studies of chimeric N proteins of λ and lambdoid phages have led to the identification of Arg-rich motifs essential for RNA binding. PCR-mediated gene fusion described here would make such constructions easier and more precise.

Method

Standard PCR

The stock reagents are prepared as follows:

> $10 \times$ PCR buffer: 100 mM Tris–HCl, pH 8.0–8.3; 500 mM KCl; 15 mM MgCl$_2$; 0.01% gelatin; this buffer is available from Perkin–Elmer Cetus (Norwalk, CT) along with the purchase of *Taq* polymerase.
>
> dNTP mix: Mixture containing 2.5 mM of each (dATP, dCTP, dGTP, dTTp) (we make it by mixing equal volumes of 10 mM stock solution of each nucleotide, available commercially). Use autoclaved Millipore (Bedford, MA) water.

Step-by-Step Procedure

1. PCR 1: It is assumed that the readers are familiar with a standard PCR protocol. In brief, use the following recipe for the first PCR (PCR 1). Make 100μl reaction mix in a 0.5-ml Eppendorf tube as follows:

> 80 μl H$_2$O
> 10 μl $10 \times$ PCR buffer
> 8 μl dNTP mix (final concentration of each nucleotide is 200 μM)
> 0.5 μl *Taq* polymerase (2.5 U)
> 50 pmol of primer A (for a 20-mer oligonucleotide of 50% GC content this equals 0.3 μg)
> 50 pmol of primer M
> 10–100 ng DNA template (usually a plasmid clone).

(If a number of PCRs are to be done using a common template and different mutagenic primers, make a master mix using the common reagents, distribute in different PCR tubes, and then add one mutagenic primer in each tube.) Vortex well to mix, and then spin briefly in a microfuge. Reopen the tube, overlay the reaction mixture with ~100 μl mineral oil to cover the surface, and then close the cap. The tube is now ready for thermal cycling. A representative set of parameters for producing a 400-bp-long megaprimer is 94°C, 5 min (initial denaturation; called "delay" in the Perkin–Elmer program); 35 cycles of denaturation (94°C, 1.5 min), annealing (2 min at appropriate temperature: see below), elongation (72°C, 45 sec); and a final elongation ("extension," called "delay" in the Perkin–Elmer program; 72°C, 1 min).

Following synthesis, the samples are maintained at 4°C (called "soak" file in the Perkin–Elmer program) for indefinite time. Some instruments lack an active cooling mechanism and keep samples at an ambient temperature of ~15-20°C by circulating tap water around the heat block, which appears to be adequate for overnight runs.

2. After PCR, remove samples from the block and add 200 μl of chloroform to each tube. The mineral oil overlay and chloroform will mix to form a single phase and sink to the bottom of the tube. Quick-spin for 30 sec in a microfuge. Collect ~80 μl of top aqueous layer taking care not to touch the chloroform, and transfer to a fresh 1.5-ml Eppendorf tube.

3. Removal of the small primers (A, M): We offer a choice of two procedures, membrane filtration and gel elctrophoresis, both of which provide a recovery of >90% of the megaprimer; use whichever is convenient.

a. Membrane filtration: We routinely use Centricon-100 (Amicon, Danvers, MA) for this purpose, which safely retains DNA 100 bp or bigger. Thus, it works best when the megaprimer is 150 bp or longer and the small primers are shorter than 40 nucleotides. Instructions for use are supplied by the manufacturer. In brief, after assembling the unit, first wash the membrane by adding 1 ml H_2O and centrifuging at 2000 rpm (Beckman J2-21, rotor JA 20, Fullerton, CA, or an equivalent centrifuge) for 10 min. Take out the assembly, discard the filtrate (from the bottom compartment), load the cleaned PCR (from step 2), add another 1.5 ml H_2O, spin again as before. Repeat these steps four times to completely remove the small primers and ions at the same time. Now collect the liquid from above the membrane by centrifuging briefly in an inverted position with the collector cup fitted at the bottom as per instructions. The volume collected will be 150–200 μl; reduce it to less than 80 μl using a Speed-Vac (takes ~10 min with a good vacuum pump). Alternately, concentrate by precipitation with ethanol as follows. If the DNA is in, say, 50 μl, add 5 μl of 3 M sodium acetate, 2–5 μg carrier tRNA, and 150 μl absolute ethanol (−20°C); mix well; spin at top speed in a microfuge at 4°C. Wash DNA pellet with 500 μl of 70% ethanol (−20°C) and carefully remove the ethanol without losing the pellet. Dry DNA pellet under vacuum (Speed-Vac, 2 min). Dissolve in 20 μl. This solution contains megaprimer and wild-type template. Use it in PCR 2 (step 4).

b. Gel electrophoresis: Prepare a standard 0.7–0.8% agarose gel in 1× TBE (10× TBE buffer: 108 g Tris base, 55 g boric acid, 9.3 g Na_2EDTA, $2H_2O$ per liter; dissolve, filter through 0.2 μm filter, and store at room temperature) containing ethidium bromide (1 μg/ml final concentration; make a 5 mg/ml stock in sterile water, store at 4°C in dark) in a mid-size horizontal apparatus; use a comb of well volume >35 μl. Cover gel with 1× TBE containing the same concentration of ethidium bromide. Reduce the volume of PCR to ~25 μl by Speed-Vac. Add 5 μl of 6x loading dye (0.25% bromophenol blue, 0.25% xylene cyanol, 30% glycerol), mix, and load in the agarose gel. Use DNA markers in a parallel lane; we routinely use the BRL 100-bp ladder (containing DNA fragments differing by 100 bp). Electrophorese at appropriate voltage (~80 V) until desired resolution is achieved between megaprimer and the small primers (~1 hr); monitor by hand-held UV light. Following electrophoresis, excise the megaprimer band with a scalpel, put it in an Eppendorf tube, freeze for 5 min in a dry ice–ethanol bath (or 15 min in a −70°C freezer), and spin for 15 min in a microcentrifuge. Collect the exudate by pipetting. Expect a recovery of 70–80% for DNA fragments ~500 bp or smaller. Use directly in step 4; removal of ethidium bromide is not necessary.

4. PCR 2: In a 0.5 ml Eppendorf tube, make 100 μl PCR mix as follows:

10 μl 10× PCR buffer
8 μl dNTP mix (final concentration of each nucleotide is 200 μM)
50 pmol of primer B
All of the recovered megaprimer from step 3 (20–50 μl)
1 μg DNA template
0.5 μl *Taq* polymerase (2.5 U)

Make up volume to 100 μl with H_2O

Overlay with oil as for PCR 1. A representative set of parameters for a 1-kb-long final product using a 400-bp-long megaprimer is 94°C, 5 min (initial denaturation; called "delay" in the Perkin–Elmer program); 35 cycles of denaturation (94°C, 1 min 30 sec), annealing (2 min at appropriate temperature: see below), and elongation (72°C, 1 min; since the megaprimer is 400 bp long, you are only synthesizing another 600 nucleotide stretch in this PCR); and a final elongation (extension, called "delay" in the Perkin–Elmer program; 72°C, 1.2 min). After the cycles, use a soak file as before.

5. Following the second PCR, remove oil and concentrate by Speed-Vac as before. Analyze by electrophoresis in an agarose gel. Run the gel long enough to resolve the full-length product (A-M-B) from the wild-type template. In a typical example, the 1-kb linear PCR product is to be resolved from a 3- to 5-kb supercoiled plasmid, which is easily achieved. Purify the PCR product by excising the band and recovering it from agarose by freeze-squeeze as described above.

6. If it is to be restricted for cloning, the DNA can be concentrated by precipitation with ethanol as described in step 3(a). Restrict and ligate to appropriate vectors using standard procedures.

Special Considerations

Annealing Temperature and Primer Design

For a given PCR, choose an appropriate annealing temperature based on the nucleotide composition and length of the annealed region at the 3′ end of the primer. A quick approximation of annealing temperature can be obtained as follows. T_m (in °C) of the annealed region is (number of A-T pairs $\times$ 2) + (number of G-C pairs $\times$ 4), i.e., 2 °C for each A-T pair and 4 °C for each G-C pair. Subtract 5 °C from T_m to obtain the annealing temperature. For example, if the annealed region has the sequence AGACATTAATGC-TAGCTG, its T_m is $11 \times 2 + 7 \times 4 = 50$ °C. Therefore, a safe yet stringent annealing temperature for PCR will be 45 °C. It is obvious that one should check the T_m of all primers to be used in a given PCR and then use the lowest number to arrive at the annealing temperature for that PCR. As a golden rule, have 15–20 nucleotides annealed at the 3′ end for optimum specificity of priming. If possible, avoid sequences that are highly rich in GC or AT; also avoid long runs of any nucleotide, since such stretches tend to anneal to complementary regions elsewhere in a nonspecific manner.

Primer–template mismatch at the very 3′ end of the primer prevents DNA synthesis; when the mismatch is three to four nucleotides away from the 3′ end, synthesis is restored. We recommend that at least the first 12–15 nucleotides at the 3′ end of the primer have uninterrupted homology with the template. Thus, mutations (substitution, insertion, or deletion) in the primer should be placed accordingly.

In addition to having homology to the respective termini of the template, primers A and B may contain unique restriction sites for cloning of the mutant product into appropriate vectors. Ensure that extra nucleotides are added to the 5′ end of the restriction sites for optimal restriction enzyme action. More detailed considerations of thermodynamic parameters in primer design can be found elsewhere (17, 18, and references therein).

A megaprimed PCR differs from a standard PCR on three accounts: the large size of the megaprimer, the double-stranded nature of the megaprimer, and the fact that it is not a synthetic oligonucleotide but a product of another PCR. These unique considerations make PCR 2 somewhat different from a standard PCR. In what follows, these considerations are discussed in detail.

Purification of Megaprimer

A variety of methods are available for the purification of DNA fragments in general, any of which can potentially be used to purify the megaprimer so long as two conditions are met: (a) complete removal of the smaller primer (primer A in Figs. 2–4), and (b) good recovery of the megaprimer. Since the megaprimer is large, a greater amount of it is required (in PCR 2) to achieve the same molar amount as that of the small primer. We usually perform two 100-μl reactions of PCR 1 and pool them together for the purification of the megaprimer.

It is claimed that the Centricon-100 filtration procedure also removes *Taq* polymerase (19); however, we have not tested this. Retention of the template does not create a problem, since the same template is going to be used in PCR 2.

Improvement of Yield in PCR 2

One modification that we routinely use in the laboratory is the use of a higher amount of template (100 ng or above) in PCR 2, i.e., when the megaprimer is being used as a primer. Quite often, this dramatically improves the yield of the final mutant product (20). This is probably due to the fact that the template as well as the nonpriming strand of the megaprimer competes for the priming strand of the megaprimer; at a higher concentration, the template may have a better chance to win the competition.

If this still fails to improve the yield, the best choice is to first analyze PCR 2 by electrophoresis in standard agarose gels. Often times, when the yield of the desired product is low, additional products are seen that differ in size from the desired one, most likely resulting from nonspecific initiation events. To recognize the desired (mutant) product in such cases, we routinely perform a standard PCR using primers A and B and the wild-type template and analyze an aliquot of this PCR (like a molecular weight marker) in a parallel lane. Following electrophoretic resolution, excise the gel fragment containing the desired (mutant) product (based on its size), purify the DNA by electroelution or freeze-squeeze, and then use it as the template in a standard PCR (PCR 3) with A and B as primers.

Problem of Nontemplated Nucleotides and Its Solution

Taq polymerase, like many other DNA polymerases, tends to add extra, nontemplated nucleotides at the 3′ end of the product strand at a certain frequency, the preferred nucleotide being A (adenylate). (This, in fact, forms the basis of the A-T cloning procedure that utilizes the terminal A and T of complementary strands as cohesive ends for ligation and, thus, does not require the use of restriction enzymes.) In the usual PCR, these nucleotides are rarely a problem since they are lost following restriction of the product. In the megaprimer procedures, however, the 3' end of the megaprimer (priming strand) is incorporated into the product. As indicated under Annealing Temperature and Primer Design, if the 3'-nontemplated residues are indeed present in the megaprimer and if that residue is a mismatch with the template, amplification in PCR 2 may not occur at all. Usually, therefore, such primers are not incorporated into the product and do no harm except to reduce the yield of the final product. Occasionally, however, they do get incorporated and generate a substitution mutation (16). Elsewhere, we have presented a variety of possible solutions to this problem (6); the one that we recommend is as follows. Briefly, try to design the megaprimer against a region of the template such that there are one or two T residues in the template strand just outside of the 3' terminus of the megaprimer. Thus, even if the megaprimer contains an extratemplated A at its 3' end, it will still be complementary to the T residue on the template and, therefore, produce no unwanted mutation.

Enzymatic Inverse PCR

General Principle

A relatively new method, termed enzymatic inverse PCR (EIPCR) has been described that can be an effective and convenient alternative to megaprimer-based methods in generating substitutions and deletions (14). The unique feature of EIPCR is the incorporation of identical class 2s restriction sites in the two primers of the PCR. Class 2s restriction enzymes (such as *Bbs*I, as opposed to the standard class 2 enzymes, e.g., *Eco*RI and *Bam*HI) cut the DNA at a short distance from their recognition sites. Thus, primers can be designed such that they contain the enzyme recognition site followed by mutations and then homology with the template (see Fig. 6). When the PCR product is restricted, the enzyme removes its entire recognition site and leaves the DNA with complementary overhangs at the termini. Thus, following ligation, the only part of the primer that becomes incorporated into the plasmid is the *NNNN* overhang which can be made to be the native sequence. Since there is no sequence specificity at the actual site of cutting, EIPCR can be used to engineer virtually any site on the template DNA. An example of this technique is shown in Fig. 6 in which five amino acid residues of PP-λ (orf221 protein phosphatase of phage λ) are deleted (21).

Notes

(a) Since this is not a megaprimer method, use the standard considerations of a PCR. The crucial part is the designing of the primers; follow the example in Fig. 6 carefully. (b) Although most class 2s enzyme will cut the product

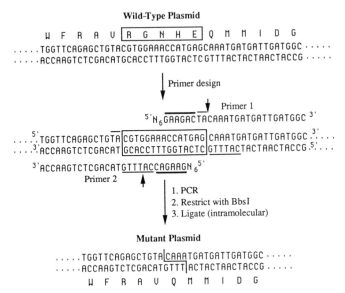

FIG. 6   Enzymatic inverse PCR. The RGNHE pentapeptide sequence of PP-λ is deleted as an example (21).

with the six extra nucleotides (N6) as shown in Fig. 6, the efficiency of restriction may be improved by adding upto nine nucleotides. (c) Other class 2s enzymes that have worked well in our hands are *Bsa*I, *Bsm*I, and *Bsp*MI. Ensure that the restriction site is absent within the template. (d) Since EIPCR involves amplification of the whole plasmid, avoid using templates that are too big. Templates up to 6 kb long work well, but smaller (e.g., pGEM, pUC) is better. Use proportional time of elongation (72°C) in PCR (~1.2 min per 1 kb) with extra time for longer products, e.g., 4 min for 3 kb, 6 min for 4 kb, 10 min for 6 kb. (e) Following PCR, purify the product by agarose gel electrophoresis as described earlier in step 3(b). The linear PCR product will have slower mobility than the closed circular template. (f) Restrict the gel-purified product with the appropriate class 2s enzyme, carry out intramolecular ligation at a lower concentration of DNA, and then transform competent cells.

Acknowledgments

Research in the author's laboratory was supported in part by a grant from the National Institutes of Health (AI 37938).

References

1. K. Kleppe, E. Ohtsuka, R. Kleppe, I. Molineux, and H. G. Khorana, *J. Mol. Biol.* **56,** 341 (1971).
2. M. Smith, *Annu. Rev. Genet.* **19,** 423 (1985).
3. D. Botstein and D. Shortle, *Science* **229,** 1193 (1985).
4. R. Wu and L. Grossman, *in* "Methods in Enzymology" (R. Wu and L. Grossman, eds.), vol. 154, p. 329. Academic Press, Orlando, FL, 1987.
5. R. K. Saiki, S. Scharf, F. Faloona, K. B. Mullis, G. T. Horn, H. A. Erlich, and N. Arnheim, *Science* **230,** 1350 (1985).
6. S. Barik, *Methods Mol. Biol.* **15,** 277 (1993).
7. A. Hemsley, N. Arnheim, M. D. Toney, G. Cortopassi, and D. J. Galas, *Nucleic Acids Res.* **17,** 6545 (1989).
8. R. Higuchi, B. Krummel, and R. K. Saiki, *Nucleic Acids Res.* **16,** 7351 (1988).
9. S. N. Ho, H. D. Hunt, R. M. Horton, J. K. Pullen, and L. R. Pease, *Gene* **77,** 51 (1989).
10. D. H. Jones and B. H. Howard, *BioTechniques* **10,** 62 (1991).
11. G. Sarkar and S. S. Sommer, *BioTechniques* **8,** 404 (1990).
12. M. Tomic, I. Sunjevaric, E. S. Savtchenko, and M. Blumenberg, *Nucleic Acids Res.* **18,** 1656 (1990).
13. F. Vallette, E. Mege, A. Reiss, and M. Adesnik, *Nucleic Acids Res.* **17,** 723 (1989).
14. W. P. C. Stemmer and S. K. Morris, *BioTechniques* **13,** 215 (1992).
15. 1993 Nobel Prize in Chemistry to Michael Smith and Kary Mullis.
16. S. Barik, unpublished, 1992.
17. R. A. McGraw, E. K. Steffe, and S. M. Baxter, *BioTechniques* **8,** 674 (1990).
18. W. Rychlik, *Methods Mol. Biol.* **15,** 31 (1993).
19. A. M. Krowczynska and M. B. Henderson, *BioTechniques* **13,** 286 (1992).
20. S. Barik and M. Galinski, *BioTechniques* **10,** 489 (1992).
21. S. Barik, *Proc. Natl. Acad. Sci. U.S.A.* **15,** 10633 (1993).

[22] Use of PCR in Analysis of 5'-Flanking Region of Androgen Receptor Gene

M. Vijay Kumar and Donald J. Tindall

Introduction

Since the first report of specific DNA amplification using polymerase chain reaction (PCR) (1–3), the technique has transformed DNA analysis both in research and clinical laboratories. Although this technique was originally utilized to amplify DNA, at present PCR is being applied to many problems in molecular biology. PCR has been used for identification and sequencing of the unknown DNA that flanks a known segment (4), genome walking (5), identification of point mutations (6), genomic footprinting (7), and mutagenesis to analyze the function of genes and their regulatory elements (8–12). In this review, we discuss some of the PCR-based mutagenesis techniques used in our laboratory during the course of analysis of the 5'-flanking region of the androgen receptor gene.

Androgen Receptor

Androgens play a central role in the development and maintenance of male reproductive organs. The effects of androgens are mediated by an intracellular androgen receptor (AR) that shares strong homology with other steroid receptors. The AR protein is involved in normal sexual differentiation and development (13, 14) and is implicated in benign prostatic hyperplasia (15–17). An understanding of the molecular pathway(s) of androgen action has been facilitated by the cloning and sequencing of cDNAs and genes for the androgen receptor (18–21). However, very little is known about the mechanism(s) which regulates its expression at the molecular level. Therefore, in order to study the regulation of the AR gene, the 5'-flanking region of the mouse AR was isolated and characterized.

Reagents

Tris-saturated phenol: Redistilled phenol (Boehringer-Mannheim Biochemical, Indianapolis, IN) is saturated with Tris by extracting first

Methods in Neurosciences, Volume 26

with an equal volume of 1 M Tris–HCl, pH 8.0, and then with
100 mM Tris–HCl, pH 8.0.

Chloroform: Chloroform and isoamyl alcohol (24:1 v/v) are mixed and
stored in dark bottles.

3 M sodium acetate, pH 5.2: Sodium acetate trihydrate (408.1 g) is
dissolved in 800 ml of water. The pH is adjusted to pH 5.2 with glacial
acetic acid and the volume is brought up to 1000 ml.

Ampicillin (stock solution): 25 mg/ml of the sodium salt of ampicillin in
water. The solution is sterilized by filteration through a 0.2 μm filter,
aliquoted, and stored at $-20°C$. The working concentration is
100 μg/ml.

PCR Amplification Reagents

10× polymerase buffer (500 mM KCl, 100 mM Tris–HCl, pH 8.3,
15 mM MgCl$_2$, 0.1% gelatin).

100 mM dATP, 100 mM dTTP, 100 mM dGTP, and 100 mM dCTP.

TE buffer: 10 mM Tris–HCl (pH 8.0), 1 mM ethylenediaminetetraacetic
acid, disodium salt (EDTA). Stored at 4°C.

Gel Electrophoresis Reagents

Agarose, ultrapure, electrophoresis grade (GIBCO BRL, Gaithersburg, MD).

TAE buffer: Working solution—40 mM Tris–acetate, 1 mM EDTA.
50× concentrated stock solution—Tris base, 242 g; glacial acetic
acid, 57.1 ml; and 500 mM EDTA (pH 8.0), 100 ml. The buffer is
made up to 1000 ml.

6× electrophoresis loading buffer: 0.25% bromophenol blue, 0.25% xylene cyanol, 40% (w/v) sucrose in water.

Ethidium bromide, 10 mg/ml. For agarose gels ethidium bromide is used
at a concentration of 0.5 μg/ml. *Note:* Ethidium bromide is a potential
carcinogen and therefore gloves should be worn while handling the
solution. Store at 4°C in a dark bottle.

Gene Clean kit (Bio 101, La Jolla, CA).

Reagents for Ligation

10× Ligation buffer: 500 mM Tris–HCl, pH 7.4, 100 mM MgCl$_2$,
200 mM DTT, 10 mM ATP, and 50 μg/ml BSA. Store at $-20°C$.

T$_4$ DNA ligase (Promega, Madison, Wisconsin).

Plasmid Purification and Sequencing Reagents

pZ523 columns (5 Prime-3 Prime Inc, Paoli PA).

10N NaOH: NaOH (200 g) is dissolved in 450 ml distilled water and brought up to 500 ml.

10% SDS: Sodium dodecyl sulfate (SDS) (10 g) is dissolved in 100 ml distilled water.

TELT solution: 50 mM Tris–HCI, pH 8.0, 62.5 mM EDTA, 2.5 M lithium chloride, 4% (v/v) Triton X-100.

fmol sequencing kit (Promega, Madison, Wisconsin).

Sequenase kit (United States Biochemical, Cleveland Ohio).

Enzymes

Restriction enzymes are purchased from Promega (Wisconsin) or BRL Life Technologies (Gaithersburg, MD). AmpliTaq polymerase (Perkin–Elemer Cetus, Norwalk, CT) or pfu polymerase (Stratagene Cloning Systems, La Jolla, CA) are used for PCR.

Vectors

pBluescript SK$^+$ phagemid (Stratagene Cloning Systems, La Jolla, CA) is used for cloning.

pBLCAT3 (25) is used for cloning PCR products upstream of the chloramphenicol acetyltransferase (CAT) cDNA. The vector is used in transient transfections.

pCRII Vector (Invitrogen Corporation, San Diego, CA) was used to clone PCR products without any enzymatic manipulation.

Oligonucleotides

We synthesized oligonucleotides on an Applied Biosystems (Foster, CA) DNA synthesizer at the Molecular Biology Core Facility, Mayo Foundation, Rochester, MN. The oligonucleotides are synthesized with the dimethyl trityl group removed from the nascent oligonucleotides. The oligonucleotides are purified using NAP-25 columns (Pharmacia, Piscataway, NJ). NAP-25 are disposable columns prepacked with Sephadex G-25. The purified oligonucleotides are dried in a Speed

Vac, and the concentration of the oligonucleotides is measured in a Beckman DU 64 spectrophotometer.

Equipment

Thermal cycler (Perkin–Elmer Cetus, Norwalk, CT).

Speed Vac (Savant Instruments Inc, Farmingdale, New York).

Horizontal gel electrophoresis apparatus (Bio-Rad Laboratories, Hercule, CA).

Electrophoresis power supply unit (Bio-Rad Laboratories, Hercules, CA).

Controlled environment incubator shaker (New Brunswick Scientific Company, Inc., Edison, NJ).

Biochiller 2000 (Fotodyne, Inc. Hartland, WI).

Microcentrifuge.

UV transilluminator.

In Vitro Mutagenesis

Prior to the advent of PCR, *in vitro* mutagenesis was carried out by chemical and/or enzymatic manipulation of DNA. With the availability of the techniques to synthesize short pieces of DNA, oligonucleotide-mediated mutagenesis became the technique of choice (22, 23), but it required the presence of convenient restriction enzyme cleavage sites on either end of the segment to be mutated thus limiting the use of this method. With the construction of vectors which were capable of producing single-stranded templates, such as the M13 vectors (24), *in vitro* mutagenesis techniques became more efficient. Although this technique was more efficient and less cumbersome than the earlier method, it still involved several steps and was very time-consuming. However, with the availability of PCR technology, it has become easier and less labor-intensive to generate site-specific insertion, deletion, or point mutations. Furthermore, unlike the earlier methods, the template for PCR need not contain convenient restriction enzyme sites, and it is not necessary to produce single-stranded templates. The DNA to be mutagenized are usually cloned in plasmids which are used without subcloning or other manipulations thus saving effort and time.

Deletion Mutagenesis

Our laboratory has been interested in studying the regulation of the androgen receptor. We have isolated and characterized a 1.5-kb fragment (-546 to $+971$, Fig. 1) in the 5' flanking region of the androgen receptor gene. In

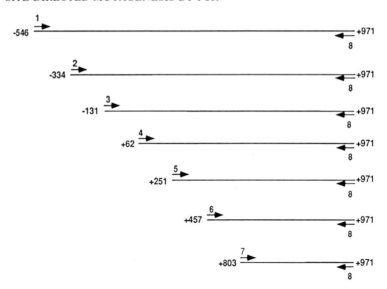

FIG. 1   Schematic representation of the construction of nested deletions using PCR. The 5′primers (oligonucleotides 1 to 7) contained 16–17 nucleotides homologous to the template with *Bam*HI and *Pst*I cleavage sites flanked by 4 nucleotides (Table I) upstream. The DNA was amplified using the same 3′ end (oligonucleotide 8) primer.

order to identify functional response elements and characterize the promoter, the PCR technique has been used to create deletion mutations. The mutants are cloned into a pBLCAT3 vector (25) upstream of the CAT gene and are then used in transient transfection assays.

Earlier approaches to the construction of deletion mutants used restriction endonucleases to cleave the DNA (26) and ligate the cleaved end back to the vector. The most important requirement of the method is the presence of a convenient restriction site at the point of mutation. Subsequent improvement in the techniques involves the use of enzymes such as exonuclease III (27), *Bal*31 (28), or DNase I (29). These techniques are time-consuming and labor-intensive and require a suitable restriction enzyme site in the proximity of deletion site. Thus, it is not possible to create deletion mutants at a desired nucleotide.

More recently, the PCR technique (see Methods) has been used to generate deletion mutations. Using this technique it is simpler to create deletions at a predetermined site by synthesizing a primer homologous to that region. Both 5′ and 3′ end deletions can be created by selecting the appropriate primer. It is also possible to create a series of nested deletions at predetermined sites by using suitable primers. Furthermore, all the deletion mutants generated by PCR can be cloned at similar restriction enzyme sites in a vector by designing the primers in such a way that the 5' ends contain convenient restriction enzyme cleavage sites.

Methods

Screening of Genomic Library

The full-length mouse androgen receptor (mAR) cDNA is used to screen an EMBL3 genomic library (Clonetech Laboratories) for the 5' flanking region using the 5'-most fragment of the cDNA (21) as a probe. From the positive clones a 1.5-kb fragment is isolated which is located upstream of the ATG start site. This fragment is cloned into the EcoRI site of a pBluescript vector. Both strands of the cloned fragment are sequenced using the Sequenase enzyme and [α-^{35}S]ATP. The sequences are further confirmed with a fmol sequencing system using Taq polymerase, [α-^{35}S]ATP, 3 μg template DNA, and 4 pmol primer for 30 cycles at 95°C (0.5 min), 50°C (0.5 min), and 72°C (1.0 min).

Primer Design

The choice of an appropriate primer is crucial for the success of the PCR. Ideally the primer should not possess secondary structures and should contain approximately 50% GC nucleotides. Preferably, both the primers should be of the same length. Their melting temperatures should be approximately similar as noted by their GC content, and they should not be complementary to each other. For the AR 5' deletion mutations, the 5' end primer, complementary to the bottom strand, consisted of 16–17 nucleotides homologous to the sequence where the deletion was desired. Upstream of the matched sequence two restriction enzyme cleavage sites (BamHI and PstI) plus 4 flanking nucleotides were present (Table I, oligonucleotides 1 to 7). The design of the 3' end primer was similar to that of the 5' end primer in which 17 nucleotides were complementary to the top strand, upstream of which were two restriction enzyme sites (XhoI and XbaI) with 4 flanking nucleotides (Table I, oligonucleotide 8). Oligonucleotides 9 and 10 (Table I) were used in the generation of site-specific mutations and are discussed below.

Amplification and Cloning of PCR Product

DNA is amplified in a 20-μl reaction mixture consisting of 2 μl 10× polymerase buffer, 200 μM each of dNTP, 2 pmol each of the primers, 1 ng of intact

TABLE I   Oligonucleotides Used in This Study

Number	Position	Sequence (5' to 3')
1	−530 to −546	ATGCGGATCCCTGCAGCCAGCTATCCTACAGGA
2	−334 to −349	ATCGGGATCCCTGCAGGGATTGGGTTCAGGAA
3	−131 to −146	ATCGGGATCCCTGCAGACTCTGCGCTAGCTTG
4	+62 to +77	ATCGGGATCCCTGCAGAACCTGGAGGCTGAGA
5	+251 to +266	ATCGGGATCCCTGCAGAGACTCAGAGGAAGCA
6	+457 to +472	ATCGGGATCCCTGCAGACATTGCAAGGAAGGC
7	+803 to +819	ATCGGGATCCCTGCAGCAAACTGTGTAAGTAGCA
8	+971 to +955	ATGCTCTAGACTCGAGCTCTTGCTCTGAAGAGT
9	+131 to + 112	ATGCTCTAGACTCGAGGGTACCAAGCTTCTGTATGGCACTGG
10	(−403 to −420) + (−449 to −466)	CTCCCTTCTGCTTGTCCTATACCTAAGAGCAATTGG

template, and 0.5 U of AmpliTaq polymerase diluted in TE. Following initial denaturation at 94°C for 1 min the DNA is amplified through 30 cycles for 1 min at 94°C, 2 min at 50°C, and 3 min at 72°C. The final extension step is carried out at 72°C for 6 min and then cooled to 4°C. Typically all the reagents are stored at −20°C except TE which is stored at 4°C. AmpliTaq polymerase, which is purchased as a more concentrated enzyme (5 U/μl), is diluted immediately before use with cold TE. Unused diluted enzyme is discarded. Whenever necessary the reaction volume is scaled up in parallel with the concentrations of the constituents.

The full-length (−546/+971) fragment (Fig. 1) is amplified using the oligonucleotides 1 and 8 (Table I). Further 5' deletions of the DNA are created by using oligonucleotides 2 to 7 (Table I) thus deleting approximately 200 nucleotides from the 5' end. All the constructs have the same 3' end since oligonucleotide 8 is used in each of the PCR reactions.

PCR products are separated on a 1.2% agarose gel which contains ethidium bromide. Electrophoresis loading buffer (3 μl) is added to the PCR product, quickly spun in a microfuge, loaded on the gel, and electrophoresed in TAE buffer at 100 V. At the end of electrophoresis, the DNA bands are visualized on a UV transilluminator. The band of interest is excised using a scalpel and collected in a 1.5-ml microfuge tube. The DNA is eluted from the agarose gel using a Gene Clean kit. The purified product is resuspended in TE and stored at −20°C. (*Note:* To avoid damaging the UV transilluminator, after visualizing the band of interest and taking a photograph, transfer the gel to a gel-casting tray, place the tray on the transilluminator, and cut through the gel using a scalpel.)

A computer analysis of the −546/+971 sequence indicated the absence of *Bam*HI and *Xho*I sites. Therefore, the purified PCR product is sequentially digested with these enzymes since the primers are designed to yield a *Bam*HI cleavage site at the 5′ end of the PCR product and an *Xho*I cleavage site at the 3′ end. After incubation of the DNA with the enzyme at 37°C, the enzyme is inactivated by incubation at 65°C for 15 min and extracted twice with equal volumes of 1:1 mixture of Tris-saturated phenol and chloroform containing isoamyl alcohol. The DNA is extracted with chloroform–isoamyl alcohol and mixed with 1/10 volume of 3 *M* sodium acetate, pH 5.2. Two volumes of cold absolute ethanol (stored at −20°C) is added and vortexed. The mixture is incubated at −20°C for 45 min to 60 min, at −70°C for 15 to 30 min, or in a slurry of dry ice and ethanol for 5 to 10 min. The precipitated DNA is pelleted by centrifugation for 5–10 min. The pellet is washed with 70% (v/v) ethanol, dried in a Speed Vac, and resuspended in TE.

The PCR product digested with *Bam*HI and *Xho*I is ligated to pBLCAT3 vector upstream of CAT cDNA (25) into *Bam*HI and *Xho*I sites. The ligation reaction is carried out at 12°C, overnight, in a Biochiller 2000 in the presence of T₄ DNA ligase. The ligated DNA is used to transform competent HB101 or DH5α *Escherichia coli* (BRL Life Technologies) and streaked on LB plates containing 100 μg/ml ampicillin. The bacterial colonies are placed in 5 ml LB broth containing 100 μg/ml ampicillin in a sterile 15-ml stoppered tube and incubated overnight at 37°C at 250 rpm. Plasmid DNA is extracted using either TELT or the NaOH minipreparation technique (30).

The DNA is digested sequentially with *Bam*HI and *Xho*I and separated on an agarose gel to confirm cloning of the PCR product into pBLCAT3 vector (Fig. 2). Figure 2 indicates the results of separation of digested DNA

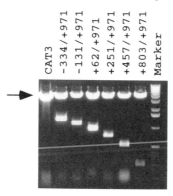

FIG. 2   Densimetric scan of an ethidium bromide-stained agarose gel. pBLCAT3 vector deletion constructs were digested sequentially with *Bam*HI and *Xho*I and separated on a 1.2% agarose gel in TAE buffer. The arrow indicates the vector at approximately 4.3 kb. The cloned products differed in size ranging from 1.3 kb (construct −334/+971) to 188 bp (+803/+971). The marker lane shows a kilobase DNA ladder from BRL Life Technologies.

on a 1.2% agarose gel. The top band in all the lanes is the vector (indicated by arrow) which is similar to the CAT3 vector in lane 1 (Fig. 2). The deletion products cloned into CAT3 vector differ from each other by approximately 200 bp ranging from 1.3 kb (construct −334/+971, Fig. 2) to 188 bp (−803/ +971).

DNA is prepared on a large scale using pZ523 columns and is used for further analysis of the 5′ flanking region including transfection of mammalian cells.

Site-Specific Mutagenesis

Deletion mutants of the 5′ flanking region of the AR gene are created as described above. PCR products are cloned into the pBLCAT3 vector and analyzed by transient transfection. These experiments suggest the presence of a suppressor element in the region −546 to −351. Computer analysis of this region revealed a putative suppressor sequence at −421/−448 (see Fig. 3). In order to determine whether the suppressor is functional, a site-specific mutagenesis technique is used to create an internal deletion of the 5′ flanking region.

With the advent of PCR technology, several methods for generating site-specific mutations have been reported. One of the earliest techniques reported for creating site-specific mutations was by Higuchi *et al.* (31). This method required two separate amplifications utilizing two mutant primers which are homologous to the sense and antisense strands. Using the 5′ flanking primer and antisense mutant primer, the 5′ end of the DNA is amplified including the region to be mutated. Similarly the 3′ end DNA is amplified using the 3′ end primer and sense strand mutant. The PCR products are used as templates for amplification using the 5′ and 3′ end primers. The amplified product, which includes the mutation, is cloned. Several variations of this technique have been reported (32–36).

In order to analyze the 5′ flanking region of the AR gene, the megaprimer technique (10) is used to create specific internal deletions of the putative suppressor. The 5′ end primer is complementary to the bottom strand and contains nucleotides corresponding to sequence −530 to −546, two restriction enzyme (*Bam*HI and *Pst*I) cleavage sites at the 5′ end, and 4 flanking nucleotides (Table I, oligonucleotide 1). Similarly the 3′ end primer (Table I, oligonucleotide 9) contains nucleotides corresponding to sequence +131 to +112, *Xho*I and *Xba*I sites, and 4 flanking nucleotides. The mutant primer is complementary to the bottom strand and consists of the sequence 5′ CTCCCTTCTGCTTGTCCTATACCTAAGAGCAATTGG 3′ (Table I, oli-

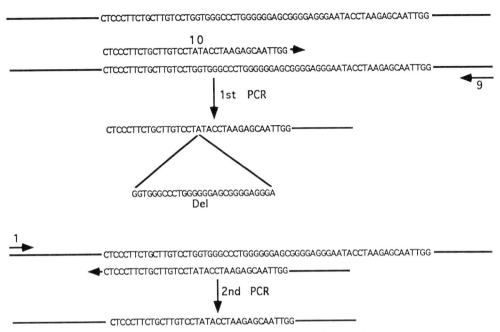

FIG. 3   Schematic representation of the use of megaprimer technique (10) to delete a putative suppressor element. Oligonucleotide 10, which was used as the 5′end primer, contained sequences corresponding to 18 nucleotides upstream of the putative suppressor and 18 nucleotides downstream of the putative suppressor. Oligonucleotide 9, which was used as 3′ end primer, contained 20 nucleotides corresponding to sequences +131 to +112, with restriction enzyme sites and 4 flanking nucleotides upstream. The sequence deleted in the first PCR has been shown as ''Del.'' The sequence −546 to +131 (without the sequence −421 to −448) was amplified by using the product of the first PCR as the 3′ end primer and oligonucleotide 1 (Table I) as the 5′ end primer. The template used for both the PCR reactions was −546 to +971.

gonucleotide 10). An oligonucleotide is synthesized in which the first 18 nucleotides (CTCCCTTCTGCTTGTCCT) are similar to the sequence on the 5′ end of the putative suppressor, and the second half of the oligonucleotide (ATACCTAAGAGCAATTGG) is similar to the sequence downstream of the putative suppressor. The first PCR reaction consists of 10 pmol each of the oligonucleotides 9 and 10 (Table I) and 1 ng of −546/+971 construct which is used as the template (Fig. 3). The PCR reaction is carried out in a 100-μl mixture for 30 cycles at 94°C (1 min), 55°C (2 min), and 72°C (3 min) using *Taq* or pfu polymerase. The PCR product is separated on a 1.2% (w/v) agarose gel. The band of interest is excised and purified using a Gene

Clean kit. The PCR product contains the sequence -403 to $+131$, but missing the sequence -421 to -448, which is deleted (Fig. 3, Del). The purified PCR product serves as a 3' end primer in the second PCR reaction wherein oligonucleotide 1 (Table I) is used as a 5' primer along with $-546/+971$ construct as the template. The second PCR product contains the sequences -546 to $+131$ without the putative suppressor (-421 to -448) (Fig. 3). The product of the second PCR is electrophoresed, and the band of interest is extracted and ligated into a pCRII vector. The ligation takes advantage of the activity of DNA polymerase wherein a single deoxyadenosine is added to the 3' end of the PCR product. This DNA could be used to clone into the pCRII vector which contains a single 3' T overhang. The ligated vector is transformed into One Shot competent *E. coli*. As the insert contains a *Bam*HI site at the 5' end and an *Xho*I site at the 3' end, the construct is sequentially digested with these two enzymes, separated on 1.2% agarose gel, and purified using a Gene Clean kit. The *Bam*HI–*Xho*I fragment is ligated into the same site of the pBLCAT3 vector. All the PCR-generated DNAs are sequenced using the fmol sequencing system to screen for possible mutations generated during PCR.

Summary

During the analysis of the 5' flanking region of the androgen receptor, we have used the PCR technique extensively to create mutations. The 5' and 3' end primers were designed to contain 16–17 nucleotides homologous to the template sequence, with restriction enzyme sites and flanking nucleotides upstream of the homologous sequences. Using these primers we have successfully created several nested deletions which were cloned into pBLCAT3 vectors and used in transient transfection analysis. On identification of a putative suppressor element we used the PCR megaprimer technique to delete a 28-bp sequence. The 5' end oligonucleotide contained 18 nucleotides corresponding to sequences upstream of the putative suppressor element and another 18 nucleotides corresponding to sequences downstream of the putative suppressor element. The putative suppressor element was deleted in two successive PCR reactions.

Acknowledgments

This research was supported by NIH Grants CA 32387, DK 47592, and HD 09140 (to DJT) and a grant from the American Foundation for Urologic Diseases in cooperation with The Connaught Foundation (to MVK). We also thank Mr. Mike Grossmann and Dr. Jonathan Lindzey for their help.

References

1. R. K. Saiki, S. Scharf, F. Faloona, K. Mullis, G. Horn, H. A. Erlich, and N. Arnheim, *Science* **230,** 1350 (1985).
2. R. K. Saiki, D. H. Gelfand, S. Stoffel, S. J. Scharf, R. Higuchi, G. T. Horn, K. B. Mullis, and H. A. Erlich, *Science* **239,** 487 (1988).
3. K. B. Mullis and F. Faloona, *in* "Methods in Enzymology" (R. Wu, ed.), Vol. 155, p. 335. Academic Press, Orlando, FL, 1987.
4. D. H. Jones and S. C. Winistorfer, *Nucleic Acids Res.* **20,** 595 (1992).
5. D. H. Jones and S. C. Winistorfer, *PCR Methods Appl.* **2,** 197 (1993).
6. L. Ugozzoli and R. B. Wallace, *Methods: Companion Methods Enzymol.* **2,** 42 (1991).
7. P. R. Mueller and B. Wold, *Methods: Companion Methods Enzymol.* **2,** 20 (1991).
8. R. M. Nelson and G. L. Long, *Anal. Biochem.* **180,** 147 (1989).
9. S. Bowman, J. A. Tischfield, and P. J. Stambrook, *Technique* **2,** 254 (1990).
10. G. Sarkar and S. S. Sommer, *BioTechniques* **8,** 404 (1990).
11. D. H. Jones and S. C. Winistorfer, *Methods: Companion Methods Enzymol.* **2,** 2 (1991).
12. L. -J. Zhao, Q. X. Zhang, and R. Padmanabhan, *in* "Methods in Enzymology" (R. Wu, ed.), Vol. 217, p. 218. Academic Press, San Diego 1993.
13. A. J. Evans and I. A. Hughes. *J. Clin. Endocrinol.* **23,** 567 (1985).
14. L. Chan, M. P. Johnson, and D. J. Tindall, *in* "Pediatric Endocrinology" (R. Collu, J. R. Ducharme, and H. Guyda, eds.), p. 81. Raven Press, New York, 1989.
15. W. W. Scott, *J. Urol.* **70,** 477 (1953).
16. J. W. White, *Ann. Surg.* **22,** 1 (1985).
17. A. T. Cabot, *Ann. Surg.* **24,** 265 (1986).
18. C. Chang, J. Kokontis, and S. Liao, *Proc. Natl. Acad. Sci. U. S. A.* **85,** 7211 (1988).
19. D. B. Lubahn, D. R. Joseph, P. M. Sullivan, H. F. Willard, F. S. French, and E. M. Wilson, *Science* **240,** 327 (1988).
20. J. -A. Tan, D. R. Joseph, V. E. Quarmby, D. B. Lubahn, M. Sar, R. E. Larson, F. S. French, and E. M. Wilson, *Mol. Endocrinol.* **2,** 1276 (1988).
21. W. W. He, L. M. Fisher, S. Sun, D. L. Bilhartz, X. Zhu, C. Y. -F. Young, D. B. Kelley, and D. J. Tindall, *Biochem. Biophys. Res. Commun.* **171,** 697 (1990).
22. M. Smith, *Annu. Rev. Genet.* **19,** 423 (1985).
23. C. A. Batt, Y. Cho, and A. C. Jamieson, *in* "Methods in Enzymology" (R. Wu, ed.), Vol. 217, p. 280. Academic Press, San Diego, 1993.
24. J. Messing, *in* "Methods in Enzymology" (R. Wu *et al.,* eds.), Vol. 101, p. 20. Academic Press, New York 1983.
25. B. Luckow and G. Schutz, *Nucleic Acids Res.* **15,** 5490 (1987).
26. R. F. Lathe, J. P. Lecocq, and R. Everett, *in* "Genetic Engineering" (R. Williamson, ed.), p. 1. Academic Press, New York, 1983.
27. S. Henikoff, *Gene* **28,** 351 (1984).
28. R. J. Legerski, J. L. Hodnett, and H. B. Gray, *Nucleic Acids Res.* **5,** 1445 (1978).
29. A. Laughon and M. Scott, *Nature (London)* **310,** 25 (1984).

30. F. M. Ausubel, R. Brent, R. E. Kingston, D. D. Moore, J. G. Seidman, J. A. Smith, and K. Struhl, "Current Protocols in Molecular Biology." Wiley (Interscience), New York, 1994.
31. R. Higuchi, B. Krummel, and R. K. Saiki, *Nucleic Acids Res.* **16,** 7351 (1988).
32. S. M. Ho, H. D. Hunt, R. M. Horton, J. K. Pullen, and L. R. Pease, *Gene* **77,** 51 (1989).
33. M. Kamman, J. Laufs, L. Schell, and B. Gronenborr, *Nucleic Acids Res.* **17,** 33 (1989).
34. S. E. Mole, R. D. Iggo, and D. P. Lane, *Nucleic Acids Res.* **17,** 3319 (1989).
35. J. Yon and M. Fried, *Nucleic Acids Res.* **17,** 4895 (1989).
36. S. Perrin and G. Gilliland, *Nucleic Acids Res.* **18,** 7433 (1990).

Section IX

Application of PCR in AIDS Research

[23] Detection of HIV-1 in Brain Tissue of Individuals with AIDS by *in Situ* Gene Amplification

Omar Bagasra and Roger J. Pomerantz

Molecular Mechanisms of HIV-1 Replication *in Vivo* and *in Vitro*

Human immunodeficiency virus type 1 (HIV-1) infects a variety of cell types in cell cultures and *in vivo* (1, 2). Two cell types which harbor HIV-1 *in vivo* are the CD4$^+$ T lymphocyte and the monocyte/macrophage (1, 2). Other cell types including microvascular endothelial cells and astrocytic glial cells may also be infected with HIV-1 *in vivo* (3–5). The CD4$^+$ lymphocyte appears to be the primary viral reservoir in the bloodstream, while the monocyte/macrophage may contain HIV-1 in solid tissues and may be the major, although not sole, focus of productive infection in the central nervous system (6–8). The monocyte/macrophage may, as well, be the first cell infected in the body (4) and act as a "Trojan Horse," concealing the virus from the immune system (1).

After internatlization, the viral core is uncoated, and the viral genome (which is RNA in nature) is transcribed into DNA by the activation of RNA-dependent DNA polymerase or reverse transcriptase (RT). This step requires RNA as a primer, RT, and two strands of HIV-1 RNA as template—all present in the viral core (9–11). Initially, RNA–DNA hybrids are formed. These hybrids are dissociated by the action of RNase H activity found in the RT. At this stage integration of HIV-1 dsDNA may not be necessary for its replication. Whether the sites of integration of HIV-1 dsDNA are random or specific is still unknown. A clinical latent phase may last from a few months to many years (9–11).

The control of HIV-1 replication involves the binding of a variety of HIV-1-encoded proteins and cellular factors, which primarily interact with long terminal repeats (LTR) in the 5′ end of the provirus (12). A viral-encoded transactivator of HIV-1 gene expression, Tat, binds to a section of RNA transcribed from the R region of the 5′ LTR, Tar, and dramatically stimulates LTR-directed transcription and, possibly, posttranscriptional events (12, 13). The HIV-1–LTR has a variety of well-described, and putative, motifs which bind cellular factors which then affect transcriptional efficiency. The HIV-1–LTR contains a TATA box, three GC-rich regions which bind the SP1 transcription factor, and two 11-base pair enhancer motifs which bind nuclear factor-κ B (NF-κB) (12, 14). Each of these regions has been demonstrated to affect HIV-1 replication significantly (12). Nuclear factor-κB, though, appears to be extremely important in the response of HIV-1 replication to a variety of exogenous stimuli (15–18). This transcription factor appears to be a family of proteins related to the *rel* oncogene and has been cloned (19, 20). Nuclear factor-κB is bound to a repressor protein, IκB, in the cytoplasm. After stimulation by a variety of agents, including phorbol esters, antigenic stimulation, tumor necrosis factor α (TNFα), and lipopolysaccharide (LPS), IκB is phosphorylated and dissociates from NF-κB (16–19, 21, 22). The unbound NF-κB then is transported to the nucleus where it binds to enhancer regions of a wide variety of viral and cellular genes, including HIV-1. The activation of NF-κB, which is extremely important but possibly not absolutely essential for HIV-1 replication (23), occurs via a variety of pathways which lead to IκB phosphorylation (22). The stimulation of the HIV-1–LTR by NF-κB has been demonstrated in a number of cellular systems (e.g., T lymphocyte and monocytic cell lines), using transient transfections of the HIV-1–LTR bound upstream of a reporter gene and through the use of HIV-1 latently infected cell lines (24–27). While phorbol esters and TNFα stimulate NF-κB activation and, thus, HIV-1 replication in T lymphocytic and monocytic cell lines, LPS has this effect only in monocytic lines (21). Interleukin 6 (IL-6) is another agent which has been demonstrated to augment HIV-1 replication only in monocyte/macrophages (28). Heterologous viral proteins, especially herpes simplex (HS) gene products, may also stimulate HIV-1–LTR-directed transcription by activating NF-κB (some directly and others via TNFα induction) and probably through other cellular intermediates (29). Other agents, such as granulocyte—macrophage colony-stimulating factor (GM-CSF), augment HIV-1 production via mechanisms not involving NF-κB (18). The HIV-1–LTR appears to be an extremely complex control region (30–34). Many of the HIV-1–LTR DNA-binding protein motifs appear to differentially interact in various cellular milieus. For example, the three SpI sites appear to be necessary for viral replication only if activated NF-κB is not present in a particular intracellular environment (35).

Viral-encoded proteins called the "*trans*-activating factor" *(tat)*, the "regulator of viral expression" *(rev)*, and a putative negative regulatory factor *(nef)* have been described (9–11, 36). The product of the *tat* gene, Tat protein, dramatically increases the expression of all genes expressed from HIV-1–LTR. Tat function requires the presence of a *cis*-acting target sequence and *trans*-acting response region or TAR, which is located downstream of the site of transcription initiation, between nucleotide +14 and +44 in the LTR. TAR function is both position- and orientation-dependent and requires the presence of an upstream promoter and enhancer (36). The 5' untranslated leader sequence transcribed from TAR is capable of forming a stable stem–loop structure, and mutations that change the sequences in the loop or disturb the stem structure greatly reduce *trans*-activation by Tat. These findings support the theory that TAR functions as an RNA target (36, 37). The *cis*-acting RNA target site for HIV-1 Tat is a 59-nucleotide RNA stem—loop structure located immediately proximal to the start site for viral mRNA transcription. Mutations that disturb the helical structure of the 27-nucleotide apical region of TAR, or that affect the pyrimidine-rich 3-nucleotide bulge, inhibit TAR function *in vivo* and also reduce the TAR–Tat interaction *in vitro*. On the contrary, mutation of the 6-nucleotide terminal loop of TAR has no measurable effect on the *in vitro* TAR–Tat interaction but significantly blocks TAR function *in vivo*. It has therefore been proposed that *trans*-activation of the HIV-1–LTR by Tat may require the specific interaction of not only Tat but also a cellular cofactor(s) with TAR (38).

The *tat* gene encodes a small 14-kDa protein that appears to be required for viral replication. Any condition that increases the levels of positive regulatory factors will enhance the level of transcription. For example, antigenic, mitogenic, and lymphokine-mediated cell activations are reported to activate dormant HIV-1. Similarly coinfection with other viruses [e.g., cytomegalovirus (CMV), Epstein–Barr virus (EBV), Herpes–Simplex virus (HSV), adenoviruses, papovaviruses, HBV, HTLV-1, and human herpes virus-6, all of which can activate HIV-1-LTR], also transactivates HIV-1 (41). The Tat protein may be taken up into infected cells *in vitro* and may enhance transcription of HIV-1 genes, apparently via TAR-mediated activation. Our laboratory has shown that in certain cells (e.g., glial cells), activation of HIV-1 can occur in TAR-negative or TAR-defective HIV-1 (40).

The *rev* gene acts on sequences found within the envelope gene of HIV-1. The *Tat* and *rev* genes are the first genes expressed at the breakdown phase of the latent stage and allow the expression of the structural genes of HIV-1 (9–11, 41, 41a, 42).

There is an expanding body of literature on the various complex and interdependent factors which control HIV-1 replication. Therefore, data have been reported which demonstrate that HIV-1 production can be stimulated by a variety of agents, the mechanisms of which lead to and maintain HIV-1 latency.

HIV-1 Latency and AIDS Dementia

The term "retroviral latency" is an imprecise term and various forms of latency may exist in cell cultures or *in vivo*. These forms of latency may occur at a variety of stages in the viral life cycle. A transient viral DNA intermediate has been described in unstimulated (i.e., without phytohemag-glutinin treatment) T lymphocytes after infection with HIV-1 (41). This was proposed to represent a form of latency prior to retroviral integration. Another model of HIV-1 latency has been described for the integrated provirus, using the U1 and ACH-2 cell lines as model systems (40). This form of HIV-1 proviral latency has been confirmed by other investigators (43) and has been demonstrated in other cell lines, including the well-differentiated monocyte/macrophage-like cell line, THP-1 (44). The virally encoded Rev protein, which rescues unspliced genomic HIV-1 RNA from the nucleus, appears to be involved in this model of proviral latency (40).

In discussing retroviral latency, one must also specifically define the level of viral expression required to be consistent with a functional definition of this term. Latency can be defined as a totally nonproductive infection or as a state with significantly lower levels of viral replication than the levels produced by the cell during maximum stimulation.

The study of HIV-1 infection and replication in the central nervous system (CNS) and its targeted cell types has been an active area of investigation since the beginning of the acquired immune deficiency syndrome (AIDS) epidemic. The AIDS dementia complex (ADC), characterized by various degrees of memory loss, ataxia, tremors, weakness, and dementia, affects over 60% of the patients with AIDS and pathological findings of HIV-1 infection of the CNS can be found in 90% of HIV-1-infected individuals at postmortem examination (45). The mechanisms involved are, as yet, poorly understood. This noninflammatory syndrome, characterized by microglial nodules (45), may be secondary to neurotoxins or (TNFα) secreted from HIV-1-infected microglial, neurotoxicity secondary to the HIV-1 envelope glycoprotein gp 120, or other factors (46–48). Importantly, the level of HIV-1 in the brain correlates with the degree of CNS dysfunction (49). Studies utilizing *in situ* hybridization and immunohistochemical techniques suggest that most productive HIV-1 infection in the CNS is in the monocyte/macrophage derivative, the microglia (3, 5, 7, 8, 50). These data do not address the hypothesis that other cell types (especially astrocytes) may be latently infected with HIV-1. Of particular note, murine retroviruses have been demonstrated to lead to abortive infection in spongiform CNS degeneration and are difficult to detect using standard methodologies (51). Small numbers of astrocytes and endothelial cells have been demonstrated to be infected with HIV-1 in earlier studies (3, 52). A study has demonstrated interleukin 6 production by astrocytes, *in vitro*, stimulates HIV-1 expression from latently infected monocytic cells and may thus play an indirect role, at least in part, in the development of ADC (53). It is also instructive to note that macrophage-tropic strains of HIV-1 have been cloned from the CNS and high levels of unintegrated HIV-1 DNA reside in CNS macrophage/microglial cells in infected individuals (54–56).

Astrocytic glial cell lines have been studied *in vitro* in relation to HIV-1 infection, as their role in ADC remains controversial. A variety of astrocytic glial cell lines (e.g., U373MG, U251MG, U138MG, U87MG) have been infected with HIV-1 in cell culture (57–60). Although some have been demonstrated to allow highly productive infection (60), many produce low levels of HIV-1 and may be latently infected, as demonstrated using PCR (61).

The concept of proviral latency in astrocytic glial cells is complex. Human fetal glial explants have been demonstrated to pass through an early phase of productive HIV-1 infection and then remain in a state of low-level persistent infection (62). Of note, the viral RNA expression patterns in these cells were not reported (62). As well, in a preliminary study, it was suggested that latent HIV-1 infection in astrocytic cells may be secondary to an increased expression of Nef (63). Nevertheless, in an important study, stable CD4 antigen transfections into neuroglioma cells led to high levels of HIV-1 expression in these cells (64). Thus, at least in some astrocytic lines, the spread and penetration of the virus within a culture may be a primary determinant of viral production.

Unlike microglial cells (65), most astrocytic glial cell lines are infected by HIV-1 in a CD4-independent manner (66–68). In addition, it remains controversial whether glial cell-tropic strains of HIV-1 exist (58, 59). As with many cell types which can be infected *in vitro* (e.g., CD8 lymphocytes, B lymphocytes, and fibroblasts), the precise documentation of HIV-1 infection of astrocytic glial cells *in vivo* requires further study (69). With few neuronal cells, apparently infected with HIV-1 *in vivo* (3, 52), although a novel receptor, galactosylceramide, has been demonstrated on neuronal and some glial cell lines (70), astrocytic glial cells remain an intriguing and critical area of investigation.

As such, studies of the molecular mechanisms of HIV-1 replication, and their possible *in vivo* correlations, in astrocytic glial cells will lead to a better understanding of both the increasingly complex cell-specific controls of HIV-1 virion production and the possible mechanisms of HIV-1-induced CNS disease states.

In Situ Polymerase Chain Reaction (IS-PCR) for Detection of HIV-1 in the Central Nervous System

The PCR (71) has proven a valuable tool for amplifying defined DNA sequences, even if they are available in only minute amounts, to obtain quantities which can be analyzed and/or sequenced. Using a variety of thermostable DNA polymerase enzymes (e.g., *Taq*, Vent, etc.), the PCR can quickly and efficiently amplify a genetic sequence utilizing an automated thermocycler (71). Thus genes or virus sequences (72, 73) present only in small samples of cells, or in a small fraction of cells in a heterogeneous population, can be traced. A specific area of study especially important for PCR has been in the area of HIV-1/AIDS research, as the actual percentage of HIV-1-infected cells in the peripheral blood has been subject of controversy (74, 75). Since HIV-1 was first described as the etiologic agent of AIDS (76), the number of cells infected *in vivo* with HIV-1 has been evaluated in patients in various clinical stages of disease (74). These studies have sought to correlate levels of HIV-1 infection with the pathogenesis and the clinical course of the disease. Various modifications of the PCR method have been used to assess quantitatively or semiquantitatively the relative frequencies of HIV-1-infected cells in peripheral blood mononuclear cells (PBMC), lymph nodes, and other cell types (76a, 77). One of the major drawbacks of the currently used standard DNA-PCR method is that the procedure does not allow the association of amplified signals of a specific genetic segment with the histological cell type(s). The ability to identify individual cells, carrying a specific gene(s) or a portion of a genetic element, under the microscope or by automated signal sensor [e.g., fluorescence activated cell sorter (FACS) or image analyzer] would be extremely useful in delineating various aspects of normal and pathological conditions. For example, this technique could be used in various leukemias and lymphomas, where specific aberrant gene sequences are associated with certain types of malignancy. As well, the HIV-1 virus has been demonstrated to infect $CD4^+$ lymphocytes, $CD8^+$ lymphocytes, monocytes, β lymphocytes, fibroblasts, and glial cells in cell culture (75, 78, 79). The ability to demonstrate nonproductive HIV-1 infection in differing cell types, *in vivo,* will be critical to the further understanding of HIV-1 pathogenesis.

Determination of HIV-1-Infected Cells before Development of *in Situ* PCR

In order to determine the percentage of PBMCs and lymph node cells infected with HIV-1, the initial studies of Haprer *et al.* (74) demonstrated that with the use of *in situ* hybridization for HIV-1-specific RNA, only 1 in 10,000 to 1 in 100,000 PBMC and lymph node cells could be identified as positive for HIV-1 *in vivo*. Of course, these findings did not rule out the possibility that HIV-1 may be present in a higher proportion of PBMC as a nonreplicating provirus. These data, though, made it difficult to understand how such a low number of HIV-1-infected cells could cause such a severe depletion of $CD4^+$ lymphocytes. Data from Lewis *et al.* (80) and Ho *et al.* (75) suggested that the number of PBMC-containing HIV-1-specific RNA is higher than initially demonstrated in patients infected with HIV-1 using limiting dilution assays. They showed that infectious HIV-1 can be isolated from an average of 1 in

400 PBMC obtained from patients with AIDS. Much higher levels were detected during acute seroconversion to HIV-1 by Darr and Clark *et al.* (81, 82). Schnittman *et al.* (77), using a combination of cell-sorting and quantitative DNA-PCR techniques, observed that in patients with AIDS, at least 1% of CD4$^+$ lymphocytes were infected with HIV-1. In asymptomatic persons seropositive for HIV-1, the range of CD4$^+$ lymphocytes harboring HIV-1 is broad (1 in 100 to 1 in 100,000). Hsia and Spector (83) using a "booster" PCR method, calculated that at least 10% of CD4$^+$ lymphocytes carry HIV-1 provirus in AIDS and symptomatic HIV-1 infection. Nevertheless, relatively lower proportions of CD4-positive lymphocytes are positive for the provirus in asymptomatic HIV-1 infection. Thus, *in situ* polymerase chain reaction (DNA-IS-PCR) for proviral sequences of HIV-1 is an important next step in precisely quantifying the proviral load in infected individuals.

Development of *in Situ* PCR Techniques

As noted above, a current limitations of PCR with isolated DNA is that the results of amplification cannot be directly associated with a specific cell type, nor can the percentage of cells that carry the target sequences be easily measured. Although the CD4$^+$ lymphocyte may be the primary reservoir of HIV-1 in the bloodstream (77), the monocyte–macrophage may be the principal reservoir in solid tissues (84). It is highly desirable to identify all cell types that carry the virus *in vivo,* as well as the cells that allow active replication of HIV-1. It would, therefore, be greatly advantageous if gene sequences could be amplified and traced *in situ* within intact cells. Other investigators have reported success in developing a DNA-IS-PCR method for the sheep lentivirus, visna, using cell suspensions (85, 86). Importantly, smears or tissue sections are readily available and are often stored for long periods, allowing reevaluation, whereas cell pellets or even viable frozen cells are rarely preserved for isolation of DNA. If it would be possible to perform the DNA-IS-PCR procedure directly on slides, visualization of altered or foreign DNA directly in the cells would allow morphological and cytochemical characterization of the cells containing the sequences in question, which would be especially helpful in heterogeneous cellular populations (85–88).

We have designed a procedure to apply the polymerase chain reaction to cell preparations on slides. We have demonstrated not only that it is possible to sufficiently amplify single-copy genes to be visualized by microscopy or microautoradiography, but also that this reaction is highly specific and allows cells containing defined gene sequences to be distinguished. It can be hypothesized that an intact fixed cell may function as a ultrasmall chamber for amplification. Once cells are heat-fixed and then permeabilized by paraform-aldehyde, and DNA-binding proteins are digested by proteinase K, the entrance of DNA polymerase, PCR primers, and other agents can be accomplished. It appears that in our DNA-IS-PCR method, after heat fixation, amplification products are retained by the nuclear and/or cytoplasmic membranes within the cell (89, 90).

The current standard DNA-PCR method in which one isolates DNA from many cells, usually 1 μg of DNA (or about 1.5×10^5 cells), for amplification, has several limitations. As stated above, one of the limitations of standard DNA-PCR is that, with isolated DNA, one cannot generally link the amplification signal to a specific cell type or easily quantify the percentage of cells which carry the target gene(s) or genetic sequence(s). One of the other main concerns of investigators, using the standard DNA-PCR method, is false-positive results due to contamination of samples by HIV-1-positive amplified genetic segments (73, 81). However, with the use of DNA-IS-PCR, such concerns are less significant. Using the DNA-IS-PCR, the intracellular DNA is amplified and remains localized in the intranuclear/intracellular areas. Therefore, even if a small fragment of DNA enters the cell, it probably will not contaminate nuclear DNA. Even in the worst case scenario, the contamination would only involve few cells instead of providing totally false-positive results as in the case of the standard DNA-PCR method, where amplified results are measured as absolute positive or negative results.

Studies of Retroviruses Using *in Situ* PCR

The technique of DNA-IS-PCR, which allows amplification of a specific DNA fragment within an intact cell, has many potentials. For example, it can be used in determining the actual peripheral blood or tissue proviral or viral load in various stages of many infections (e.g., cytomegalovirus, Epstein–Barr virus) and in evaluating the efficacy of various therapeutic interventions. One of its many potential uses is to determine the tumor load, especially in various human leukemias and lymphomas where selective chromosomal rearrangements and genetic alterations are known to be associated with a specific malignancy. In addition, early intracellular viral events, especially in the case of a retrovirus, can be quantified during the course of viral infections.

One of the important uses of the DNA-IS-PCR technique may thus be in evaluating retroviral entry and replication. Currently, there are several hypotheses regarding the early molecular events following HIV-1 entry into target cells. A hypothesis was forwarded to Zack *et al.* (91) who postulated that HIV-1 entry is unrestricted into CD4$^+$ T lymphocytes, but completion of reverse transcription and proviral integration is limited only to cells which are stimulated, whereas in nonstimulated primary T lymphocytes HIV-1 is not completely reverse-transcribed. This partial HIV-1 DNA intermediate can persist in these quiescent cells for a short period. In immortalized T lymphocytic cells lines a full-length HIV-1 provirus is reverse-transcribed but viral latency is regulated by temporal programming of HIV-1-specific RNA species (92). Bukrinsky *et al.* (93) have demonstrated full-length uninte-grated HIV-1 proviral DNA in unstimulated peripheral blood lymphocytes which integrate only after cellular activation. Utilizing various specific primer pairs and probes, studies are underway to investigate the molecular pathogen-esis of HIV-1 infection *in vivo*, using DNA-IS-PCR technology.

In Situ PCR Method

By adapting a modified PCR *in situ*, we have demonstrated the percentage of PBMC infected with HIV-1. In these experiments, the cells used are PBMC isolated from whole blood using Ficoll–Hypaque gradient centrifugation, as well as various cell lines. U1 (94) is a subclone of the monocytoid U937 cell (95), which is chronically infected with HIV-1 and carries two copies of integrated proviral HIV-1 per cell. The ACH-2 cell line (96) is a subclone of a variant of the CEM T lymphocyte cell line which carries a single copy of HIV-1 provirus per cell. SUP-T1/HIV-1 is a chronically infected derivative of the SUP-T1 cell line, a T lymphocytic cell line which expresses a very high density of CD4 antigen (97). To perform DNA-IS-PCR on glass slides (Fig. 1), cells (1×10^6 cells/ml) to be examined are seeded into the wells (1×10^5 cells per well) of specifically designed heavy Teflon-coated (HTC) slides and allowed to settle through sedimentation via gravity. Cells are fixed first on a heat block at 105°C for 90 sec and then in 2% paraformaldehyde for 1 hr or longer. Paraformaldehyde is inactivated by washing the slides with $3\times$ phosphate-buffered saline (PBS), and then endogenous peroxidase activity is removed by quenching the specimens with a 3% hydrogen peroxide overnight at 37°C. Then specimens are treated with proteinase K (1 μg/ml) for 2 hr at 55°C. Proteinase K is inactivated by placing the slides on a heat block at 96°C for 2 min and finally the slides are washed in distilled water and air-dried. The PCR reaction mixture, with T*aq* polymerase, is added to the top two wells of each slide. A PCR mixture lacking the primers is added to the bottom well. These slides are covered with coverslips, which are sealed with a clear nail polish. The slides are placed on an automatic ther-mocycler. The amplification is carried out at 94/45/72°C for 1 min for 30 cycles. After PCR, the slides are placed in 100% alcohol for 2 hr, the cov-erslips are removed, and the slides are washed with $2\times$ SSC. Amplification

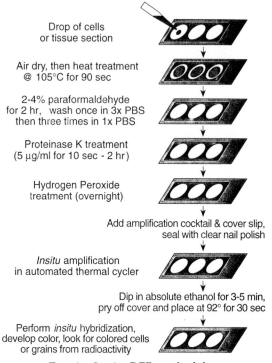

Drop of cells
or tissue section

Air dry, then heat treatment
@ 105°C for 90 sec

2-4% paraformaldehyde
for 2 hr, wash once in 3x PBS
then three times in 1x PBS

Proteinase K treatment
(5 µg/ml for 10 sec - 2 hr)

Hydrogen Peroxide
treatment (overnight)

Add amplification cocktail & cover slip,
seal with clear nail polish

In situ amplification
in automated thermal cycler

Dip in absolute ethanol for 3-5 min,
pry off cover and place at 92° for 30 sec

Perform *insitu* hybridization,
develop color, look for colored cells
or grains from radioactivity

FIG. 1   *In situ* PCR methodology.

products are detected by a biotinylated oligonucleotide according to the *in situ* hybridization method. For HIV-1, the primers and probe can be from various sections of the HIV-1 genome (89, 90). After hybridization the slides are thoroughly washed and then incubated with streptavidin–peroxidase complex for 1 hr at 37°C. After incubation, the color is developed with 3′-amino-9′-ethylene carbazole ((132-32) $C_{14}H_{14}N_2$) in the presence of 0.3% hydrogen peroxide in 50 mM acetate buffer. Positive staining cells, using biotinylated probes, stained brownish red, whereas negative cells usually appear colorless or slightly pink. Of note, these conditions of fixation and amplification corrected our initial problem with leakage of amplified products from cells. In addition, we have demonstrated similar results utilizing fluoresceinated and ^{32}P-labeled probes (89, 90).

The sensitivity of the DNA-IS-PCR technique was further tested with the ACH-2 and U1 cells. When ACH-2 and U1 cells were subjected to DNA-IS-PCR, all cells were positive at the same degree of intensity. When the ACH-2 cells were mixed in varying proportions with uninfected CEM cells, the results were those expected and no leakage of amplified products with contamination of uninfected cells was demonstrated (89, 90).

In addition, experiments using DNA-IS-PCR were conducted to evaluate the theoretical possibility that HIV-1 virions may encapsulate some proviral DNA, which could contaminate uninfected cells during DNA-IS-PCR. Cells from a productively HIV-1-infected T lymphocytic cell line SUP-T1 were mixed in various ratios with uninfected cells from a T lymphocytic cell line H9 (44), as the ACH-2 cells and uninfected CEM cells had been mixed, and the predicted ratios of infected to uninfected cells were observed after DNA-IS-PCR. Thus, if there was virion-associated proviral DNA, it did not contaminate HIV-1-negative cells during this procedure (89, 90).

These experiments demonstrate that *in situ* amplification can be accomplished in cell populations known to carry only one copy of the HIV-1 provirus per cell. This modification of gene amplification makes DNA-IS-PCR more sensitive than many standard PCR methods for examining DNA (76b, 77). The reason(s) for the unusually high sensitivity of the DNA-IS-PCR is not fully clear. It is possible that in the standard DNA-PCR one is diluting the positive genetic element in a sea of nucleic acids. As well, poorly described cellular factors may inhibit amplification (98). In addition, these data demonstrate that with this technique, amplified DNA does not leak out of infected cells and contaminate uninfected cells. In the other DNA-IS-PCR techniques, where signal leakage was described (89, 90), it usually manifests as nonspecific perimembranous staining. With our technique, such staining has not been observed.

Frequency of Peripheral Blood Mononuclear Cells Positive for HIV-1 Sequences Assessed by DNA-*in Situ* PCR

Using this DNA-IS-PCR technique, we reported the percentages of PBMC infected with HIV-1 (89). We demonstrated that relatively higher percentages of PBMC (10–15%) carry HIV-1 in infected individuals than those previously demonstrated by some other groups (74, 75). Our observation that the numbers of PBMC harboring HIV-1 provirus are significantly higher than the levels of infectious HIV-1 cells per mononuclear cell in coculture assays (75) suggest that some copies of the HIV-1 provirus may be either defective or maintained in cells that are not activated in cell cultures to produce virions. As such, the evaluation of proviral latency and defective viral genomes *in vivo* remains an important area in the study of the complex pathogenesis of HIV-1 infection. Certainly, as the sensitivity to detect HIV-1 *in vivo* has improved, the understanding of its molecular pathogenesis has continued to evolve. Several laboratories have independently confirmed our initial report that up to 13% of PBMC are infected in the late stages of HIV-1 infection (83, 88, 99, 100).

Utilizing our IS-PCR technique, we have demonstrated HIV-1 in low levels of peripheral blood monocytes (mean—1%) of HIV-1-infected individuals. Although tissue-bound macrophages, in HIV-1-infected persons, are known to harbor HIV-1 proviral DNA *in vivo,* whether peripheral blood monocytes contain provirus is quite controversial (84). Using the IS-PCR technique, we have now demonstrated HIV-1 provirus in 8 of the 11 HIV-1-infected subjects evaluated. Monocytes from 4 HIV-1-seronegative hosts were not positive for provirus. Of note, the morphology for the proviral positive cells in these preparations were classic for monocyte/macrophages (84).

To address further the issue of proviral-positive cells in PBMC of HIV-1-infected individuals, using IS-PCR, we have proceeded with subset analyses. Fluorescent-activated cell sorting could not be utilized as our IS-PCR requires nonfixed cells to be applied and heat-fixed to special slides and live HIV-1-infected cells cannot be used in most FACS equipment. As well, cell panning was inefficient and distorted cellular morphology. Nevertheless, we were able to utilize immunomagnetic bead separation to give highly specific separation of CD4$^+$ lymphocytes from other PBMC. Of note, mixing experiments using HIV-1-infected and uninfected Sup-T1 cells, as described for the initial studies (89, 90), utilizing CD4-immunomagnetic beads and IS-PCR, yielded expected results. Thus, leakage of amplified products was not a problem utilizing immunomagnetic beads prior to IS-PCR (specificity control). As well, IS-PCR could be used to evaluate cells after beads were dissociated or with beads still attached, as beads are easily distinguished from cells and did not alter the IS-PCR procedure (89, 90).

We evaluated PBMC from 42 HIV-1-infected individuals, using IS-PCR both before and after bead separation. These are different patients from those used in our initial studies. Seronegative controls were evaluated in all experiments. Importantly, the mean levels of HIV-1-positive unfractionated PBMC were similar in each stage of disease among patients in this series of experiments, as compared to the previous study (89). Only rare cells in the unbound fraction, using immunomagnetic beads for CD4, were positive (<1%) for HIV-1 by IS-PCR. These cells appeared to be morphologically monocytoid. Thus, this analysis agrees with previous studies (86, 88, 89, 100) that the major reservoir of HIV-1 in PBMC *in vivo,* with the exception of low levels in some monocyte populations, is the CD4$^+$ lymphocyte. The CD4$^+$ lymphocyte fraction revealed HIV-1-positive cells in the range of 0.2 to 69%. The mean levels of CD4$^+$ lymphocytes in stages 2 and 4 patients were statistically different (Student's *t* test: $p < 0.001$). All studies were done blinded and at least twice. Thus, these important new data further point to the utility of IS-PCR in the investigations of HIV-1 levels *in vivo* (101).

Detection of HIV-1 in Brain Tissues

As most standard techniques which determine HIV-1 infection of cells either are not sensitive enough (e.g., *in situ* hybridization and immunohistochemistry) to detect low productivity or latent infections or do not measure HIV-1 infection in specific intact cells (e.g., standard DNA-PCR), our laboratory has begun to evaluate brain tissue using our *in situ* PCR technique. Using brain tissue, obtained at Thomas Jefferson University, from two HIV-1-infected individuals with severe AIDS-dementia complex, we have preliminary data regarding HIV-1 infection of CNS cell types *in vivo*.

As demonstrated in Fig. 2, numerous CNS cells were demonstrated to be positive for HIV-1-specific DNA by *in situ* PCR. Brain tissue from an HIV-1-seronegative individual revealed no positively staining cells. Although methodological alterations are planned to allow better definition of cellular morphology, certain cells in these samples revealed a morphology which may be more consistent with astrocytes than monocyte/macrophages. These data are quite preliminary and require further study. Of note, though, the *in situ* PCR revealed a 100-fold higher level of HIV-1-positive CNS cells in this sample as compared to those from standard *in situ* hybridization. A similar level of HIV-1-infected cells has been demonstrated in a second patient with CNS lymphoma using *in situ* PCR (Fig 2).

These studies are analogous to our investigations of HIV-1 proviral-positive cells in peripheral blood. It is critical to note that immunohistochemistry measures only highly productive infections leading to high levels of viral protein expression, while standard *in situ* hybridization techniques measure HIV-1-specific RNA. As has been demonstrated in PBLs (88–90, 99, 100), using standard quantitative DNA-PCR and now using our *in situ* PCR technique, standard *in situ* hybridization grossly underestimates the number of HIV-1-infected cells. These findings may have significant implications for HIV-1 infection of the CNS. As such, our laboratory has begun to utilize the *in situ* PCR technique to investigate which cells in the CNS of individuals, in various clinical HIV-1 disease states, harbor the HIV-1 provirus.

Conclusions

The technique of DNA-IS-PCR allows a specific DNA fragment to be amplified within the intact cell. This technique has great potential for determining the actual proviral load in peripheral blood and CNS tissues at various stages of HIV-1 infection and for evaluating the efficacy of various therapeutic interventions. This technique should allow for the direct localization of other

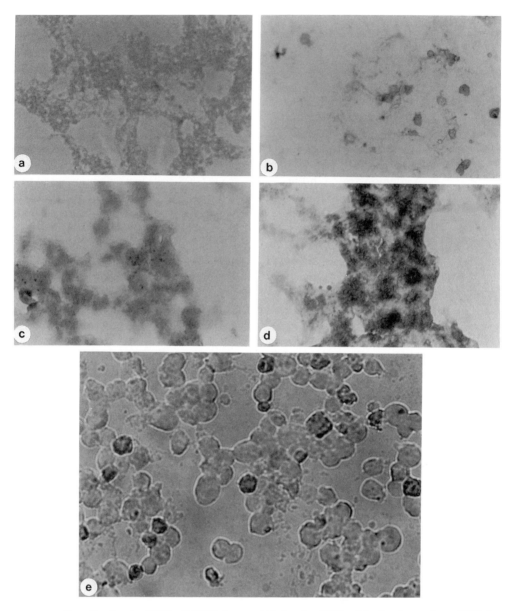

FIG. 2   *In situ* PCR of CNS tissue. (A) *In situ* PCR of brain tissue from HIV-1-seronegative individual. (Magnification: ×296). (B and C) *In situ* PCR of brain tissue from patient with AIDS dementia complex. (D) *In situ* PCR of brain tissue from a HIV-1-positive patient with CNS lymphoma. (E) Positive controls for IS-DNA-PCR: a 1:10 mixture of ACH-2 cells with CEM cells.

viruses and DNA sequences present in one to a few copies per cell. Although great strides have been made in the past few years, the technology of DNA-IS-PCR is clearly still in its infancy. Further modifications of this powerful technique will allow a continued increase in the sensitivity, specificity, and reproducibility of DNA-IS-PCR. Although a variety of genetic sequences, such as papillomavirus, cytomegalovirus, visna virus, HIV-1, HLA-DQα, and various cellular genes (98–100), have been studied using DNA-IS-PCR, unlimited others await investigation. Thus, DNA-IS-PCR should allow the study of various key aspects of disease pathogenesis, especially in infectious diseases and oncology.

Acknowledgments

The authors thank Drs. Gerald Nuovo and Ashley Haase for helpful discussions and Ms. Rita M. Victor for excellent secretarial assistance.

References

1. D. D. Ho, R. J. Pomerantz, and J. C. Kaplan, *N. Engl. J. Med.* **317,** 278 (1987).
2. A. S. Fauci, *Science* **239,** 617 (1988).
3. C. A. Wiley, R. D. Schrier, J. A. Nelson, P. W. Lampert, and M. B. A. Oldstone, *Proc. Natl. Acad. Sci. U.S.A.* **83,** 7089 (1986).
4. R. J. Pomerantz, S. M. de la Monte, S. P. Donegan, T. R. Rota, M. W. Vogt, D. E. Craven, and M. S. Hirsch, *Ann. Intern. Med.* **108,** 321 (1988).
5. D. H. Gabuzda, D. D. Ho, S. M. de la Monte, M. S. Hirsch, T. R. Rota, and R. A. Sobel, *Ann. Neurol.* **20,** 289 (1986).
6. S. M. Schnittman, M. C. Psallidopoulos, H. C., Lane, L. Thompson, M. Baseler, F. Massari, C. H. Fox, N. P. Salzman, and A. S. Fauci, *Science* **245,** 305 (1989).
7. S. Koenig, H. E. Gendelman, J. M. Orenstein, M. C. Dal Canto, G. H. Pezeshkpour, M. Yungbluth, F. Janotta, A. Aksamit, M. A. Martin, and A. S. Fauci, *Science* **233,** 1089 (1986)
8. S. Gartner, P. Markovits, D. Z. Markovitz, M. H. Kaplan, R. C. Gallo, and M. Popovic, *Science* **233,** 214 (1986).
9. A. S. Fauci, *Science* **239,** 617 (1988).
10. A. T. Haase, *Nature (London)* **322,** 130 (1986).
11. Y. N. Vanishar and F. Wong-Staal, *Annu. Rev. Biol.* **60,** 577 (1991).
12. B. R. Cullen and W. C. Greene, *Cell (Cambridge, Mass.)* **58,** 423 (1989).
13. P. A. Sharp and R. A. Marciniak, *Cell* **59,** 229 (1989).
14. K. A. Jones, J. T. Kadonaga, P. A. Luciw, and R. Tjian, *Science* **232,** 755 (1986).
15. M. J. Lenardo and D. Baltimore, *Cell (Cambridge, Mass.)* **58,** 227 (1989).
16. G. Nabel and D. Baltimore, *Nature (London)* **326,** 712 (1987).

17. E. J. Duh, W. J. Maury, T. M. Folks, A. S. Fauci, and A. B. Rabson, *Proc. Natl. Acad. Sci. U.S.A.* **86,** 5974 (1989).

18. L. Osborn, S. Kunkel, and G. J. Nabel, *Proc. Natl. Acad. Sci. U.S.A.* **86,** 2336 (1989).

19. M. Kieran, V. Blank, F. Logeat, J. Vandekerckhove, F. Lottspeich, O. LeBail, M. B. Urban, P. Kourilsky, P. A. Baeurle, and A. Israel, *Cell (Cambridge, Mass.)* **62,** 1007 (1990).

20. S. Gosh, A. M. Gifford, L. R. Riviere, P. Tempst, G. P. Nolan, and D. Baltimore, *Cell (Cambridge, Mass.)* **62,** 1019 (1990).

21. R. J. Pomerantz, M. B. Feinberg, D. Trono, and D. Baltimore, *J. Exp. Med.* **172,** 253 (1990).

22. S. Ghosh and D. Baltimore, *Nature (London)* **344,** 678 (1990).

23. J. Leonard, C. Parrott, A. J. Buckler-White, W. Turner, E. K. Ross, M. A. Martin, and A. B. Rabson, *J. Virol.* **63,** 4919 (1989).

24. T. Folks, J. Justement, A. Kinter, C. A. Dinarello, and A. S. Fauci, *Science* **238,** 800 (1987).

25. T. M. Folks, K. A. Clouse, J. Justement, A. Rabson, E. Duh, J. H. Kehrl, and A. S. Fauci, *Proc. Natl. Acad. Sci. U.S.A.* **86,** 2365 (1989).

26. K. A. Clouse, D. Powell, I. Washington, G. Poli, K. Strebel, W. Farrar, B. Barstad, J. Kovacs, A. S. Fauci, and T. M. Folks, *J. Immunol.* **142,** 431 (1989).

27. G. E. Griffin, K. Leung, T. M. Folks, S. Kunkel, and G. J. Nabel, *Nature (London)* **339,** 70 (1989).

28. W. Phares, B. Franza, and W. Herr, *J. Virol.* **66,** 1490 (1992).

29. J. M. Gimble, E. Duh, J. M. Ostrove, H. E. Gendelman, E. E. Max, and A. B. Rabson, *J. Virol.* **62,** 4104 (1988).

30. S. L. Zeichner, J. Y. H. Kim, and J. C. Alwine, *J. Virol.* **65,** 2436 (1991).

31. J. A. Garcia, F. K. Wu, R. Mitsuyasu, and R. B. Gaynor, *EMBO J.* **12,** 3761 (1987).

32. W. Foon, J. Garcia, R. Mitsuyasu, and R. Gaynor, *J. Virol.* **62,** 218 (1988).

33. D. Harrich, J. Garcia, F. Wu, R. Mitsuyasu, J. Gonzalez, and R. Gaynor, *J. Virol.* **63,** 2585 (1989).

34. C. Parrott, T. Seidner, E. Duh, J. Leonard, T. S. Theodore, A. Bukler-White, M. A. Martin, and A. B. Rabson, *J. Virol.* **65,** 1414 (1991).

35. E. K. Ross, A. J. Buckler-White, A. B. Rabson, G. Englund, and M. A. Martin, *J. Virol.* **65,** 4350 (1991).

36. K. Yeon-Soo and A. T. Panganiban, *J. Virol.* **67,** 3739 (1993).

37. R. J. Pomeratz, O. Bagasra, and D. Baltimore, *Cur. Opin. Immunol.* **4,** 475 (1993).

38. S. J. Madore and B. R. Cullen, *J. Virol.* **67,** 3703 (1993).

39. O. Bagasra, S. D. Wright, T. Seshamma, J. Oakes, and R. J. Pomerantz, *Proc. Natl. Acad. Sci. U.S.A.* **89,** 6285.

40. M. Roederer, F. J. T. Stall, P. A. Raju, S. W. Ela, and L. A. Herzenberg, *Proc. Natl. Acad. Sci. U.S.A.* **87,** 4884 (1990).

41. W. C. Green and B. R. Cullen, *Cell (Cambridge, Mass.)* **1,** 195 (1990).

41a. Y-S. Kim and R. Risser, *J. Virol.* **67,** 239 (1993).

42. M. H. Malin and B. R. Cullen, *Mol. Cell. Biol.* **13**, 6180, 1993.

43. A. L. Kinter, G. Poli, W. Maury, T. M. Folks, and A. S. Fauci, *J. Virol.* **64**, 4306 (1990).

44. J. A. Zack, S. J. Arrigo, S. R. Weitsman, A. S. Go, A. Haislip, and I. S. Y. Chen, *Cell (Cambridge, Mass.)* **61**, 213 (1990).

45. R. J. Pomerantz, D. Trono, M. B. Feinberg, and D. Baltimore, *Cell (Cambridge, Mass.)* **62**, 1271 (1990).

46. N. Michael, P. Morrow, J. Mosca, M. A. Vahey, D. S. Burke, and R. R. Redfield, *J. Virol.* **65**, 1291 (1991).

47. J. A. Mikovits, M. Raziuddin, M. Gona, M. Ruta, N. C. Lohrey, H. F. Kung, and F. W. Russetti, *J. Exp.Med.* **171**, 1705 (1990).

48. R. W. Price, B. Brew, J. Sidtis, M. Rosenblum, A. C. Scheck, and P. Cleary, *Science* **239**, 586 (1988).

49. D. Giulian, K. Vaca, and C. A. Noonan, *Science* **250**, 1593 (1990).

50. E. B. Dreyer, P. K. Kaiser, J. T. Offermann, and S. A. Lipton, *Science* **248**, 364 (1990).

51. J. Pulliam, B. G. Herndier, N. M. Tang, and M. S. McGrath, *J. Clin. Invest.* **87**, 503 (1991).

52. B. Weiser, N. Peress, D. La Neve, D. J. Eilbott, R. Seidman, and H. Burger, *Proc. Natl. Acad. Sci. U.S.A.* **87**, 3997 (1990).

53. B. A. Watkins, H. H. Dorn, W. B. Kelly, R. C. Armstrong, B. J. Potts, F. Michaels, C. V. Kufta, and M. Dubois-Dalcq, *Science* **249**, 549 (1990).

54. A. H. Sharpe. J. J. Hunter, P. Chassler, and R. Jaenisch, *Nature (London)* **246**, 181 (1990).

55. F. Gyorkey, J. L. Melnick, and P. Gyorkey, *J. Infect. Dis.* **155**, 870 (1987).

56. L. Vitkovic, G. P. Wood, E. O. Major, and A. S. Fauci, *AIDS Res. Hum. Retroviruses* **7**, 723 (1991).

57. S. Pang, Y. Koyanagi, S. Miles, C. Wiley, H. V. Vinters, and I. S. Y. Chen. *Nature (London)* **343**, 85 (1990).

58. Y. Koyanagi, S. Miles, R. T. Mitsuyasu, J. E. Merrill, H. V. Vinters, and I. S. Y. Chen, *Science* **236**, 819 (1987).

59. W. A. O'Brien, Y. Koyanagi, A. Namazie, J-Q. Zhao, A. Diagne, K. Idler, J. A. Zack, and I. S. Y. Chen, *Nature (London)* **348**, 69 (1990).

60. F. Chiodi, S. Fuerstenberg, M. Gidlund, B. Asjo, and E. M. Fenyo, *J. Virol.* **61**, 1244 (1987).

61. C. Cheng-Mayer, J. T. Rutka, M. L. Rosenblum, T. McHugh, D. P. Stites, and J. A. Levy, *Proc. Natl. Acad. Sci. U.S.A.* **84**, 3526 (1987).

62. S. Dewhurst, K. Sakai, J. Bresser, M. Stevenson, M. J. Evinger-Hodges, and D. J. Volsky, *J. Virol.* **61**, 3774 (1987).

63. S. Dewhurst, K. Sakai, X. H. Zhang, A. Wasiak, and D. J. Volsky, *J. Virol.* **62**, 151 (1988).

64. B. Keys, J. Albert, J. Kovamees, and F. Chiodi, *Virology* **183**, 834 (1991).

65. C. Tornatore, A. Nath, K. Amemiya, and E. O. Major, *J.Virol.* **65**, 6094 (1991).

66. R. Brack-Werner, A. Kleinschmidt, A. Ludvigsen, W. Mellert, M. Neumann, R. Herrmann, M. C. L. Khim, A. Burny, N. Muller-Lantzsch, D. Stavrou, and V. Erfle, *AIDS* **6**, 273 (1992).

67. B. Volsky, K. Sakai, M. M. Reddy, and D. J. Volsky, *Virology* **186,** 303 (1992).
68. S. Swingler, A. Easton, and A. Morris, *AIDS Res. Hum. Retroviruses* **8,** 487 (1992).
69. M. Shahabuddin, B. Volsky, H. Kim, K. Sakai, and D. Volsky, *Pathobiology* **60,** 195 (1992).
70. C. A. Jordan, B. A. Watkins, C. Kufta, and M. Dubois-Dalcq, *J. Virol.* **65,** 736 (1991).
71. J. Bell, *Immunol. Today* **10,** 351 (1989).
72. F. F. Chehab, X. Xiao, Y. W. Kan, and T. S. Yen, *Med. Pathol.* **2,** 75 (1989).
73. S. Kwok, M. A. Innis, D. H. Gelfand, J. J. Sninsky, T. J. White, and M. O. Troy, eds., ''PCR Protocols: A Guide to Methods and Applications'' *Academic Press,* San Diego, 1989.
74. M. E. Harper, L. M. Marselle, R. C. Gallo, and F. Wong-Staal, *Proc. Natl. Acad. Sci. U.S.A.* **83,** 772 (1986).
75. D. D. Ho, T. Moudgil, and M. Alam, *N. Engl. J. Med.* **321,** 1621 (1989).
76. Barre-Sinoussi, J. C. Chermann, F. Rey, et al., *Science* **220,** 868 (1983).
76a. G. H. Keller, D. P. Huang, and M. D. Manak, *Anal. Biochem.* **177,** 27 (1989).
77. S. M. Schnittman, M. C. Psallidopoulos, H. C. Lane, and A. S. Fauci, *Science* **245,** 305 (1989).
78. C. Cheng-Mayer, J. T. Rutka, M. L. Rosenblum, T. McHugh, D. P. Stites, and J. A. Levy, *Proc. Natl. Acad. Sci. U.S.A.* **84,** 3526 (1987).
79. L. Montagnier, J. Gruest, and S. Chamasret, *Science* **225,** 63 (1984).
80. D. E. Lewis, M. Minshall, N. P. Wray, S. W. Paddock, L. C. Smith, and M. M. Crane, *J. Infect. Dis.* **162,** 1373 (1990).
81. S. J. Clark, M. S. Saag, W. D. Decker, et al., *N. Engl. J. Med.* **324,** 954 (1991).
82. E. S. Daar. T. Moudgil, R. D. Meyer, and D. D. Ho, *N. Engl. J. Med.* **324,** 961 (1991).
83. K. Hsia and S. A. Spector, *J. Infect. Dis.* **164,** 470 (1991).
84. O. Bagasra and R. J. Pomerantz, *AIDS Res. Hum. Retroviruses.* **9,** 69 (1993).
85. A. T. Haase, E. F. Retzel, and K. A. Staskus, *Proc. Natl. Acad. Sci. U.S.A.* **87,** 4971 (1990).
86. K. A. Staskus, L. Couch, P. Herman, E. F. Retzel, M. Zupancic, J. List, and A. T. Haase, *Microb. Pathog.* **11,** 67 (1991).
87. G. J. Nuovo, F. Galley, R. Hom, P. MacConnell, S. Comite, and W. Bloch, *in* ''PCR Methods and Applications.'' **2,** 305 (1993).
88. G. J. Nuovo, P. MacConnell, A. Forde, and P. Delvenne, *Am. J. Pathol.* **139,** 847 (1991).
89. O. Bagasra, T. Seshamma, and R. J. Pomerantz, *J. Immunol. Methods* **158,** 131 (1993).
90. O. Bagasra, S. P. Hauptman, H. W. Lischner, M. Sachs, and R. J. Pomerantz, *N. Engl. J. Med.* **326,** 1385 (1992).
91. J. A. Zack, S. R. Weitsman, A. S. Go, A. Haislip, and I. S. Y. Chen, *Cell (Cambridge, Mass.)* **61,** 212 (1990)
92. S. Kim, R. Byrn, J. Groopman, and D. Baltimore, *J. Virol.* **63,** 3708 (1989).
93. M. I. Bukrinsky, T. L. Stanwick, M. P. Dempsey, and M. Stevenson, *Science* **254,** 423 (1991).

94. T. Folks, J. Justement, A. Kinter, C. A. Dinarello, and A. S. Fauci, *Science* **238,** 800 (1987).
95. C. Sundström and K. Nilsson, *Int. J. Cancer* **17,** 565 (1976).
96. K. A. Clouse, D. Powell, I. Washington, G. Poli, K. Strebel, W. Farrar, B. Burstad, J. Kovacs, A. S. Fauci, and T. M. Folks, *J. Immounol.* **142,** 431 (1989).
97. J. A. Hoxie, J. D. Alpers, J. L. Rackowsk, R. Huebner, B. S. Haggart, A. J. Cederbaum, and J. C. Reed, *Science* **234,** 1123 (1986).
98. J. P. Clewley, *J. Virol. Methods* **25,** 179 (1989).
99. J. Embretson, M. Zupancic, J. L. Ribas, A. Burke, P. Racz, K. Tenner-Racz, and A. T. Haase, *Nature (London)* **362,** 359 (1992).
100. B. K. Patterson, M. Till, P. Otto, C. Goolsby, M. R. Furtado, L. J. McBride, and S. M. Wolinsky, *Science* **260,** 976 (1993).
101. O. Bagasra, T. Seshamma, J. W. Oakes, and R. J. Pomerantz, *AIDS* **7,** 1419 (1993).

[24] Estimation of Genetic Heterogeneity in Primate T-Cell Lymphoma/Leukemia Viruses by PCR

D. K. Dube, S. Dube, M. P. Sherman, J. Love,
N. K. Saksena, W. J. Harrington, Jr., J. F. Ferrer,
L. Papsidero, L. Dyster, R. Yanagihara, A. E. Williams,
J. B. Glaser, V. M. A. Herve, F. Barre-Sinoussi,
B. S. Blumberg, and B. J. Poiesz

Introduction

The primate T-cell lymphoma/leukemia viruses (PTLV) are a subgroup of retroviruses, which includes human T-cell lymphoma/leukemia viruses types I and II (HTLV-I and HTLV-II) and simian T-cell leukemia virus (STLV-I) (1–3). HTLV-I is the etiologic agent of adult T-cell leukemia/lymphoma (ATL) (4), HTLV-I-associated myelopathy (HAM), and HTLV-I-associated polymyositis (5–9). HTLV-II has been detected and isolated in several patients with unusual T-cell neoplasias (2, 10–13). However, no specific malignancy has yet to be linked unequivocally with HTLV-II infection. We (14, 15) and others (16, 17) have reported the sole presence of HTLV-II in patients with a spastic ataxic illness similar to HTLV-I-associated myelopathy. STLV-I has been etiologically associated with lymphoid neoplastic diseases in monkeys (18–20). The PTLV are a group of plus-sense and single-stranded RNA-containing viruses. The PTLV and bovine leukemia virus (BLV), the etiologic agent of enzootic bovine leukemia (21), form an unnamed genus of retroviruses. One of the characteristics of these four type C viruses is the presence of a conserved epitope in their core proteins. This epitope is absent from all other retroviruses, including HIV-1 and HIV-2 (22). Furthermore, each of the members of this subgroup has in its genome a unique region (the *pX* gene) 3′ to the *env* gene which is absent from the genome of other C-type retroviruses. The *pX* gene encodes a protein, Tax, which transactivates viral and host genes and is thought to play an essential role in viral expression, replication, and pathogenicity (23, 24). In addition, the PTLV also possess a Rex protein coding region as well as some newly defined ORFs in the *pX* gene (25) (Fig. 1).

Methods in Neurosciences, Volume 26

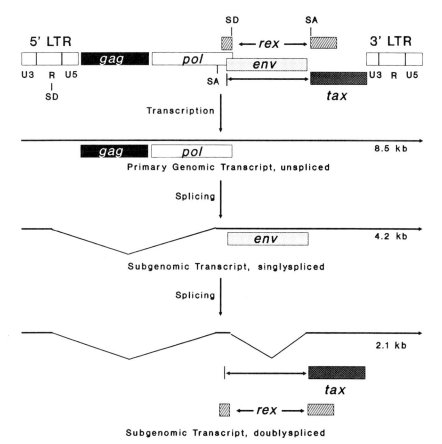

FIG. 1   HTLV-I proviral DNA structure with the respective genes and RNA transcripts shown. The gag and pol proteins are translated off of the primary unspliced RNA transcript. The env proteins are translated off of the singly spliced RNA and the regulatory proteins Tax and Rex are translated off of the smaller multiply spliced RNA.

Multiple isolates of each of the members of the PTLV have been characterized. The genomic diversity found among HTLV-I isolates from asymptomatic carriers and patients with ATL and HAM from throughout the world exhibits no correlation with disease, but, rather, depends on their geographic origin (26–29). A variant of HTLV-I has been discovered from isolated peoples of Melanesia (30). This variant of HTLV-I was found to be highly divergent from all previously known strains (31–33). Further sequence analyses of HTLV-I from Melanesia and those from Australian aborigines indicated that they are closely related to each other (34). Multiple variants of STLV-I are also well-established (20, 35, 36). Sequence analyses demonstrate that an STLV-I strain from an Indonesian pig-tailed monkey (*Macaca nemestrina*) is the most variable PTLV of all of the STLV-I and HTLV-I isolates characterized to date (37). We have reported a new STLV-I from a naturally infected tantalus monkey from Central Africa (35). Sequence analyses of its *LTR, gag, pol, env,* and *pX* (Orf II) genes indicated that this isolate, STLV-I (Tan 90), is 6% divergent from the prototype HTLV-I (ATK) and is the most divergent African STLV-I characterized to date (36).

The two original isolates of HTLV-II (MoT and NRA) were obtained from patients with atypical hairy cell leukemia and CD8$^+$ leukemia, respectively (2, 38). There are at least two major subtypes (A and B) of HTLV-II in the New World; the MoT isolate belongs to subtype A, while NRA belongs to subtype B (39, 40). The majority of North Americans infected with HTLV-II, including IVDU in whom the virus is endemic, are infected with subtype A (40). HTLV-II has also been found to be endemic among Amerindians (40–42) and sequence analyses of isolates obtained from Paleo-Amerindians, including the Seminole from Florida, the Guayami from Panama, and the Toba from Argentina, indicate that they belong to the B subtype (40–42). There have also been reports suggesting that HTLV-II may be endemic to Africa, although no sequence data were provided (43–45). An HTLV-II type A isolate has been identified in a Ghanian prostitute (46), but it is unclear whether this strain is endemic to Ghanians. So far, no STLV-II equivalent has been detected in Old World monkeys. However, the isolation of a virus, provisionally designated STLV-II, from a New World monkey has been reported (47).

Application of PCR for Epidemiological Studies and Phylogenetic Analyses

Epidemiological Studies

The technique of gene amplification by polymerase chain reaction (PCR) (48, 49) has revolutionized the fields of molecular biology and retrovirology because of its power to produce many copies of a desired, previously undetectable nucleic acid target. The initial identification and characterization of human retroviruses involved a long and laborious process that relied on the purification of growth factors and on reverse transcriptase (RT) assays which were relatively insensitive because these viruses are not very productive in their infected hosts (1, 2, 50). Since retroviruses are often in low copy number in an infected host, a PCR-based system was desirable not only to detect *in vivo* infections, but also to gain insights about viral pathogenesis and to characterize prototype, variant, and potential new retroviral isolates.

The use of PCR has allowed us, not only to detect rapidly and to distinguish between the different PTLV (7, 12, 14, 15, 32), but also to study their biology and to analyze many gene regions from multiple viral sources (28, 33, 35, 36, 40, 41, 51). We have detected HTLV-I proviral DNA sequences from fixed tissues of seropositive patients using PCR (29, 52, 53). We have also designed and used several primers to successfully amplify BLV from peripheral blood mononuclear cells (PBMCs) of infected cattle (54, 55). Further, we have been able to examine minute amounts of archival and prospective sera for the presence of PTLV nucleic acid by using sequential RNA and DNA-directed PCR (36, 55). Also, we have employed RNA-directed PCR (RT-PCR) to identify and characterize the negative strand or antisense RNA produced by HTLV-I *in vivo* or *ex vivo,* which is discussed in greater detail in Chapter 25 in this volume. Finally, we have elucidated the evolutionary relationships among members of the PTLV subgroup through the use of PCR by cloning and sequencing selected regions throughout the proviral genome (56).

Because of the importance of reverse transcription in the retroviral life cycle there are regions of highly conserved sequence within the *pol* gene of the PTLV. However, some regions of the *pol* gene of the PTLV are highly divergent also. The divergence between the entire *pol* sequences of prototypes HTLV-I and HTLV-II is 37%, very close to the variation found in the complete proviral DNA. For PCR amplification of the generic PTLV genome, the primer pair SK110 and SK111 was chosen from the very conserved regions of the *pol* gene (32, 40, 52). As a result, this primer pair can be used to amplify all PTLV genomes whose sequences are known to date (40, 56). However, the region of the *pol* gene flanked by SK110/SK111 is very interesting and unique. The generic detector oligonucleotide, SK115, can hybridize to any PTLV DNA amplified by SK110/SK111, whereas detector oligonucleotide SK112 can detect all HTLV-I and STLV-I, but not HTLV-II, and the detector SK188 can detect all HTLV-II but not HTLV-I and STLV-I (Fig. 2). We have also been successful in developing a rapid enzymatic nonisotopic detection system for SK110/SK111 products (57) (Fig. 3). Furthermore, HTLV-II can be subtyped by simply digesting the amplified DNA (SK110/SK111) with the restriction enzymes *Hin*fI and *Mse*I which specifically cleave the amplified DNA from the A and B subtypes, respectively (Fig. 4). Besides SK110/SK111, we employ a number of other primer pair and detector systems for the detection and diagnosis of PTLV infection. A list of such primer pairs are given in Table I.

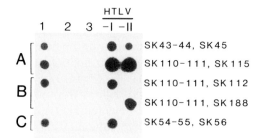

FIG. 2   Dot-blot DNA hybridization analyses of PCR-amplified DNA. Lane 1 is DNA from unknown patient. Lanes 2 and 3 are DNA from HTLV-I/II seronegative volunteer blood donors. Known HTLV-I- and HTLV-II-positive controls are shown. (STLV-I samples would give results similar to HTLV-I in these examples). The primer pair SK43/SK44 and probe SK45 can amplify and detect both HTLV-I and HTLV-II pX DNA. The primer pair SK54/SK55 and probe SK56 can detect HTLV-I *pol* DNA only. The primer pair SK110/SK111 amplifies both HTLV-I and HTLV-II *pol* DNA, which can be generically detected with the probe SK115. The probes SK112 and SK188 can specifically detect only HTLV-I or HTLV-II DNA, respectively, using the same primers. The unknown case in lane 1 types out as HTLV-I.

Phylogenetic Analysis

We mentioned above that virus-encoded reverse transcriptase is essential for the completion of the retroviral life cycle. Although evidence of multiple recombinations of *env* sequences among distantly related retroviruses exists, *pol* sequences have been shown to reflect their phylogenetic relationship

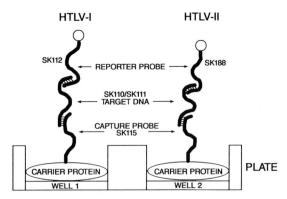

FIG. 3   A schematic illustrating the nonisotopic HTLV-I or HTLV-II EOA assays to detect *pol* sequences amplified with the primer pair SK110/SK111.

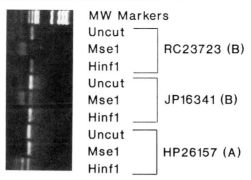

MW Markers
Uncut ⌐
Mse1   ⎤ RC23723 (B)
Hinf1 ⌐
Uncut ⌐
Mse1   ⎤ JP16341 (B)
Hinf1 ⌐
Uncut ⌐
Mse1   ⎤ HP26157 (A)
Hinf1 ⌐

FIG. 4 Ethidium bromide-stained gel of HTLV-II-positive DNA amplified with the primer pair SK110/SK111 with or without digestion with the restriction endonucleases *Mse*I, which digests HTLV-IIB sequences only, or *Hin*fI, which digests HTLV-IIA sequences only. As can be seen, this type of quick analysis can easily discriminate between an HTLV-II type A or B isolate.

more reliably (58). We have already established that DNA amplification by PCR with the primer pair SK110/SK111 [also call HTIIP (4735–4756)+/ HTIIP(4920–4897) −], which is homologous to a region conserved in the *pol* genes of all the PTLV and flanks a region of both conservation and variability, can be used to detect and analyze PTLV isolates for sequence diversity quickly. In fact, linear regression analyses of a comparison of individual percentage homology among published HTLV-I, HTLV-II, STLV-I, and other retroviral isolates over the complete genome or LTR sequences vs the sequences amplified by primer pair SK110/SK111 indicate that the sequence heterogeneity in the DNA flanked by this primer pair reflects the overall sequence diversity for the entire genome among all retroviruses including the PTLV (40) (Fig. 5). Hence, simply sequencing the 140 bp flanked by SK110/SK111 can allow for facile phylogenetic comparisons among the PTLV and other retroviruses.

We describe herein the detailed methods on the application of PCR to the detection, characterization, and phylogenetic analyses of prototype and variant PTLV.

Materials and Methods

Patient Samples

Peripheral blood samples are obtained from different HTLV-I and HTLV-II-infected humans and STLV-I-infected primates. Some of the patients are

TABLE I Generic and Specific Primer Pairs and Detectors for Amplification and Detection of PTLVs

Oligonucleotide and genomic location	Gene	Type	Sequences
HTIL (124–143) +	LTR	HTLV-I/primer	AAGGCTCTGACGTCTCCCCC
HTIL (797–775) −	LTR	HTLV-I/primer	ATCCCGGACGAGCCCCCAACTGT
HTIL (724–768) +	LTR	HTLV-I/detector	GGAGCCAGCGACAGCCCA TCCTATAGCACTCTCAGGAGAGAAATT
HTIIL (26–47) +	LTR	HTLV-II/primer	CCAGCCACCCAGGGCGAGTCAT
HTIIL (351–329) −	LTR	HTLV-II/primer	GTCTCCGTGACCAGAGGGTCGGT
HTIIL (257–278) +	LTR	HTLV-II/primer	TTGCCTAGTCAAAATAAAGAT
HTIIL (624–606)	LTR	HTLV-II/primer	CGGCGTTGAGGTTTCGTTT
HTIG (1215–1235) +	*gag*	HTLV-I/primer	CTGCAGTCATGCATCCACATGGTG
HTIG (1560–1537) −	*gag*	HTLV-I/primer	AGTTGCTGGTATTCTCGCCTTAAT
HTIG (1388–1411) +	*gag*	HTLV-I/detector	CTGCAGTACCTTTGCTCCTCCCTC
HTIIG (779–799) +	*gag*	HTLV-II/primer	GGGATTTGAATTCCTCCATCC
HTIIG (942–916) −	*gag*	HTLV-II/primer	GCTGCTGGAAGTCGAAATCGGAGGGCC
HTIIG (860–898) +	*gag*	HTLV-II/detector	GCTATCAACCCACCACTGGCTTAACTT TCTCCAGGCTGC
HTIP (4757–4778) +	*pol*	Generic/primer	CCCTACAATCCAACCAGCTCAG
HTIP (4942–4919) −	*pol*	Generic/primer	GTGGTGAAGCTGCCATCGGGTTTT
HTIP (4870–4895) +	*pol*	Generic/detector	CATAGCCCTATGGACAATCAACCACC
HTIP (4825–4850) +	*pol*	HTLV-I/detector	GTACTTTACTGACAAACCCGACCTAC
HTIIP (4735–4756) +	*pol*	Generic/primer	CCATACAACCCCACCAGCTCAG
HTIIP (4920–4897) −	*pol*	Generic/primer	GTGGTGGATTTGCCATCGGGTTTT
HTIIP (4848–4873) +	*pol*	Generic/detector	GAAAGCCCTTTGGACTCTCAATCAGC
HTIIP (4880–4898) +	*pol*	HTLV-II/detector	TCATGAACCCCAGTGGTAA
HTIpX (7358–7377) +	pX	Generic/primer	CGGATACCCAGTCTACGTGT
HTIpX (7516–7496) −	pX	Generic/primer	GAGCCGATAACGCGTCCATCG
HTIpX (7447–7486) +	pX	Generic/detector	ACGCCCTACTGGCCACCTGTCCAGA GCATCAGATCACCTG

infected with both HTLV-I and HTLV-II. Most patients enrolled in our study were from the metropolitan New York City and South Florida areas, but several other patients from throughout the United States were tested as well. Other patients were Toba and Mataco Indians who are descendants of the Guarani subgroup of South American Indians who inhabit the Gran Chaco tropical forest in Bolivia, Paraguay, and Argentina. Like the Guaymi Indians in Panama, the Toba and Mataco fled from the early European explorers. They lead a primitive lifestyle and show very little evidence of contact or genetic admixture with Europeans or Africans. Additional samples were obtained from Melanesians, including the very primitive and equally isolated Hagahai of Papua New Guinea (30). Finally, archival plasma samples from

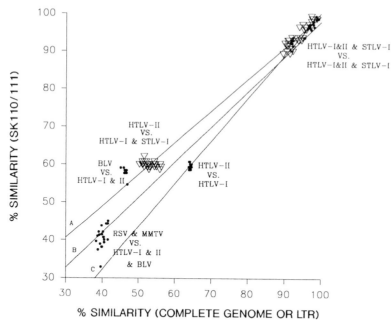

FIG. 5   Linear regression analyses comparing the percentage similarity of the 140-bp sequences flanked by primers SK110/SK111 with the percentage similarity of the complete genomes or LTR sequences of different PTLV isolates as well as BLV, Rous sarcoma virus (RSV), and mouse mammary tumor virus (MMTV) isolates. Line A ($r = 0.995$) compares the SK110/SK111 sequences to the LTR sequences of all of the PTLV (▼). Line B ($r = 0.973$) compares the SK110/SK111 sequences with the complete genomes of all of the isolates save for the STLV-I isolates for which no complete genomes are published (·). Line C ($r = 0.999$) compares the SK110/SK111 sequences and complete genomes of just the HTLV-I and HTLV-II sequences only (·). As can be seen, the BLV vs HTLV-I and HTLV-II comparisons are significantly above line B, while the HTLV-II vs HTLV-I comparisons are below line B. This suggests a possible recombination between BLV and HTLV-II sometime in the distant past, a fact that has also been noted by others (58) using different techniques.

Northeastern Zaire (55) were studied as well as blood samples from 14 species of wild nonhuman primates collected in Central and Western Africa (36).

Peripheral Blood Mononuclear Cells (PBMC)

Blood samples are obtained using heparin (10 U/ml) as the anticoagulant. Blood samples from different patients or animals are first screened for HTLV-

I/II antibodies using a whole viral antigen enzyme-linked immunosorbent assay (ELISA) (7). Seropositives are confirmed by Western blot analyses using USPHS criteria (59). After centrifugation on Ficoll–Hypaque PBM are washed twice in HBSS. DNA is extracted either directly from these cells or after they had been cultured. Cells from patients with HTLV-I are grown directly with phytohemagglutinin and interleukin-2 (1).

Extraction of DNA

Chromosomal DNA is isolated by sodium dodecyl sulfate (SDS)/proteinase K digestion of cells, followed by phenol and chloroform extraction as described earlier (40). DNA from cultured samples is dialyzed against $1\times$ TE through at least three changes of buffer. The concentration of DNA is determined spectrophotometrically. Alternatively, 10^6 PBM are directly lysed (52) by adding them to 25 μl of lysis solution A [100 mM KCI, 10 mM Tris (pH 8.3), and 2.5 mM MgCI$_2$]. Immediately prior to use lysis solution B is prepared [10 mM Tris (pH 8.3), 2.5 mM MgCI$_2$, 1% Tween-20, 1% nonidet P-40 (NP-40), and proteinase K (5 mg/ml)]. Twenty-five milliliters of solution B is then added to the cells in solution A and they are incubated for 1 hr at 60°C. The proteinase K is then inactivated by boiling the sample for 30 min. The sample is spun and the supernatant is decanted and used for subsequent PCR reaction.

Extraction of RNA

A total of 500 μl of plasma samples is centrifuged at 3000g for 2 min at 4°C. The precipitate is referred to as cryoprecipitate and has been found to inhibit subsequent PCR reactions. The supernatant is then centrifuged at 13,000g for 50 min. The supernatant is discarded and the RNA is extracted from the sediment containing virions using acid guanidinium thiocyanate–phenol/chloroform procedure as described earlier (60). The final RNA pellet is suspended in 24 μl of RNase-free, gene screen-filtered, deionized H$_2$O.

Protocols

Stock Solutions and Reagents for PCR and Hybridization

10× *Taq* Buffer   The final solution contains 0.5 M KCI in 0.1 M Tris–HCl (pH 8.3), sterilized through a 0.22-μm filter (Corning).

10× MgCI₂	0.25 *M*, filter-sterilized.
20× SSPE	Dissolve 174 g NaCI; 24 g NaH₂PO₄, and 7.4 g Na₂EDTA; adjust pH to 7.4 with NaOH; and bring the final volume to 1 liter.
1× TE	10 m*M* Tris–HCI (pH 7.5) containing 1 m*M* Na-EDTA. Filter through Genescreen Plus filter.
dNTP mix	dATP, dGTP, dCTP, and dUTP or dTTP are procured from Pharmacia LKB Biotechnology (Piscataway, NJ) as 100 m*M* stocks. Mix 30 μl of each of the four dNTPs and bring the volume to 1 ml with sterile nuclease-free water. The final concentration of each of the dNTPs in the mixture is 3.0 m*M*.
Amplification primers	Prepare 10 μ*M* solution (10 pmol/μl) for each of the primers to be used for amplification with high-quality sterile water.
Denaturation solution	0.5 *M* NaOH containing 1.5 *M* NaCI.
Neutralizing solution	0.5 *M* Tris–HCI (pH 7.5) containing 1.5 *M* NaCI.
Hybridization solution	Mix the following solutions: 5 ml formamide (Sigma Chemical Co. St. Louis, MO) 2 ml of 5 *M* NaCI 2 ml of 50% dextran sulfate 500 μl of 20% SDS 250 μl of salmon testes DNA (2 mg/ml) sonicated and denatured (Sigma Chemical Co.) 250 μl of H₂O
10× TBE	Total volume 10 ml 108 g Trizma base 55 g boric acid 9.3 g Na₂ EDTA
Reverse transcriptase	Moloney murine leukemia virus reverse transcriptase (M-MLV RT) (GIBCO/BRL, Life Technologies, Inc. Gaithersburg, MD)
Taq DNA polymerase	Roche Molecular Systems.
10x RT reaction buffer	500 m*M* Tris–HCI (pH 8.3); 750 m*M* KCI; 100 mM DTT; 30 m*M* MgCI₂; and 6 m*M* each of dGTP, dATP, dCTP and dTTP

PCR Setup

This procedure outlines the methods for the amplification of HTLV-I and HTLV-II proviral DNA isolated from the fresh PBM as well as from cultured cells. The conditions were optimized for a variety of primer pairs as listed in Table I.

1. In a 0.5-ml microfuge tube, add 1 μg of DNA and bring to a volume of 50 μl with nuclease-free water.
2. Add 50 μl of reaction cocktail containing following:

   10 μl of *Taq* buffer
   10 μl of MgCI$_2$ (0.025 M)
   10 pmol of upstream primer
   10 pmol of downstream primer
   17.0 μg bovine serum albumin (BSA)
   6 μl of dNTP solution
   2.0 units of *Taq* polymerase
   Nuclease-free H$_2$O to a final volume of 50 μl

Close the caps of the tubes and microfuge very briefly

3. Add 75 μl of light mineral oil slowly to each of the tubes.
4. Place the tubes in a thermocycler (Perkin–Elmer Cetus, Norwalk, CT).

Cycle as follows.

   Denature at 94°C for 30 sec
   Anneal at 54°C for 30 sec
   Extend at 68°C for 30 sec (or 60 sec if the size of the amplified DNA is larger than 400 bp)

Samples are amplfied for 30–60 cycles. At the completion of the cycles, the DNA is extended for an additional 10 min at 68°C. If the samples are treated with uracil glycosylase prior to amplification for sterilizing carryover DNA(61), the tubes in the thermocycler must be held at 72°C after completion of the desired cycles. Alternatively, 100 μl chloroform–isoamyl alcohol (24 : 1,v/v) (CIAA) must be added to each of the tubes immediately after completion of amplification. Otherwise, the uracil glycosylase, which can survive the brief thermal denaturation steps, will digest the amplified DNA containing dUMP. Uracil glycosylase is not active at 72°C. Hence, the amplified DNA can be preserved at 72°C if the soak temperature in the thermocycler is set at this temperature. The chloroform–isoamyl alcohol mixture denatures the uracil glycosylase.

Reverse Transcriptase PCR Assay

The RT-PCR assay is performed as published previously (62). Viral RNA is transcribed to cDNA using M-M uLV RT (GIBCO, BRL). Twelve microliters of RNA sample in a 1.5-ml microfuge tube is first heated at 93°C for 3 min and is put into an ice bucket for 2 min. The tube containing RNA is microfuged briefly. Eighteen microliters of RT reaction mixture is added to the tube. The total 30-μl reaction mixture is incubated first at 55°C for 5 min and subsequently at 42°C for 20 min. Seventy microliters of PCR reaction mix is added to the RT reaction mixture. The final concentration of the PCR reaction mixture is 10 mM Tris–HCl (pH 8.3), 2.5 mM MgCl$_2$, 50 mM KCl, 180 μM of each dNTP (in PCR reaction mix dUTP is used instead of dTTP), 20 pmol each of the primer pair SK110 and SK111, and 3 units of recombinant *Taq* polymerase. Two drops of mineral oil (Sigma) are layered over the mixture. Amplification is carried out for 30–60 cycles. The program we use for such an amplification is as follows:

1. One cycle: 5 min at 68°C,
2. Two cycles: 2 min at 94°C, 0.5 min at 53°C, and 0.5 min at 60°C,
3. 30–60 cycles: 0.66 min at 94°C, 0.5 min at 53°C, and 0.5 min at 68°C.

Detection of Amplified DNA by Liquid, Southern Blot, or Enzyme Oligonucleotide Assay Hybridization

Liquid Hybridization

This is a procedure whereby a ^{32}P end-labeled oligonucleotide detector hybridizes in solution to one of the two strands of the amplified DNA. The hybrid is separated from the unhybridized ^{32}P-labeled oligonucleotides by SDS–polyacrylamide gel electrophoresis (PAGE) and is finally autoradiographed. The directions of this procedure are as follows:

1. 150-μl of chloroform–isoamyl alcohol mixture (24 : 1 is added to each of the tubes. The tubes re shaken vigorously. The tubes are then allowed to set until three layers are visible. The upper thin layer is the mineral oil. The bottom heavy layer is the organic layer, whereas the amplified DNA remains in the middle aqueous layer as a bubble.

2. 30 μl of the DNA-containing aqueous layer is taken out carefully and is placed in a 0.5-ml liquid hybridization mix containing ^{32}P-labeled oligonucleotide probe (250,000 cpm).

3. The mixture is heated in a boiling water bath for 5 min and then incubated at 55°C for 30 min.

4. 5 µl (1/10th volume) of gel-loading dye is added to each of the tubes.

5. The samples are then loaded on a 8% SDS-polyacrylamide gel. The electrophoresis is carried out at 200 V using 1x TBE as running buffer until the bromophenol blue dye approaches the bottom of the gel (approximately 60 min).

6. After the run is over, one of the two glass plates is taken off and the gel is blotted with tissue. Finally, the gel on the top of the second glass plate is wrapped with Saran wrap and is exposed to the X-ray film (Kodak Rochester, NY XAR-5) for 2 hr (or even overnight) at room temperature.

Southern Blot Analysis

As an alternative to liquid hybridization, Southern blot analysis is carried out to analyze amplified DNA. By Southern blot analysis one can accurately estimate the size of the amplified DNA. Hence, it is an advantage over liquid hybridization. The following procedures are followed:

1. 18 µl of the aqueous layer containing amplified DNA is taken in a 0.5-ml Eppendorf tube and 2 µl of 10x loading dye is added to it.

2. The samples are then loaded into 1.5% agarose gel in 1x TBE.

3. In one of the wells, we always load 1 µg of marker DNA (100 bp ladder from GIBCO/BRL).

4. Electrophoresis is carried out at 100 V. The gel is stained first with ethidium bromide (1 µg/ml) for 15 min and is subsequently destained for 15 min in distilled water.

5. A photograph of the gel is taken using a Polaroid camera (Fotodyne) on a UV transilluminator.

6. The gel is then soaked in 0.4 M NaOH solution for 15 min. The DNA is transferred onto Genescreen Plus nylon filter following the standard protocol overnight. The filter is washed with 2x SSPE and dried following the manufacturer's protocol.

7. Prehybridization is carried out for 2 hr at 42°C in 5–10 ml of hyb/prehyb buffer. The ^{32}P-labeled oligonucleotide probe (containing 10^6 cpm) is added and the hybridization is carried out at 42°C overnight. The blots are washed with 2x SSPE containing 0.5% SDS at 55°C for 10 min. The washing is repeated two or three times. The filters are then wrapped with Saran wrap and exposed to an X-ray film in a cassette with intensifying screen at −70°C.

Enzyme Oligonucleotide Assay (EOA)

Analysis of PCR-amplified material is carried out using Gene Detective HTLV-I and HTLV-II *pol* EOA kits (Cellular Products, Inc., Buffalo, NY)(57). Briefly, the DNA samples are heat-denatured and then simultaneously hybridized to a solid-phase capture probe (SK 115) and a solution-phase reporter probe (either SK 112 or SK 188). Following hybridization at 37°C for 75 to 90 min, the microwells are washed, strepavidin-conjugated alkaline phosphatase is added, and, after washing again, substrate (*p*-nitrophenyl phosphate) is added to each well for 2 hr. Then the absorbance at 405 nm is determined for each microwell. A reactive threshold value (RTV) for each experiment is determined by adding 0.075 OD_{405} units to the means optical density of the negative control wells. A sample whose OD_{405} is greater than or equal to the RTV is considered reactive.

Cloning and Sequencing of Amplified DNA

The linker sequence 5' ACAGGTACCTGCAGATCTAGA 3', which contains *Kpn*I and *Bam*HI sites, and 5' TACGAGCTCGCGAATTCATGA 3', which contains *Sst*I and *Eco*RI sites, are synthesized at the 5' ends of the positive- and negative-strand primers, respectively (32). The amplified DNA is digested with *Sst*I and *Kpn*I enzymes and is then ligated to the M13mp18 vector digested with the same enzymes as described elsewhere (32, 35, 40). The ligated DNA is used to transfect *Escherichia coli* DH5αF' by standard protocols and plated with isopropyl-β-D-thiogalactopyranoside (IPTG) and (5'-bromo-4-chloro-3-indoyl-β-D-galactopyranoside (X-Gal). In the instances in which dUMP is incorporated into PCR products, *E. coli* KT8052, which does not produce uracil *N*-glycosidase, is utilized (63). Alternatively, the amplified double-stranded DNA is ligated to the plasmid vector of the TA cloning system (Invitrogen Corp., Omar, UT) (33). Selection of the clones is carried out by plaque hybridization using ³²P-labeled probe as described earlier (40). Single-stranded DNA template is prepared and used for nucleotide sequencing using the dideoxy chain termination technique (64). For double-stranded DNA sequencing, DNA template is prepared by a method described elsewhere (65).

Sequence Alignment and Dendogram Analyses

The use of nonviral, nonhuman linker sequences at the 5' end of the primers has another feature besides facilitating cloning. It allows us to mark the ends of all amplified DNA is our laboratory with these "signature" sequences, enabling us to detect the presence of small amounts of contaminating amplified DNA using "signature" nonviral, nonhuman primers complementary to the terminal linker sequences (66). The nucleotide sequences of the 140-bp PTLV DNA amplified by primer-pair SK110/SK111 were aligned and compared to each other (67, 68) (Fig. 6). The PAUP program (69) was used

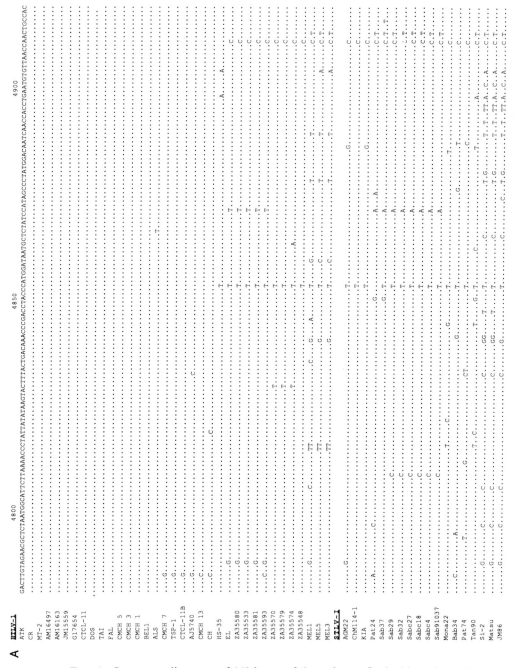

FIG. 6 Sequence alignment of 140 bases of the *pol* gene flanked by primers SK110 and SK111 from various PTLV isolates. Conserved bases are indicated by a (·). Prototype sequences for HTLV-I (A) and HTLV-II (B) are shown.

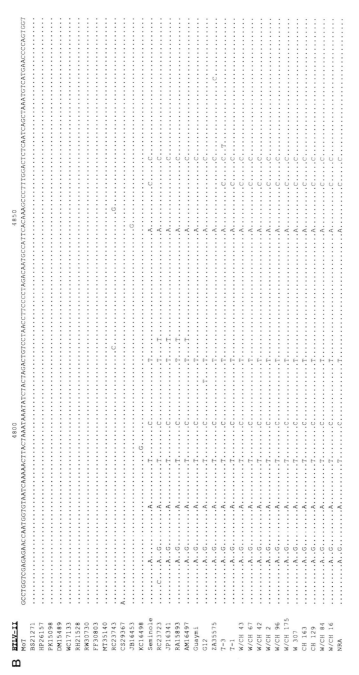

Fig. 6   (continued)

to compare new and previously published BLV, HTLV-I, STLV-I, and HTLV-II *pol* sequences (4, 10, 32, 35, 36, 40–42, 46, 55, 70–75). Dendrograms were constructed to delineate the evolutionary relationships among these different virus isolates (Fig. 7). Bootstrap (76) estimation of phylogenetic variability using 20 replications was performed on the trees generated by the PAUP program, and a consensus tree indicating the most likely branch points among the PTLV was generated. Furthermore, in order to evaluate the relative rate (40) of divergence of the *pol* sequences among various PTLV, three comparisons were made. First, the divergence between all HTLV-I and STLV-I isolates and BLV was compared with the divergence of all HTLV-II isolates and BLV. Second, the rate of divergence of the two HTLV-II substrains from BLV was determined. Finally, the rate of divergence of the two HTLV-II substrains from all HTLV-I and STLV-I isolates was determined. Statistical analyses were performed by the χ^2 technique.

Results and Conclusions

Polymerase chain reaction using the primer pair SK110/SK111 has proven to be a sensitive and specific means to detect PTLV infection. We have utilized this technique to diagnose thousands of PTLV infections from human and nonhuman samples worldwide. We have been able to detect all of the substrains of HTLV-I, STLV-I, and HTLV-II represented in Fig. 7 using this assay. However, in order to achieve close to 100% sensitivity using PBMC, we have had to use an input of up to 4 μg of DNA and to perform 45 cycles of PCR. This fact is probably due to the presence of inhibitors of PCR present in some samples, the presence of degeneracies in the SK110 or SK111 sequences of some isolates, and the relativity low copy number of PTLV proviral DNA *in vivo*. The sensitivity of the technique decreases when paraffin-embedded fixed tissue is used, often requiring multiple attempts on the same sample. The detection rate of sequential RNA and DNA-directed PCR on material pelleted from plasma approximates 50%, presumably because of the low level of expression of the PTLV relative to human immunodeficiency virus, which we can detect close to 100% of the time using the same format. We have noted no difference in sensitivity using the liquid hybridization, Southern blot, or nonisotopic solid-phase EOA detection format, with the latter being more convenient and less expensive.

Historically, the exquisite sensitivity of PCR has made it extremely susceptible to false-positives due to contamination of amplified material. We have obviated this by absolute separation of pre- and post-PCR personnel, rooms, and reagents and, also, by using dUTP in our amplification system and

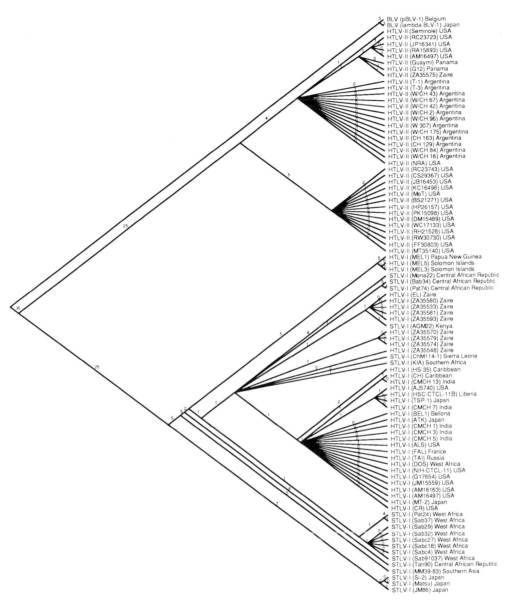

FIG. 7   A cladogram showing the phylogenetic relationships among the 140 bp of the *pol* gene flanked by SK110/SK111 of various PTLV isolates compared to two BLV isolates used as an outgroup. The country of origin of each isolate and the number of common base changes on each branch are shown.

performing sterilization with uracil-N-glycosylase (UNG) prior to PCR. We can validate the integrity of our results by performing PCR using "signature primers" to detect the presence of PCR "carryover" and ultimately by sequencing the amplified products.

Polymerase chain reaction has also increased the efficiency of sequence analyses of the PTLV. We are currently utilizing a system of overlapping primer pairs to amplify, clone, and sequence contiguous portions of the entire genomes of representative isolates of the major substrains of the PTLV. However, as is illustrated in Fig. 5, the 140 bases flanked by the primers SK110/SK111 can reliably predict the genetic relationships among the entire genomes of the PTLV. Hence, a considerable amount of molecular epidemiological information can be gleaned from phylograms comparing the *pol* sequences amplified by SK110/SK111. As can be seen (Fig. 7), the PTLV diverged from the ancestor to modern BLV a long time ago with the HTLV-I/STLV-I subgroup separating from the HTLV-II subgroup a considerable time later. There are two major substrains of HTLV-II (A and B) one of which (B) is endemic to the Paleo Amerindians of North, Central, and South America.

The type B substrain is also found in nonnative Americans as well as a Zairean patient. The close homology of these latter HTLV-II isolates to those found in the isolated groups of Central and South America suggests that it has been recently disseminated into other racial groups around the World. The endemic racial group for the type A HTLV-II isolates is uncertain at this time. The HTLV-I/STLV-I phylogram is perhaps more complex but separates into roughly two major substrains Asian/Austronesian and African. In modern time it is predominantly the West African HTLV-I substrain that has been desseminated around the world.

There are no significant differences in the rate of divergence to BLV between the HTLV-I/STLV-I isolates and the HTLV-II isolates and the rate of divergence to HTLV-I/STLV-I between the two HTLV-II substrains. These facts indicate that the rate of mutation among the PTLV has remained relatively constant over time and that genetic distances between them are linear with respect to time. Hence, given the long periods of separation between the endemic human and nonhuman hosts represented in Fig. 7, the PTLV were introduced into human and nonhuman primates many millenia ago and/or multiple times over the past 60,000 years. It is entirely possible that, rather than one single introduction into primates, multiple transmissions of variant BLV strains from different animals sources (e.g., bovids or ungulates) have occurred in the past. Also, when one examines the HTLV-I and STLV-I sequences it is quite clear that they do not cluster according to host species, indicating that a considerable amount of cross species transmission has occurred even up until the recent past.

The diversity among the HTLV-I/STLV-I isolates is much greater than that among the HTLV-II isolates, indicating that the HTLV-I/STLV-I strain has either been in primates for a longer period of time or not enough HTLV-II isolates have been examined. In fact, given the apparent equivalent mutation rates among the PTLV and assuming that their natural hosts are not extinct, it would seem probable that more extensive analyses of bovid and primate samples should yield a more diverse phylogram for both BLV and HTLV-II.

To date, it is somewhat uncertain as to whether the incidence of PTLV-associated diseases differs with respect to viral or host genetics. Clearly there is a difference between HTLV-I/STLV-I and HTLV-II. Presumably, there could be clinically relevant differences among the substrains of a particular viral strain or if a particular viral substrain endemic to one genetic host group (e.g., Melanesians or Toba Indians) was introduced into a new genetic strain of humans (e.g., Europeans) in whom the virus is not endemic. Only careful clinical trials with well-characterized isolates can resolve these issues. The use of PCR-based detection and characterization formats should facilitate such prospective studies.

References

1. B. J. Poiesz, F. H. Ruscetti, A. F. Gazdar, P. A. Bunn, J. D. Minna, and R. C. Gallo, *Proc. Natl. Acad. Sci. U.S.A.* **77**, 7415 (1980).
2. V. S. Kalyanaraman, M. G. Sarangadharan, I. Miyoshi, D. Blayney, D. Golde, and R. C. Gallo, *Science* **218**, 571 (1982).
3. T. Watanabe, M. Seiki, H. Tsujimoto, I. Miyoshi, M. Haymi, and M. Yoshida, *Virology* **144**, 59 (1985).
4. M. Seiki, S. Hattori, Y. Hirayama, and M. Yoshida, *Proc. Natl. Acad. Sci. U.S.A.* **80**, 3618 (1983).
5. A. Gessain, J. C. Vernant, L. Maurs, F. Barrin, O. Gout, A. Glender, and G. de-Thé, *Lancet* **2**, 407 (1985).
6. M. R. Osame, K. Usuku, S. Izumo, N. Ijichi, H. Amitani, A. Igata, M. Matsumoto, and M. Tara, *Lancet* **1**, 1031 (1986).
7. S. Bhagavati, G. Ehrlich, R. W. Kula, S. Kwok, J. J. Sninsky, V. Udani, and B. J. Poiesz, *N. Engl. J. Med.* **318**, 1141 (1988).
8. M. Mochizuki, T. Watanabe, K. Yamaguchi, K. Tajima, K. Yoshimura, S. Nakashima, M. Shirao, S. Araki, N. Miyata, S. Mori, and K. Takatsuki, *J. Infect. Dis.* **166**, 943 (1992).
9. O. S. C. Morgan, C. Mora, P. Rodgers-Johnson, and G. Chen, *Lancet* **2**, 1184 (1989).
10. K. Shimotono, Y. Takahashi, N. Shimuzu, T. Gojoboni, D. W. Golde, I. S. Y. Chen, M. Mieva, and T. Sugimura, *Proc. Natl. Acad. Sci. U.S.A.* **82**, 3101 (1985).

11. J. D. Rosenblatt, J. V. Giorgi, D. W. Golde, J. Ben Ezra, A. Wu, G. D. Winberg, J. Glaspy, W. Wacksman, and I. S. Y. Chen, *Blood* **71,** 363 (1988).

12. T. P. Loughran, T. Coyle, M. P. Sherman, G. Starkbaum, G. D. Ehrlich, F. W. Ruscetti, and B. J. Poiesz, *Blood* **80,** 1116 (1992).

13. D. Zucker-Franklin, W. C. Hooper, and B. L. Evatt, *Blood* **80,** 1537 (1992).

14. W. J. Harrington, B. Sheremata, B. Hjelle, D. K. Dubé, P. Bradshaw, S. K. H. Foung, S. Snodgrass, G. Toedter, L. Cabral, and B. J. Poiesz, *Ann. Neurol.* **33,** 411 (1993).

15. W. Sheremata, W. Harrington, Jr., P. Bradshaw, S. Foung, S. P. Raffanti, J. R. Berger, S. Snodgrass, L. Resnick, and B. Poiesz, *Virus Res.* **29,** 71 (1993).

16. B. Hjelle, O. Appenzellen, R. Mills, S. Alexander, N. Torrez-Matinez, R. W. Jahnke, and G. Ross, *Lancet* **339,** 645 (1992).

17. S. Jacobson, T. Lehky, M. Nishimura, S. Robinson, D. E. McFarlin, and S. Dhib-Jalbut, *Ann. Neurol.* **33,** 392 (1993).

18. T. Homma, P. J. Kaki, N. W. J. King, Jr., R. D. Hunt, M. J. O'Connell, N. L. Letvin, M. D. Daniel, and R. C. Desrosiers, *Science* **225,** 716 (1984).

19. T. Tsujimoto, Y. Noda, K. Ishikawa, H. Nakamura, M. Fukasawa, I. Sakakibara, A. Sasagawa, S. Honjo, and M. Hajauri, *Cancer Res.* **47,** 269 (1987).

20. H. Schatzl, L. Yakoleva, B. Lapin, D. Rose, L. Inzhia, K. Gaedigk-Nitschko, F. Deinhardt, and K. von der Helm, *Leukemia* **6,** 158 (1992).

21. J. F. Ferrer, *Adv. Vet. Sci. Comp. Med.* **24,** 1 (1980).

22. R. O. Zandomeni, M. Carrera-Zandomeni, G. Esteban, and J. F. Ferrer, *J. Gen. Virol.* **72,** 2113 (1991).

23. J. G. Sodroski, C. A. Rosen, and W. A. Haseltine, *Science* **225,** 381 (1986).

24. M. P. Sherman, D. K. Dubé, N. K. Saksena, and B. J. Poiesz, *in* "Leukemia: Advances in Research and Treatment" (E. J. Freireich and H. Kankayian, eds.), p. 79. Kluwer Academic Publishers, Nowell, MA, 1993.

25. V. Ciminale, G. N. Palavkis, D. Derse, C. P. Cunningham, and B. K. Felber, *J. Virol.* **66,** 1736 (1992).

26. F. Komurian, F. Pelloquin, and G. De-Thé, *J. Virol.* **65,** 3770 (1991).

27. S. Daenke, S. Nightingale, K. Cruickshank, and C. R. M. Bangham, *J. Virol.* **64,** 1278 (1990).

28. G. D. Ehrlich, J. Andrews, M. P. Sherman, S. J. Greenberg, and B. J. Poiesz, *Virology* **186,** 619 (1992).

29. M. P. Sherman, S. Dubé, T. P. Spicer, T. D. Kane, J. G. Love, N. K. Saksena, R. Iannone, C. J. Gibbs, Jr., R. Yanagihara, D. K. Dubé, and B. J. Poiesz, *Cancer Res.* **53,** 6067 (1993).

30. R. Yanagihara, C. L. Jenkins, S. S. Alexander, C. A. Mora, and R. M. Garruto, *J. Infect. Dis.* **162,** 649 (1990).

31. A. Gessain, R. Yanagihara, G. Franchini, R. M. Garruto, C. L. Jenkins, A. B. Ajdukiewiez, R. C. Gallo, and C. Gajdusek, *Proc. Natl. Acad. Sci. U.S.A.* **88,** 7694 (1991).

32. M. P. Sherman, N. K. Saksena, D. K. Dubé, R. Yanagihara, and B. J. Poiesz, *J. Virol.* **66,** 2556 (1992).

33. N. K. Saksena, M. P. Sherman, R. Yanagihara, D. K. Dubé, and B. Poiesz, *Virology* **189,** 1 (1993).

34. I. Bastian, J. Gardner, D. Webb, and I. Gardner, *J. Virol.* **67,** 843 (1993).

35. N. K. Saksena, V. Hervé, M. P. Sherman, J. P. Durand, C. Mathiot, M. Muller, J. L. Love, F. B. Sinoussi, D. K. Dubé, and B. J. Poiesz, *Virology* **193,** 312 (1993).

36. N. K. Saksena, V. Hervé, J. P. Durand, B. LeGuenno, O. M. Diop, J. P. Digoutte, C. Mathiot, M. C. Muller, J. L. Love, S. Dubé, M. P. Sherman, P. M. Benz, S. Erensoy, A. Galot-Luong, G. Galat, B. Paul, D. K. Dubé, F. Barre-Sinoussi, and B. J. Poiesz, *Virology* **198,** 297 (1994).

37. T. Watanabe, M. Seiki, Y. Hirayama, and M. Yoshida, *Virology* **148,** 385 (1986).

38. J. D. Rosenblatt, D. H. Golde, H. Wachsman, J. V. Giorgi, A. Jacobs, G. M. Schmidt, S. Quan, J. C. Gasson, and I. S. Y. Chen, *N. Engl. J. Med.* **315,** 372 (1986).

39. W. W. Hall, H. Takahashi, C. Liu, M. H. Kaplan, O. Scheewind, S. Ijichi, K. Nagashima, and R. C. Gallo, *J. Virol.* **66,** 2456 (1992).

40. D. K. Dubé, M. P. Sherman, N. K. Saksena, V. Bryz-Gornia, J. Mendelsohn, J. Love, C. B. Arnold, T. Spicer, S. Dubé, J. B. Glaser, A. E. Williams, M. Nishimura, S. Jacobsen, J. F. Ferrer, N. DelPino, S. Guiruelas, and B. J. Poiesz, *J. Virol.* **67,** 1175 (1993).

41. J. F. Ferrer, N. del Pino, M. P. Sherman, E. Esteban, S. Quiruelas, M. A. Basombrio, S. Dubé, D. K. Dube, E. Pimental, A. Segovia, and B. J. Poiesz, *Virology* **197,** 576 (1993).

42. D. Pardi, W. M. Switzer, K. G. Hadlock, J. E. Kaplan, R. B. Lal, and T. M. Folks, *J. Virol.* **67,** 4659 (1993).

43. E. Delaporte, N. Monplaisir, J. Louwagie, M. Peters, Y. Martin-Prevel, J. P. Louis, A. Trebucq, L. Bedjabaga, S. Ossari, C. Honoré, B. Larouge, L. d'Auriol, G. Vandergraen, and P. Piot, *Int. J. Can* **49,** 373 (1991).

44. P. Goubau, J. Desmyter, J. Ghesquiere, and B. Kasereka, *Nature (London)* **359,** 201 (1992).

45. P. Goubau, H. Liu, G. G. DeLange, A. Vandomme, and J. Desmyter, *AIDS Res. Hum. Retro. Viruses* **9,** 709 (1993).

46. T. Igaraski, M. Yamashita, T. Muria, M. Osei-Kwasi, N. K. Aysi, H. Shiraki, T. Kurimura, and M. Hayami, *AIDS Res. Hum. Retroviruses* **9,** 1039 (1993).

47. Y. M. A. Chen, P. J. Kanki, Y. J. Jang, R. J. Montale, K. P. Samuel, T. S. Papas, and C. W. Wu, *Cold Spring Harbor Retroviruses Meet.,* 2 abstr. No. 2 (1993).

48. R. K. Saiki, S. Seharf, F. Faloona, K. B. Mullis, G. T. Horn, H. A. Erlich, and N. Arnheim, *Science* **230,** 1350 (1985).

49. R. K. Saiki, D. H. Gelfand, S. Stoffel, S. J. Scharf, R. Higuchi, G. T. Horn, F. B. Mullis, and H. A. Ehrlich, *Science* **239,** 487 (1987).

50. F. Barré-Sinoussi, J. C. Chermann, F. Rey, M. T. Nugeyre, S. Chamaret, J. Gruest, C. Dauguet, C. Axlir-Blin, F. Vezinet-Brun, C. Rouzious, W. Rozenbaum, and L. Montaignier, *Science* **220,** 868 (1983).

51. M. A. Abbott, B. J. Poiesz, B. C. Byrne, S. Kwok, J. J. Sninsky, and G. D. Ehrlich, *J. Infect. Dis.* **158,** 1158 (1988).

52. S. Kwok, G. D. Ehrlich, B. J. Poiesz, R. Kalish, and J. Sninsky, *Blood* **72,** 1117 (1988).

53. R. Iannone, M. P. Sherman, P. E. B. Rodgers-Johnson, M. A. Beilke, C. A. Mora, R. M. Amin, S. R. Tinsley, L. P. Papsidero, B. J. Poiesz, and C. J. Gibbs, Jr., *J. Acquired Immun. Defic. Syndr.* **5,** 810 (1992).

54. M. P. Sherman, G. D. Ehrlich, J. F. Ferrer, J. J. Sninsky, R. Zandomeni, N. L. Dock, and B. J. Poiesz, *J. Clin. Microbiol.* **30,** 185 (1992).

55. D. K. Dubé, S. Dubé, S. Erensoy, B. Jones, V. Bryz-Gornia, T. Spicer, J. Love, N. Saksena, M. F. Lechat, D. I. Shrager, H. Dosik, J. Glaser, W. Levis, W. Blattner, R. Montagna, B. S. Blumberg, and B. J. Poiesz, *Virology* **202,** 379 (1994).

56. B. J. Poiesz, M. P. Sherman, N. K. Saksena, D. K. Dubé, S. Dubé, J. Gavalchin, N. Fan, M. J. Lane, and B. Paul, *in* "Frontiers of Infectious Diseases: Focus on HIV (H. C. Neu, J. Levy, and R. Weiss, eds.), (Churchill-Livingstone, London, p. 189, 1993).

57. L. M. Dyster, L. Abbott, V. Bryz-Gornia, B. J. Poiesz, and L. D. Papsidero, *J. Clin. Microbiol.* **32,** 547 (1994).

58. R. F. Doolittle, D. F. Feng, M. S. Johnson, and M. A. McClure, *Q. Rev. Biol.* **64,** 1 (1989).

59. D. W. Anderson, J. S. Epstein, T. H. Lee, M. D. Lairmone, C. Saxinger, V. S. Kalyanaraman, D. Slamon, W. Parks, B. J. Poiesz, L. T. Pierik, H. Lee, R. Montagna, P. A. Roche, A. Williams, and W. Blattner, *Blood* **74,** 2585 (1989).

60. P. Chromozinski and N. Saceki, *Anal. Biochem.* **162,** 156 (1987).

61. M. C. Longo, M. S. Beringer, and J. L. Hartley, *Gene* **93,** 125 (1990).

62. B. C. Byrne, J. J. Li, J. Sninsky, and B. J. Poiesz, *Nucl. Acids Res.* **16,** 4165 (1988).

63. T. A. Kunkel, J. D. Roberts, and R. A. Zakour, *in* "Methods in Enzymology" (R. Wu and L. Grossman, eds.), vol. 154, p. 367. Academic Press, Oakland, FL, 1987.

64. F. Sanger, S. Nicklen, and A. R. Coulson, *Proc. Natl. Acad. Sci. U.S.A.* **74,** 5463(1977).

65. D. K. Dubé and L. A. Loeb, *Biochemistry* **28,** 5703 (1989).

66. L. Z. Abbott, T. Spicer, V. Bryz-Gornia, S. Kwok, J. Sninsky, and B. J. Poiesz, *J. Virol. Methods* **46,** 51 (1994).

67. J. Devereux, P. Haebirtli, and O. Smithies, *Nucleic Acids Res.* **12,** 387 (1984).

68. S. B. Needleman and C. D. Wunsch, *J. Mol. Biol.* **48,** 443 (1970).

69. D. L. Swofford, "Phylogenetic Analysis Using Parsimony Version 3.05." Computer program distributed by the Illinois Natural History Survey, Champaign, 1991.

70. K. T. A. Malik, J. Even, and A. Karpas, *J. Gen. Virol.* **69,** 1695 (1988).

71. E. Paine, J. Garcia, T. C. Philpott, G. Shaw, and L. Ratner, *Virology* **182,** 111 (1991).

72. J. Deschamps, R. Kettman, and A. Burny, *J. Virol.* **40,** 605 (1981).

73. A. Evangelista, S. Maroushek, H. Minnigan, A. Larson, E. Retzel, A. Haase, D. Gonzalez-Dunia, D. McFarlin, E. Mingoli, E. S. Jacobsen, M. Osame, and S. Sonada, *Microb. Pathog.* **8,** (1990).

74. A. Gessain, E. Boeri, R. Yanagihara, R. C. Gallo, and G. Franchini, *J. Virol.* **67,** 1015 (1993).

75. H. Lee, K. B. Idler, P. Swanson, J. J. Aparicio, K. K. Chen, J. P. Lax, M. Nguyen, T. Mann, G. Leckie, A. Zanetti, G. Marinocci, I. S. Y. Chen, and J. D. Rosenblatt, *AIDS Res. Hum. Retroviruses* **196,** 57 (1993).

76. A. Zharkikh, and L. Weng-Hsiung, *J. Mol. Evol.* **35,** 356 (1992).

[25] Use of PCR in Detection of Antisense Transcripts in HTLV-I-Infected Patients and Human T-Cell Lines

S. Dube, B. Paul, V. Bryz-Gornia, C. Stephens,
S. Erensoy, D. K. Dube, and B. J. Poiesz

Introduction

Classically, human retroviruses, including human T-cell lymphoma/leukemia virus type I (HTLV-I), contain diploid copies of positive [(+)] or sense strand RNA as their genome (1–4). On infection of the target cell this RNA is reverse-transcribed into double-stranded proviral DNA which integrates into the host chromosomal DNA and/or exists as unintegrated viral DNA serving as template for subsequent viral RNA transcription (5). The issue of negative strand or antisense viral or host cellular RNA synthesis in retrovirus-infected cells has been raised by several investigators (6–9). We were also interested in whether the HTLV-I produces negative strand antisense message in infected cell lines as well as in fresh peripheral blood mononuclear cells (PBMC) from HTLV-I-infected patients. In this review we describe a sensitive and specific PCR-based method to detect both (+) and (−) strand HTLV-I transcript in DNase-treated, poly(A) RNA from HTLV-I-infected cell cultures, via reverse transcriptase-directed polymerase chain reaction (RT-PCR) using the thermostable enzyme from *thermus thermophilus*, rTth (10), and various primer oligonucleotides in sequential fashion.

Materials and Methods

Cell Cultures

An interleukin 2 (AJ5740) (IL-2)-dependent, HTLV-I-infected, T-cell culture, HSC-CTCL AJ-5740 (AJ-574) (11) is grown from the peripheral PBMCs of a HAM/TSP patient; an IL-2-dependent, HTLV-I-infected T cell line, HSC-CTCL-11B, is grown from the PBMCs of a patient with ATL (12). The cell lines are maintained in RPMI 1640 with 10% fetal bovine serum (FBS), 1% penicillin-streptomycin (PS) (GIBCO, Grand Island, NY), 10% IL-2 (Cellular

Products, Buffalo, NY), and 40 U/ml rIL-2 (Cetus, Emeryville, CA). The cultures are expanded approximately three times per week with feeding twice a week.

Serology

Sera from various HTLV-I-infected patients (described in the *in vivo* studies below) are evaluated for the presence of antibodies to human retroviruses using commercially available enzyme-linked immunosorbent assays (ELISA) and Western blot assays (13, 14) (Cellular Products).

Organic Extraction of DNA from Peripheral Blood Mononuclear Cells (PBMCs)

The PBMCs from HTLV-I-seropositive patients are lysed and extracted as described previously (15). DNA concentrations are then determined by spectrophotometric analyses and serially diluted to represent 1000, 100, 10, and 1 copies of HTLV-I DNA in 1 μg of uninfected control DNA. All preamplification maneuvers are performed using positive-displacement pipettes (Rainin, Woburn, MA) in a separate room from where the postamplification maneuvers are performed. To avoid contamination by amplified products, pre- and postamplification maneuvers, rooms, and personnel are separated. In addition, the Gene Amp PCR Carryover Prevention kit (Perkin–Elmer Cetus, Norwalk, CT) is used for the *in vivo* studies. This is a procedure which makes PCR products susceptible to degradation by substituting dTTP with dUTP in the PCR reaction mix and treating subsequent amplifications with the enzyme uracil N-glycosylase (UNG) prior to heating and cooling cycles (16). One unit of enzyme is added directly to the PCR mixture and any potential contaminating amplified products containing dUTP are digested prior to the RT step by incubating at 37°C for 1 min. During the RT step and prior to amplification, all samples are maintained at 72°C, such that subsequent products (cDNAs with dUMPs) are protected from UNG digestion. After PCR all samples are incubated at 72°C to prevent product degradation until they are treated with 150 μl chloroform–isoamyl alcohol (CIAA) and used for subsequent analyses.

RNA Extraction for Reverse Transcriptase-PCR Analyses

Ex Vivo Studies

Poly(A) RNA is extracted from 2×10^8 cells using the Fast Track mRNA Isolation kit (Invitrogen, Omar, UT), as per the manufacturer's instructions.

In Vivo Studies

Due to the low numbers of HTLV-I-infected cells in individual patients, poly(A) mRNA from a total of 3×10^6 cells is extracted using the Micro Fast Track mRNA Isolation kit (Invitrogen), as per the manufacturer's instructions.

DNase Treatment

All poly(A) mRNAs are treated with 30 U of RQ1 DNase (Promega, Madison, WI) in the presence of 10 mM MgCL$_2$, 40 U of RNasin (Promega) and incubated at 37°C for 1 hr. The samples are then extracted with equal volumes of phenol/CIAA and the aqueous phase is then precipitated overnight in 0.3 M sodium acetate and 95% ethanol. Prior to RT-PCR analyses, samples are microfuged for at least 45 min at 4°C.

Primers and Probes

Oligonucleotides are synthesized using the Applied Biosystem PCR-mate (Applied Biosystems, Foster City, CA) and purified by reverse-phase chromatography. All primers and probes are listed in Table I.

TABLE I   Summary of Reverse Transcriptase-PCR Reactions Generated from (+) and (−) Strand AJ-5740 RNA Using a Battery of Primer Pairs across the HTLV-I Genome

Primers	Probe	bp	Size (bp)	Region	Possible target messages
CPSS7/CPSS8	CPS6	534–702	188	5′ LTR	us[a]
1RP110/1RP111	SK112	4757–4942	185	*pol*	us[a]
359219/ss9294	S9229	5270–5540	270	*env*	us[a],ssl[b]
CP-1/CP-2	CP3	(427–471/4992–5125)		pX-exon 1/2 splice site	ssl[b], ds[d]
SK43/SK44	SK45	7358–7516	158	pX-exon3	us[a],ssl[b],ss2[c],ds[d]
MPS39/MPS40	SK44	7473–7889	416	pX-exon3	us[a],ssl[b],ss2[c],ds[d]
pXB-1/CP-10	pXA2	7761–8222	461	pX-exon3	us[a],ssl[b],ss2[c],ds[d]

[a] us, unspliced (8.5 kb) genomic.
[b] ssl, single-spliced (4.2 kb).
[c] ss2, single-spliced (1.9 kb).
[d] ds, double-spliced (2.1 kb *tax/rex*) and (approx. 3.1 kb *rof/tof* message) poly(A) RNA were extracted from AJ-5740 cells; DNased mRNA equivalent of $2.5 - 10^6$ cells was used in each RT-PCR reaction and amplified for 45 cycles.

The strategy for detecting $(+)$ or $(-)$ strand RNA is shown in Fig. 1. Poly(A) RNA is first reverse-transcribed into cDNA and then amplified using the DNA polymerase *rTth* (Roche Molecular Systems, Alameda, CA). The DNA products generated, depending on their length, are subjected to 40 (long) or 45 (short) amplification cycles consisting of denaturation at 94°C for 1 min or 40 sec, followed by annealing at 53°C for 1 min or 30 sec and followed by extension at 70°C for 2 min or 68°C for 30 sec, respectively. Products are then detected either by liquid hybridization and subsequent gel retardation on 8% (w/v) PAGE or by Southern blot hybridization on 1.5% (w/v) agarose gels using the appropriate ^{32}P end-labeled probe. In order to show that the products are indeed derived from the specific target strands of RNA, the following conditions and controls are employed for the various RT-PCR analyses.

i. *No primer.* To control for both residual DNA contamination in the RNA sample and the phenomenon of $(+)$ strand RNA autopriming, no primer is added during reverse transcription. The negative results in this control thus confirm that the sample is free of DNA. By corollary, this result also confirms that the products in the reactions that did contain strand-specific primers during the RT step (steps ii and iii) are both RNA-derived and strand specific.

ii. *Positive $(+)$ primer.* Only the $(+)$ primer is added for reverse transcription. Any product synthesized is thus derived from $(-)$ strand mRNA only.

iii. *Negative $(-)$ primer.* Only $(-)$ primer is added for reverse transcription. Any product synthesized is thus derived from $(+)$ strand mRNA only.

iv. *Reverse transcriptase inactivation control (RTIC)/DNA control.* To control for both DNA contamination as well as the possibility of false-positive $(+)$ strand amplification due to residual RT activity prior to amplification, the enzyme in the presence of one of the primers is shifted directly into the DNA-dependent mode and then added to the sample. A negative result in this control would confirm both that the sample consists of RNA only (and is therefore RT-dependent) and that the enzyme is completely switched to its DNA-dependent mode confirming its template specificity.

v. *Primer/H_2O control.* To control for contamination of reagents due to carryover of HTLV-I DNA, no nucleic acid is added in this negative control sample and it is subjected to conventional DNA-dependent PCR.

vi. *Red Cross normal (RCN).* To assure that the pCR products are indeed HTLV-I specific and not derived from human genomic or mitochondrial nucleic acid, organically extracted DNA and RNA, from the PBMCs of

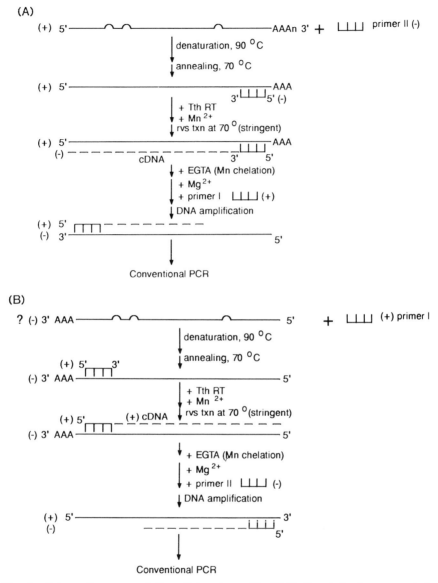

FIG. 1   Schematic representation of strand-specific, RNA-directed polymerase chain reaction (RT-PCR). Schematic representation of (+) strand RNA (A) and (−) strand RNA (B) subjected to RT-PCR analyses with the *Thermus thermophilus (rTth)* DNA polymerase. (A) When (+) strand RNA is detected, (−) primer is used during reverse transcription (rvs txn) and (+) primer during PCR amplification. (B) Conversely, when (−) strand RNA is detected, (+) primer is used during reverse transcription.

uninfected volunteer blood donors, is used as a negative control and subjected to conventional RT-PCR and DNA-dependent PCR.

vii. *HTLV-I-positive DNA*. Organically extracted DNA from the AJ-5740 cell line is used as a positive control for the DNA-dependent component of the RT-PCR reaction.

The validity of the RT-PCR assays is absolutely dependent on our use of the *rTth* enzyme which is capable of copying either RNA or DNA exclusively, depending on the presence of Mn^{2+} or Mg^{2+}, respectively. This feature obviates the possibility that positive results observed in the RT-PCR reactions targeted against ($-$) strand RNA could be due to residual reverse transcriptase activity when the assay is converted to the DNA-dependent PCR mode. Indeed, if residual reverse transcriptase activity was still present, the subsequent addition of the second primer directed against the ($+$) strand could result in pseudo ($-$) strand RT-PCR products. This problem was exactly what we encountered when we utilized Moloney murine leukemia virus (M-MLV) or Superscript RT. In these assays we found that neither enzymatic activity could be completely eliminated by heat inactivation (data not shown). However, such was not the case when the *rTth* enzyme was shifted from the RNA-dependent to the DNA-dependent mode.

To test this concept we utilized the HTLV-I *pol*-specific primers IRP110/IRP111 (Fig. 2) to synthesize ($+$) strand HTLV-I RNA (17) (Fig. 3) which was utilized as template in strand-specific RT-PCR assays. As can be seen (Fig. 4), the ($+$) strand synthetic RNA is detected only when the ($-$) strand primer IRP111 is utilized first to generate cDNA.

To confirm that amplification is occurring via RT-specific priming, a primer pair, CP-1/CP-2, and probe, CP-3, were selected that would allow for the

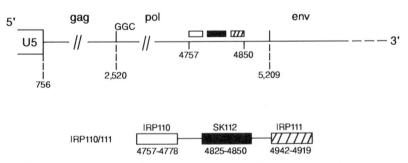

FIG. 2 Schematic representation of primers. IRP110/IRP111 and probe SK112, specific for the *pol* region of the HTLV-I genome, are used to detect genomic RNA and DNA. The location of the primers on the genomic DNA is as indicated.

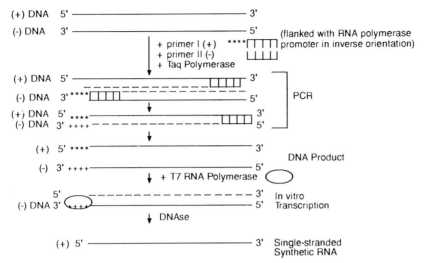

FIG. 3 Strategy for preparation of single-stranded (ss), synthetic, target RNA. Synthesis of (+) strand, synthetic RNA is schematically represented. First, DNA containing the region to be transcribed is amplified using the (+) primer I which is linked to the T7 RNA polymerase promoter sequence in inverse orientation (depicted as **** at its 5′ end), the (−) primer II, which lacks the linker, and *Taq* polymerase. The (−) strand, DNA amplification product now has at its corresponding 3′ end the T7 RNA polymerase promoter sequence in the correct orientation (depicted as + + + +) such that it can now be used in an *in vitro* transcription reaction with T7 RNA polymerase (open circle) to produce complementary, ss, synthetic RNA. The contaminating DNA is then removed from the reaction mixture by treatment with 30 U of DNase (refer to Materials and Methods for details) leaving only (+) strand, synthetic RNA product.

preferential detection of spliced RNA (Fig. 5). Synthetic RNA corresponding to the CP-1/CP-2 RT-PCR-derived amplicon was prepared as above and could be detected in an RT-PCR assay only when CP-2 was used to prime the RT reaction (data not shown).

RNA Preparation for Northern Blot Analyses

RNA Extraction

Total RNA is extracted from cells, as per published techniques (18) and is subsequently affinity-purified for poly(A) selection on oligo(dT)-cellulose columns. The aliquots are then quantitated for poly(A) RNA spectrophoto-

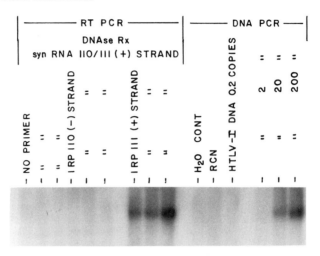

FIG. 4   Strand specificity of the RT-PCR reactions using the *rTth* DNA polymerase. Autoradiograph of liquid hybridization analyses of RT-PCR and DNA-PCR generated amplification products using primers IRP110/IRP111 and the detector SK112, which are specific for the HTLV-I *pol* gene. Target nucleic acids include HTLV-I (+) strand, synthetic RNA synthesized as described under Materials and Methods; a dilution of HTLV-I-infected human DNA; HTLV-I-uninfected DNA from a volunteer blood donor (RCN), and a negative control containing no nucleic acid (H$_2$O cont). The RT-PCR reactions were performed in triplicate to control for any artifacts of autopriming, under conditions as stated under Materials and Methods.

metrically and the indicated amounts are used for each of the Northern blot analyses. Desired aliquots are then precipitated with 1/10 volume of 3 M sodium acetate and 2.5 vol of 95% ethanol. Before they are used as targets, RNA samples are analyzed for DNA contamination by DNA-PCR using *Taq* polymerase (Cetus), and DNA-free samples are used in the following Northern blot analyses.

Strand-Specific DNA and RNA Probes

Strand-specific DNA probes are synthesized using primers SSK43 and SSK44 in a PCR amplification reaction with the resulting 180-bp fragment being directed to the *pX ORFII* (19) region of the HTLV-I genome (Fig. 6). As a further control, a (+) strand oligonucleotide, SK45, in the same region is also ^{32}P end-labeled and used as a probe.

For the synthesis of single-strand RNA probes DNA products from the RT-PCR amplification using primers CP-1/CP-2 are cloned into the TA cloning vector (Invitrogen) which contains the T7 RNA polymerase promoter

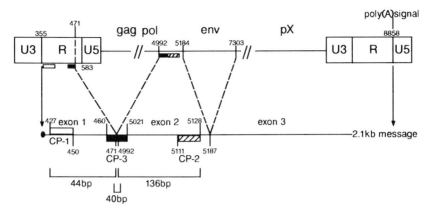

FIG. 5 Schematic representation of primers. CP-1/CP-2 and probe CP-3 used to detect HTLV-I specific, spliced messages. The probe, CP-3, is specific for the splice junction contained within the CP1/CP2 region. Their positions on the genomic and spliced RNA are approximately 4.5 and 180 bp apart, respectively.

sequence in a strand-specific orientation. Plasmid DNA is then extracted and used in an *in vitro* transcription assay using T7 RNA polymerase (Stratagene) to synthesize single-stranded RNA. The transcribed RNA is radiolabeled by direct incorporation of $[^{32}P]UMP$, as per the manufacturer's instruc-

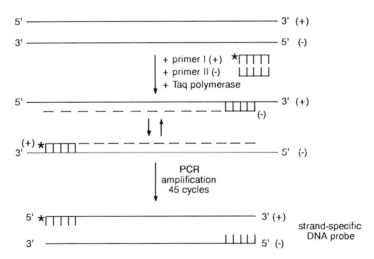

FIG. 6 Strategy for preparation of strand-specific DNA probes. The (+) primer I is ^{32}P end-labeled (*) and used in a PCR amplification reaction along with the unlabeled (−) primer II, the corresponding DNA target, and *Taq* DNA polymerase.

tions. The product is then treated with DNase, extracted with phenol/chloroform, precipitated with ethanol, and used as a probe for RNA blot hybridization.

All probes synthesized for RNA analyses are tested for strand specificity by hybridization with the synthetic single-strand SK43/SK44 or CP-1/CP-2 RNA (Figs. 7a and b).

Northern Blot Analyses and Hybridization

Poly(A) RNA from cultured cells is denatured and subjected to electrophoresis on 0.9% agarose gels containing formaldehyde (20). Blots are hybridized overnight with heat-denatured (95°C for 7 min), HTLV-I-specific, (+) strand, ^{32}P-labeled DNA or RNA probes in 50% deionized formamide, 10% dextran sulfate, 1 M NaCl, 1% sodium dodecyl sulfate (SDS), and 10 mg/ml of salmon sperm DNA, 42°C, and then washed at 65°C for 30 min in 0.1x SSPE and 1% SDS and exposed on film at −70°C for 16–24 hr. Before reprobing, the filters are stripped by boiling in 0.1x SSPE, 1% (w/v) SDS for 20–30 min and reexposed for 24 hr to rule out the possibility of residual radioactivity. The blot is then rehybridized with the complementary, (−) strand probe, washed, and reexposed under similar conditions. In the case where strand-specific DNA probes are utilized the blot is again stripped, reexposed (to exclude the presence of residual radioactivity), and rehybridized with a different (+) strand ^{32}P-labeled oligonucleotide probe.

Results

Detection of Negative- and Positive-Strand HTLV-1 mRNA by Reverse Transcriptase-PCR Amplification of AJ-5740 mRNA

Genomic Message

Reverse transcriptase-PCR amplification of cellular, AJ-5740, poly(A) RNA with the HTLV-I *pol* gene-specific primers, IRP-110 and IRP-111, and hybridization of the products with the probe, SK112, detected both (−) and (+) strand, genomic, and viral RNA (Fig. 8).

Spliced Messages

Similarly, both (−) and (+) strand, spliced, HTLV- 1 mRNAs were detected in this cell line using the primers, CP-1 and CP-2, and the splice junction-specific probe, CP-3 (Fig. 9). In this experiment, the fact that the (−) and (+) strand amplification products are of the same size (180 bp) and both

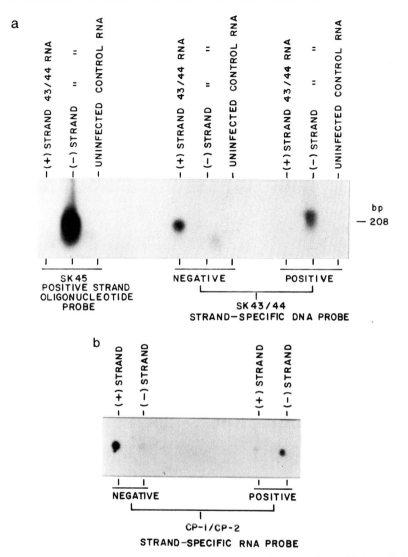

FIG. 7   RNA hybridization analyses to demonstrate the strand specificity of the DNA and single-strand, synthetic RNA probes that are complementary to either (+) or (−) strand HTLV-I messages. (a) Northern blot analyses to demonstrate strand-specific hybridization of the (+) strand oligonucleotide probe, SK45, and the synthetic SK43/44 PCR-amplified DNA probes. (b) Dot-blot analyses to demonstrate the strand specificity of the synthetic CP-1/CP-2 RNA probes. The CP-1/CP-2 RNA probes are labeled by the direct incorporation of [α-^{32}P]UTP as described under Materials and Methods.

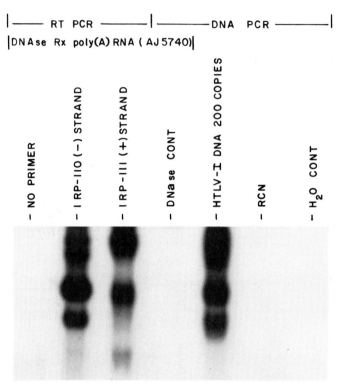

FIG. 8   Strand-directed RT-PCR analyses of AJ-5740 poly(A) RNA to detect genomic, (+) and (−) strand RNA. Autoradiograph of a liquid hybridization of DNA
products from an RT-PCR amplification using primers 1RP-110/1RP-111 and probe
SK112 specific for the *pol* region of the HTLV-I genomic DNA and RNA.

hybridize with CP-3 indicates that the (−) and (+) strand RNA sequences
must be approximate complements of each other. No product was detected
when HTLV-I (AJ-5740) DNA (even up to an input of 10^5 copies) was analyzed via PCR with the same primers and probe thereby confirming that
there are no DNA intermediates corresponding to the spliced messages (data
not shown).

Both (+) and (−) strand sequences were detected in the AJ5740 and
CTCL-11B cell lines using all of the primers and probes listed in Table I.
To optimize the detection of both genomic and spliced messages we varied
some of the parameters of the RT-PCR reactions including primer concentration, method of RNA extraction, and input RNA. Southern blot analyses
with the labeled detector CP-3 or SK112 indicated that the sensitivity of the

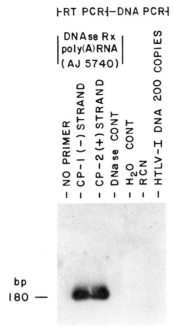

FIG. 9 Strand-directed RT-PCR analyses of AJ-5740 poly(A) RNA to detect HTLV-I-specific, spliced, (+) and (−) strand RNA. Autoradiograph of Southern blot hybridization of DNA product from an RT-PCR amplification using primers CP-1/CP-2 specific for spliced messages and the corresponding splice junction-specific probe CP-3.

assay increases with increasing concentrations of the primers and is maximum at 50 pm (Figs. 9 and 10). In the modified version of sample extraction following the elution of poly(A) RNA (see above) the eluate was immediately adjusted to 10 mM MgCl$_2$ and treated with 30 U of RQ1 DNase in the presence of 40 U of RNasin at 37°C for 1 hr. The reaction was then terminated by phenol/chloroform extraction followed by salt/ethanol precipitation in the presence of 20 μg of glycogen. This resulted in one less precipitation step and higher yield (data not shown). Further, signal intensity maximized at an input of RNA from 4 × 10^6 cells extracted as above (data not shown).

Northern Blot Analyses

The detection of HTLV-I (−) strand RNA by RT-PCR was further confirmed by Northern blot analyses of poly(A) RNA from AJ-5740 cells and uninfected PBMCs using strand-specific probes (Figs. 10 and 11). As can be seen most

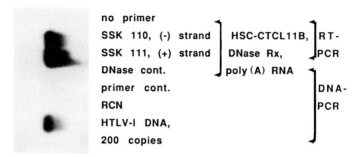

no primer

SSK 110, (-) strand   HSC-CTCL11B,   RT-

SSK 111, (+) strand   DNase Rx,   PCR

DNase cont.   poly (A) RNA

primer cont.   DNA-

RCN   PCR

HTLV-I DNA,

200 copies

↑ 234 bp

FIG. 10   Strand-specific RT-PCR analyses of HSC-CTCL11B poly(A) RNA to detect genomic, (+) and (−) strand HTLV-I RNA. Autoradiograph of a Southern blot hybridization of DNA products from an RT-PCR amplification using primers SSK110/ SSK111 and probe SK112 specific for the *pol* region of the HTLV-I genomic DNA and RNA.

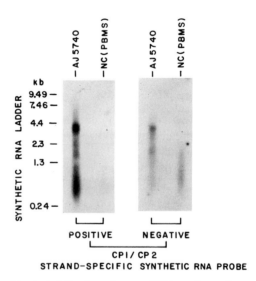

FIG. 11   Northern blot hybridization of target RNA as above, but with strand-specific CP-1/CP-2 (+) and (−), synthetic RNAs as probes to detect both (−) and (+) strand, singly and multiply spliced HTLV-I mRNAs, respectively, in the poly(A) RNA from AJ-5740 cells.

HTLV-I RNA in this and other HTLV-I-positive cell lines (data not shown) is spliced and the sizes of the RNA detected are the same regardless of whether they are positive strand or negative strand.

In Vivo Presence of (−) Strand RNA: Genomic RNA

To examine whether antisense viral RNA could be detected in fresh human PBMC, we analyzed the RNA extracted from three HTLV-I-infected patients (one each of whom was either asymptomatic or suffered from ATL or TSP/ HAM). The PBMCs of all three patients had detectable levels of both (+) and (−) strand HTLV-I RNA, albeit in relatively different amounts (Fig. 12).

Optimization of Strand-Specific Reverse Transcriptase-PCR for in Vivo Detection

Having obtained preliminary data on the *in vivo* presence of genomic antisense message and with a view to detecting both genomic and spliced messages *in vivo* on a larger scale, we decided to optimize some of the parameters of the RT-PCR reactions. In order to further enhance the sensitivity of the assay, the primer concentrations, the method of sample extraction, and the amount of input RNA, were varied.

Primer Concentrations

Concentrations of 10, 15, 25, and 50 pmol of the primers CP1 and CP2 were used for RT-PCR analyses on poly(A) RNA from AJ-5740 cells to detect HTLV-I-specific, spliced messages. Southern blot analyses with the labeled detector, CP-3, indicated that the sensitivity of the assay increases with increasing concentrations of the primers and is maximum at 50 pmol (data not shown). The usual controls were employed to confirm that the results were indeed HTLV-I-spliced RNA specific and derived from strand-specific RT-PCR reactions.

Yet another control was performed to demonstrate that the RT-PCR reactions were indeed still strand specific at 50 pmol of primer concentration (Fig. 13). Thus, RT-PCR reactions were performed using synthetic, single-strand, (+) target RNA and *pol* region primers, SSK 110/111 and probe SK-112. As can be seen, only (+) strand-derived products of expected size were observed on Southern blot analyses, thereby confirming the validity of the strand-specific RT-PCR reactions. Thus subsequent optimizations were performed at 50 pmol of primer concentration.

Sample Extraction and Input RNA

After the primer concentrations were optimized, the method for poly(A) RNA extraction of patient RNA (refer to Materials and Methods for *in vivo* RNA extraction) was modified slightly. In the modified version, after the

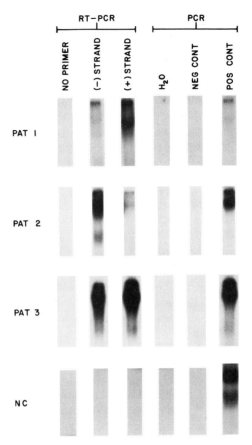

FIG. 12 *In vivo* detection of genomic, (−) and (+) strand HTLV-I RNA by RT-PCR analyses. Autoradiograph of a liquid hybridization of DNA products from the RT-PCR amplification of poly(A) RNA from fresh PBMCs of three HTLV-I-infected patients (PAT 1,2,3) and an uninfected control individual (NC). PAT 1 and 3 presented with TSP and ATL, respectively, while PAT 2 was asymptomatic.

poly(A) RNA is eluted, the salt concentration of the eluate is immediately adjusted to 10 mM MgCl$_2$ and treated with 30 U of RQ1 DNase (Promega) in the presence of 40 U of RNasin (Promega) at 37°C for 1 hr. The reaction is then terminated by phenol/chloroform extraction followed by salt/ethanol precipitation in the presence of 20 μg of glycogen (Invitrogen). In the control experiments, the eluate is first precipitated with salt/ethanol and glycogen and then resuspended in 10 mM MgCl$_2$ buffer and treated with DNase (as above). Thus one precipitation step is reduced, resulting in increased sensitiv-

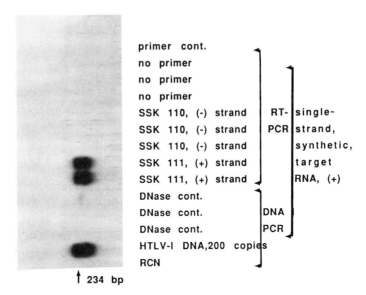

primer cont.
no primer
no primer
no primer
SSK 110, (-) strand | RT- | single-
SSK 110, (-) strand | PCR | strand,
SSK 110, (-) strand | | synthetic,
SSK 111, (+) strand | | target
SSK 111, (+) strand | | RNA, (+)
DNase cont.
DNase cont. | DNA
DNase cont. | PCR
HTLV-I DNA,200 copies
RCN

↑ 234 bp

Detector : SK-112

FIG. 13 To revalidate the strand specificity of the RT-PCR reactions at 50 pmol of primer. Autoradiograph of a Southern blot hybridization analyses of RT-PCR and DNA-PCR products using primers SSK110/SSK111 and the detector SK112, which are specific for the HTLV-I *pol* gene. Target nucleic acids include HTLV-I (+) strand, synthetic RNA, synthesized as described under Materials and Methods; a dilution of HTLV-I-infected human DNA; HTLV-I uninfected DNA from a volunteer blood donor (RCN); and a negative control containing no nucleic acid (H₂O cont, not shown).

ity of detection (Fig. 14). As expected, when the input was increased from the poly(A) RNA extracted from 1×10^6 cells to 4×10^6 cells, an increased amount of product was detected (Fig. 14).

Significance

The above data indicate that natural antisence viral messages are present in both cultured and fresh HTLV-I-infected lymphocytes. The consequences of this phenomenon could be extremely important, in that it would represent another regulatory step in the HTLV-I life cycle. An obvious function would be that (−) strand RNA could act as antisense message, thereby interfering with viral replication and/or protein translation (21). These potentially nega-

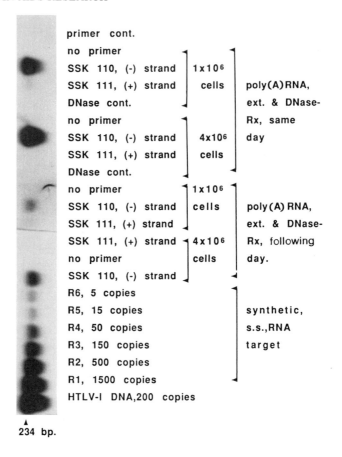

primer cont.
no primer ⎤
SSK 110, (-) strand │ 1x10⁶
SSK 111, (+) strand │ cells   poly(A)RNA,
DNase cont. ⎦   ext. & DNase-
no primer ⎤   Rx, same
SSK 110, (-) strand │ 4x10⁶   day
SSK 111, (+) strand │ cells
DNase cont. ⎦
no primer ⎤ 1x10⁶
SSK 110, (-) strand │ cells   poly(A) RNA,
SSK 111, (+) strand ⎦   ext. & DNase-
SSK 111, (+) strand ⎤ 4x10⁶   Rx, following
no primer │ cells   day.
SSK 110, (-) strand ⎦
R6, 5 copies ⎤
R5, 15 copies │ synthetic,
R4, 50 copies │ s.s.,RNA
R3, 150 copies │ target
R2, 500 copies │
R1, 1500 copies ⎦
HTLV-I DNA,200 copies

▲
234 bp.

Detector : SK-112.

FIG. 14 Optimization of *in vivo* detection of (−) and (+) strand HTLV-I RNA by varying the number of nucleic acid precipitations and the input RNA in the RT-PCR analyses. Autoradiograph of a Southern blot hybridization of DNA products of a RT-PCR amplification using poly(A) RNA from the fresh PBMs of a HTLV-I-infected patient diagnosed with TSP and primers specific to the *pol* region of the HTLV-I genome. The RNA was amplified using the primers SSK110/SSK111 and probe SK 112 and amplified for 45 cycles in each RT-PCR reaction with 50 pmol of the primer. Synthetic, single-strand RNA of positive polarity (R1–R6), defined by the same primers, R1–6, was used as a quantitative control for the assay. Their relative copy numbers are as indicated.

tive regulatory effects would be consistent with the results of the low expression and infectivity of HTLV-I obtained from our, as well as other, laboratories and may be one of the reasons HTLV-I is a poor replicator *in vivo*. Alternatively, the presence of ($-$) strand HTLV-I messages could control or amplify gene expression by making double-stranded, RNase-resistant, duplex molecules thereby altering the half-life of the messages. These duplexes could then act as, or protect, template resulting in increased RNA copies and greater protein synthesis over time (22, 23).

As stated earlier, analyses of the ($-$) strand HTLV-I RNA sequences indicate the presence of several potential open reading frames encoding for what would be novel HTLV-I proteins. These and other possibilities will require further investigation in order to understand fully the role of ($-$) strand message in HTLV-infected cells. The techniques outlined herein should facilitate such investigation.

References

1. W. S. Robinson, H. L. Robinson, and P. H. Duesberg, *Proc. Natl. Acad. Sci. U.S.A.* **54,** 137 (1967).
2. J. M. Bishop, *Annu. Rev. Biochem.* **47,** 35 (1978).
3. M. S. Reitz, B. J. Poiesz, F. W. Ruscetti, and R. C. Gallo, *Proc. Natl. Acad. U.S.A.* **78,** 1887 (1981).
4. M. Seiki, S. Hattori, Y. Kirayama, and M. Yoshida, *Proc. Natl. Acad. Sci. U.S.A.* **80,** 3618 (1983).
5. R. Weiss, N. Teich, H. Varmus, and J. Coffin, *in* "RNA Tumor Viruses," 2nd ed., p. 261. Cold Spring Harbor Lab. Cold Spring Harbor, NY, 1985.
6. D. Larocca, L. A. Chao, M. H. Seto, and T. K. Brunck, *Biochem. Biophys. Res. Commun.* **163,** 1006 (1989).
7. B. J. Poiesz, M. P. Sherman, N. K. Saksena, D. K. Dubé, S. Dubé, J. Gavalchin, N. Fan, M. J. Lane, and B. Paul, *in* "Frontiers of Infectious Diseases: Focus on HIV" (H. C. Neu, J. Levy, and R. Weiss, eds.), p. 189. Churchill-Livingstone, London, 1993.
8. M. L. Bukrinsky, and A. F. Etkin, *AIDS Res. Hum. Retroviruses* **6,** 425 (1990).
9. N. L. Michael, M. T. Vahey, L. D'Arcy, P. K. Ehrenberg, J. D. Mosca, J. Rappaport, and R. R. Redfield, *J. Virol.* **68,** 979 (1994).
10. T. W. Myers and D. H. Gelfand, *Am. Chem. Soc.* **30,** 7666 (1991).
11. S. Bhagavati, G. Ehrlich, R. W. Kula, S. Kwok, J. Sninsky, V. Udani, and B. J. Poiesz, *N. Engl. J. Med.* **318,** 1141 (1988).
12. G. D. Ehrlich, J. B. Glasser, K. Lavigne, D. Quan, D. Mildvan, J. J. Sninsky, S. Kwok, L. Papsidero, and B. J. Poiesz, *Blood* **74,** 1658 (1989).
13. S. Kwok, G. Ehrlich, B. Poiesz, R. Kalish, and J. Sninsky, *Blood* **72,** 1117 (1988).
14. L. Papsidero, F. Swartzwelder, M. Sheu, R. Montagna, G. Ehrlich, J. Sninsky, H. Dosik, S. Bhagavati, and B. Poiesz, *J. Clin. Microbiol.* **28,** 949 (1990).

15. D. K. Dubé, M. P. Sherman, N. K. Saksena, V. Bryz-Gornia, J. Mendelson, J. Love, C. B. Arnold, T. Spicer, S. Dubé, J. B. Glaser, A. E. Williams, M. Nishimura, S. Jacobsen, J. F. Ferrer, N. DelPino, S. Guiruelas, and B. J. Poiesz, *J. Virol.* **67,** 1175 (1993).
16. M. C. Longo, M. S. Beringer, and J. L. Hartley, *Gene* **93,** 125 (1990).
17. E. Fahy, D. Y. Kwok, and T. R. Geingeras, *PCR Methods Appl.,* p. 25 (1991).
18. P. Chromozinski, and N. Saceki, *Anal. Biochem.* **162,** 156 (1987).
19. M. Seiki, A. Hikikoshi, T. Taniguchi, and M. Yoshida, *Science* **228,** 1532 (1985).
20. L. A. Davis, M. D. Dibner, and J. F. Batley, *Basic Methods Mol. Biol.,* p. 143 (1986).
21. M. Matsukura, G. Zon, K. Shinosuka et al., *Proc. Natl. Acad. Sci. U.S.A.* **86,** 4244 (1989).
22. V. Volloch, *Proc. Natl. Acad. Sci. U.S.A.* **83,** 1208 (1986).
23. V. Volloch, B. Schweitzer, X. Zhang, and S. Rits, *Proc. Natl. Acad. Sci. U.S.A.* **88,** 10671 (1991).

Section X

Miscellaneous Uses of PCR

[26] Direct Chemiluminescent Sequencing of Double-Stranded PCR Products

Andrea M. Douglas and Bentley A. Atchison

Introduction

The polymerase chain reaction (PCR) is an *in vitro* method that enables the exponential enzymatic synthesis of a targeted segment of DNA (1). Thus, PCR provides a rapid, highly sensitive, and specific means of nucleic acid detection and isolation. Direct sequencing of DNA produced by a PCR has consequently received much attention of late. However, there are a number of difficulties associated with direct sequencing of PCR products. These include the presence of nonspecific amplification products and the excess primers and deoxyribonucleoside triphosphates (dNTPs) carried over from the amplification to the sequencing reaction. In addition, the small size of the DNA template in relatively high concentration results in rapid reannealing of the doublestranded DNA. Numerous methods have been described which attempt to overcome the inherent difficulties associated with sequencing of double-stranded PCR products (2–5). These methods, however, are not widely used mainly because of the difficulty in obtaining reproducible sequencing ladders and because of the complexity of the protocols.

In an attempt to avoid the problem of rapid reassociation of the double-stranded DNA template, single-stranded DNA templates can be prepared. However, many experiments are usually required in order to optimize the production of single-stranded templates whether by assymetric PCR (2), by the use of biotinylated primers (5), or by preferential enzymatic degradation of one strand (3). The variability in the quality and quantity of template obtained, in practice, causes a major problem.

Because of the simplicity associated with the direct sequencing of double-stranded DNA, we developed a protocol to overcome the problem of the reassociation of template DNA and the consequent reduction of signal intensity (6). Cycle sequencing has previously been found to enhance band intensity (7), and, therefore, this method was incorporated into our protocol. Essentially, our protocol incorporates PCR not only in the initial amplification step but also for the sequencing of the PCR product. The DNA is thus sequenced from both ends simultaneously using the same primers, enzymes, buffers, and thermal profiles in both the specific amplification and the sequencing stages. As a result, the variability of the sequencing resulting from the need to prepare single-stranded templates is overcome and only one preparation is required in order to sequence both DNA strands. This is particularly important when encountering regions of strong secondary structure, which can often be overcome by sequencing the opposite strand of the template DNA.

When performing PCR sequencing, the purity of the double-stranded template is critical to successful sequencing of products. Of particular importance is the removal of excess dNTPs and primers prior to the sequencing reaction. Our protocol overcomes this alleviating the need for complex purification procedures. Simple modifications to the initial PCR conditions, to minimize the amount of dNTPs remaining at the end of the initial amplification step, abolish the need to purify the DNA template of excess dNTPs. Similarly, the requirement of purification of PCR primers is not necessary as the same primers are used in the initial PCR and sequencing reactions. Sequencing of a specific strand is accomplished by probing for one of the primers used in the PCR with a labeled probe complementary to the primer. This condition also allows the pooling of a number of products on the one gel and, thus "multiplex" sequencing. Spurious bands, if present in sequencing reactions, may be removed simply by probing to an internal region of the sequenced PCR fragment.

Our protocol uses chemiluminescent detection which has several advantages over radioactive detection methods (8, 9). All radioactive detection methods introduce handling and disposal concerns and generally require exposure times ranging from several hours to days as opposed to an average of 1 hr for chemiluminescent detection. Biotin-labeled oligonucleotides and sequencing reactions are also not subjected to decay, radiolysis, or light bleaching. In addition the chemiluminescent detection method described here offers a chemiluminescent detection system which is a more cost-efficient alternative to the more commonly used radioactive detection techniques.

Materials and Methods

Overall Scheme of Sequencing Method

A specific fragment of genomic DNA is amplified by PCR to produce a suitable template for sequencing. Portions of this PCR reaction are then added to dideoxyribonucleoside triphosphate (ddNTP) termination mixes for sequencing using the primers already present in the initial PCR reaction. Under these conditions sequencing reactions occur from both ends of the PCR product. Specific sequences from either end of the PCR product are detected by probing for each of the strands in turn, using probes complementary, or internal, to the PCR primers, in combination with a chemiluminescent detection procedure.

Oligonucleotide Synthesis

Oligonucleotide primers are synthesized on an Applied Biosystems Model 391 DNA synthesizer and purified on oligonucleotide purification cartridges (Applied Biosystems, Foster City, CA) according to the manufacturer's instructions. Alternatively, there are a number of commercial suppliers of purified oligonucleotides.

DNA Extraction

Human genomic DNA is purified by a simple and inexpensive salting-out procedure (10); however, it should be noted that the method of extraction of the DNA is not critical to the sequencing procedure.

One-milliliter samples of blood (collected into EDTA sequestrene tubes) are diluted with 1 ml of $2\times$ lysis buffer ($1\times$ lysis buffer is 11% sucrose, 10 mM MgCl$_2$, 10mM Tris–HCl, pH 7.5, 1% Triton X-100) and leucocytes pelleted by centrifugation (10 min, 3800 rpm). The cell pellet is then washed with 5 ml of $1\times$ lysis buffer and used immediately for DNA purification.

Cell pellets are resuspended by vortexing in 900 μl TEN buffer (10 mM Tris–HCl, pH 8.2, 2 mM EDTA, 400 mM NaCl) followed by the addition of 100 μl 10% sodium dodecyl sulfate (SDS). This mixture is then incubated in a shaking water bath at 55°C for 1 hr (with occasional disruption of the cell pellet with an inoculation loop). After incubation, 250 μl saturated NaCl is added and the mixture shaken vigorously for 15 sec. Proteins are then removed by centrifugation (10 min, 3000 rpm). Two volumes of ethanol are added to the supernatant and the DNA is collected onto an inoculation loop. The DNA is rinsed in 70% ethanol and then dissolved in TE buffer (10 mM Tris–HCl, pH 8,1 mM EDTA) at 55°C for 2 hr. DNA is then reprecipitated by the addition of 0.5 volume of 7.5 M ammonium acetate, pH 7.5, and 2 volumes of ethanol. After being washed with 70% ethanol and airdried, the DNA is dissolved in TE at 55°C.

PCR Conditions

Segments of human genomic DNA (100 ng) are amplified in 100-μl reactions of the following reagents: 200 ng (0.3 μM) of each primer, 20 μM of each dNTP (Boehringer-Mannheim, Indianapolis, IN), 2.5 units AmpliTaq (Perkin–Elmer Cetus, Norwalk, CT), 50 mM KCl, 10 mM Tris–HCl, pH 8.3, and 1.5 mM MgCl$_2$. The reaction is overlaid with 50 μl mineral oil. After an initial denaturation step of 5 min at 94°C, PCR is performed (Perkin–Elmer thermal cycler Model 480) for 35 cycles, each consisting of 1 min denaturation at 94°C, 1 min annealing at 60°C, and 2 min polymerization at 72°C.

It should be noted that PCR conditions, including components and thermal profiles, must be optimized for each system amplified to produce the strongest and most specific product possible. However, it is critical that the dNTP concentration be kept to a minimum.

DNA Sequencing Conditions

After PCR 16 μl of the reaction mixture is added to 5 units AmpliTaq (1 μl), 1 μl of 10× PCR buffer (100 mM Tris–HCl, pH 8.3, 500 mM KCl, 15 mM MgCl$_2$), and 100 ng (2 μl) of the relevant sequencing primer(s). The reaction mix is then dispersed into four 5-μl aliquots and mixed with 5 μl of the respective ddNTP termination mixes (Perkin–Elmer). The termination mixes all contain 20 μM of each dNTP and the following concentrations of the relevant ddNTPs: G mix, 60 μM ddGTP; A mix, 800 μM ddATP; T mix, 1200 μM ddTTP; C mix, 400 μM ddCTP. The reactions, overlaid with 5 μl mineral oil, are then taken through a further 10 cycles of cycle sequencing with the same thermal profile as in the initial PCR, before being stopped with 4 μl of formamide stop solution (deionized formamide containing 0.3% bromophenol blue, 0.3% xylene cyanol, and 0.37% disodium EDTA, pH 7.0).

Electrophoresis

Sequencing reaction products are denatured at 95°C for 2 min before being stored at 72°C prior to electrophoresis. Samples (2–10 μl) of each reaction (depending on the number of products to be loaded into a sequencing gel well) are loaded on a 5–8% polyacrylamide gel (19 acrylamide : 1 bisacrylamide) in TBE (134 mM Tris–HCl, 44.5 mM boric acid, 2.7 mM EDTA, pH 8.7) and 7.7 M urea and electrophoresed at 42 W for 3-5 hr in a Bio-Rad Sequi-Gen apparatus (Hercules, CA). Gels are 40 cm long, 21 cm wide, and 0.4 mm thick. The electrophoresis conditions and the polyacrylamide concentration of the gel depend on the length of the PCR fragment being sequenced.

Transferring the DNA

DNA can be transferred from the gel onto the nylon membrane (Immobilon-S-membrane supplied by Millipore, Bedford, MA), by a Southern transfer method or by a vacuum blotting procedure. Vacuum blotting is more efficient and generally produces sharper sequencing bands.

Southern Transfer

The Southern transfer is essentially a variation of the procedure described in the Millipore Plex Luminescent Detection kit procedure manual. Following electrophoresis, the gel is lifted from the glass plate with dry blotting paper cut slightly smaller than the gel size. Membrane, prewet in transfer buffer (0.5× TBE, pH 8.7), is then lowered onto the gel and trimmed to remove excess membrane and gel. The paper/gel/membrane sandwich is then centered onto a plastic frame slightly smaller than the gel size on the wicking surface of blotting paper prewet in 0.5× TBE. A second plastic frame is placed on the membrane and overlaid with a stack of weighted absorbent paper. Southern transfer is performed overnight using 0.5× TBE.

Vacuum Transfer

The paper/gel/membrane sandwich is centered onto the surface of a Bio-Rad Model 543 gel dryer, with the membrane surface down. Transfer is initiated by connecting the apparatus to an Edwards Speedivac 2 vacuum pump (Crawley, UK) operating at approximately 10 Pascals. Transfer is completed in 1 hr.

Drying the Membrane and Fixation of DNA

The membrane is completely dried in an oven at 60°C for 30 min–1 hr prior to the cross-linking procedure. DNA is UV cross-linked onto the membrane using a 254-nm UV light (300 μ W/cm^2) for 2–2.5 min.

Preparation of Biotin-Labeled Probes

Oligonucleotides complementary or internal to the sequencing primers are biotin-labeled in preparation to be used as probes. The end-labeling reaction incorporating dUTP-biotin is performed with terminal transferase (TdT) (Boehringer-Mannheim). Then 10 μl 5× TdT reaction buffer (1 M potassium cacodylate, 125 mM Tris–HCl, 1.25 mg/ml BSA, pH 6.6), 5 μl 25mM CoCl$_2$,

2.5 μl 0.4 mM dUTP-biotin,7.5 μl 0.4 mM dTTP, and 600 ng (24 μl) of primer are mixed together. A total of 30 units (1 μl) TdT is then added and the mixture incubated at 37°C for 15–30 min. The reaction is stopped by the addition of 10 μl 100 mM EDTA, pH 8.0.

Hybridization and Chemiluminescent Detection

The hybridization, washing, and detection steps are all performed in a plastic bottle (13 cm diameter $\times$ 20 cm length) within a rotating incubator, using the Millipore Plex Luminescent Detection kit (Millipore, Bedford, MA). The procedure used is a slight variation to the manufacturer's instructions. As washing is more efficient in rotating bottles than in hybridization bags the amounts of solutions used and times of incubation required are considerably less than those recommended.

Hybridization is performed for 1 hr and hybridization temperatures are generally found to be optimal at approximately 15°C below T_m of the labeled primer. After DNA fixation, the membrane is placed into the bottle and 60 ml of prehybridization solution [125 mM NaCl, 17 mM Na$_2$HPO$_4$, 8 mM NaH$_2$PO$_4$, 173 mM SDS, 12.5 mM polyethylene glycol (PEG), pH 7.2] added. After incubation for 5 min at the desired hybridization temperature, the prehybridization mix is replaced with 600 ng of labeled primer in 30 ml of prehybridization solution and incubated for 60 min at the hybridization temperature.

After hybridization all subsequent washing steps are performed at room temperature. The membrane is washed three times for 3 min each in a 1:10 dilution of blocking solution (blocking solution is 125 mM NaCl, 17 mM Na$_2$HPO$_4$, 8 mM NaH$_2$PO$_4$, 173 mM SDS, pH 7.2) and then blocked with 60 ml of blocking solution for 5 min prior to a 5-min incubation with 17 ml of 10 μg streptavidin/ml blocking solution. The membrane is then washed twice for 5 min in 1:10 blocking solution, incubated for 5 min in blocking solution and 5 min with 17 ml of 5 μg biotin-AP/ml blocking solution, and washed twice in wash solution II (10 mM Tris–HCl, 10 mM NaCl, 1 mM MgCl$_2$, pH 9.5) for 5 min each. The membrane is then incubated with 100 μl Lumigen-PPD reagent in 10 ml 1 X diluent (2-amino-2-methyl propanol buffer, pH 9.6) for 5 min prior to being exposed, between two plastic sheets, to HT-U medical X-ray film (Agfa Curix, Belgium) for 30 min-1 hour.

For subsequent probing the membrane is stripped by a 15-min incubation in 1:10 blocking solution at 60°C, followed by two washes at room temperature for 8 min in 1:10 blocking solution. The membrane can be stored indefinitely in the 1:10 blocking solution.

Performing Direct Double-Stranded Sequencing

It is critical that the concentration of dNTPs be kept to a minimum in the initial PCR, so that there are little or no remaining dNTPs to alter the dNTP : ddNTP ratio in the sequencing reaction. As can be seen in Fig. 1 sequencing of PCR products with 200 μM dNTPs in the initial PCR results in a sequence with nonspecific terminations in all four lanes. Minimizing the dNTP concentration to the lowest possible, while still producing a strong PCR product, along with a slight increase in PCR cycle number can overcome the problem of remaining dNTPs. (One should note the importance of decreasing the $MgCl_2$ concentration in the initial PCR when decreasing dNTP

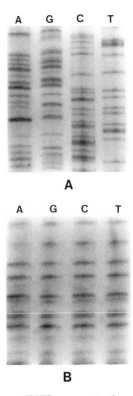

FIG. 1   Comparison of different dNTP concentrations in the initial PCR. Sequence ladders produced when (A) 20μM dNTPs and (B) 200 μM dNTPs were used in the initial PCR. Nonspecific termination results when 200 μM dNTPs were used in the initial PCR as can be seen from the banding in all four lanes. DNA in the sequencing gels was Southern transferred to nylon membrane for detection.

concentration in order to optimize product yield.) In practice, each PCR/ sequencing reaction will be different as the utilization of the dNTPs will largely depend on the PCR efficiency and the cycle number used. However, in our hands, the use of 20 μM dNTPs has been optimal with several different products ranging in size from 80–450 bases.

Figure 2 shows a DNA sequence obtained by the above protocol. A 354-base region of the cytochrome P450 gene (11) was amplified and sequenced and the sequencing ladder detected with probes complementary to the se-

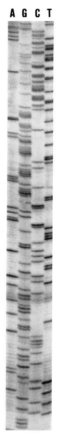

FIG. 2   Direct sequencing of the cytochrome P450 double-stranded PCR product under optimal conditions. The sequence shown (from base 2031 to base 1843 with the reverse primer) was generated by the direct sequencing protocol, before being vacuum-transferred onto Immobilon-S-membrane and subsequently detected by the Lumigen-PPD (Millipore, Bedford, MA) substrate. Reproduced with permission from Douglas *et al.* (6). © 1993 Eaton Publishing.

quencing primers. Typically 250–300 bases of this sequence could be read from the one gel and up to three different PCR fragments (six probings) have been placed into the one well on a sequencing gel and each probed by this procedure.

When a specific 1211-base fragment from a region of the cytochrome P450 gene was amplified by this sequencing protocol the sequence ladder contained some very strong "compressions" (i.e., intense bands in all four tracks) and, thus, reduced the amount of sequence that could be accurately read. These compressions were not due to the commonly described gel (12) or sequencing artifacts which result from strong secondary DNA structure (13), but rather from nonspecific PCR products interfering with sequence ladder detection. As can be seen from Fig. 3, probing this fragment with a labeled primer internal to the sequencing primers reduced the number of false bands. The detection of these nonspecific PCR products was also found when sequencing

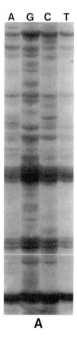

A G C T

A

Fig. 3 Direct sequencing of the cytochrome P450 1211-base PCR product. The sequence shown was generated by the direct sequencing protocol, before being vacuum-transferred onto Immobilon-S-membrane and subsequently detected by the Lumigen-PPD substrate. The membrane was probed with a probe (A) complementary to and (B) internal to the sequencing primer.

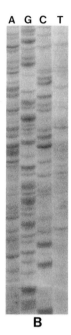

FIG. 3   (*continued*)

a 1078-base fragment of the apolipoprotein AI gene (14). The problem of the artifact bands was also alleviated by internal probing.

As a consequence of the problems that can be encountered when directly sequencing products greater than 1000 bases, it is recommended that PCR products less than 600 bases be amplified. Although sequencing larger fragments seems attractive as fewer PCR systems have to be initially optimized, the direct sequencing of smaller fragments is essentially more efficient for a number of reasons.

1) Optimization of the initial PCR is simpler with smaller fragments.

2) PCR is more efficient with smaller fragments and thus produces stronger sequencing ladder signals: background nonspecific termination products do not interfere with these sequencing ladders. If nonspecific PCR products are produced they can usually be eliminated by probing internal to the primer.

3) The number of bases that can be read from the one gel is limited to approximately 300. It is, therefore, more efficient to load more than one PCR product into one well and perform multiplex PCR, rather than running

more than one gel for each section of a larger PCR product (probing only entails approximately 2.5–3 hr work versus 6–10 hr for the entire electrophoresis procedure). That is, for a 900-base sequence, rather than amplifying and sequencing one 900-base product, and needing three electrophoreses to resolve all bases, it is more efficient to amplify three PCR products (approximately 300 bases each) and load the three sequenced products into the one well. Only one electrophoresis run is then required and three separate probings will detect all 900 bases.

References

1. R. K. Saiki, S. Scharf, F. Faloona, K. B. Mullis, G. T. Horn, H. A. Erlich, and N. Arnheim, *Science* **230**, 1350 (1985).
2. U. B. Gyllensten and H. A. Erlich, *Proc. Natl. Acad. Sci. U.S.A.* **85**, 7652 (1988).
3. R. G. Higuchi and H. Ochman, *Nucleic Acids Res.* **17**, 5865 (1989).
4. N. Kusukawa, T. Uemori, K. Asada, and I. Kato, *BioTechniques* **9**, 66 (1990).
5. L. G. Mitchell and C. R. Merril, *Anal. Biochem.* **178**, 239 (1989).
6. A. M. Douglas, A. M. Georgalis, and B. A. Atchison, *BioTechniques* **14**, 824 (1993).
7. A. M. Carothers, G. Urlaub, J. Mucha, D. Grunberger, and L. A. Chasin, *BioTechniques* **7**, 494 (1989).
8. S. Beck, T. O'Keefe, J. M. Coull, and H. Koster, *Nucleic Acids Res.* **12**, 5115 (1989).
9. A. Creasey, L. D'Angio, Jr., T. S. Dunne, C. Kissinger, T. O'Keefe, H. Perry-O'Keefe, L. S. Moran, M. Roskey, I. Schildkrant, L. E. Sears, and B. Slatko, *BioTechniques* **11**, 102 (1991).
10. A. M. Douglas, A. M. Georgalis, L. R. Benton, K. L. Canavan, and B. A. Atchison, *Anal. Biochem.* **201**, 362 (1992).
11. S. Kimura, M. Umeno, R. C. Skoda, U. A. Meyer, and F. J. Gonzalez, *Am. J. Hum. Genet.* **45**, 889 (1989).
12. M. A. D. Brow, *in* "PCR Protocols: A Guide to Methods and Applications" (M. A. Innis, D. H. Gelfand, J. J. Sninsky, and T. H. White, eds), p. 189. Academic Press, San Diego, 1990.
13. P. J. Barr, R. M. Thayer, P. Laybourn, R. C. Najarian, F. Seela, and D. R. Tolan, *BioTechniques* **4**, 428 (1986).
14. J. J. Seilhamer, A. A. Protter, P. Frossand, and B. Levy-Wilson, *DNA* **3**, 309 (1984).

[27] Use of PCR to Determine Genomic DNA Target Sites for Zinc Finger Protein Expressed in Mouse Cerebellum

Annette Christoph and Hans-Jürgen Thiesen

Introduction

The central nervous system is the most complex organ that has evolved (Chaudhari and Hahn, 1983; Sutcliffe, 1988). Steps of spatial and temporal organ specification leading from neuroectodermal cells to adult brain tissues require the expression of stage-specific genes (Fraser *et al.*, 1990). Transcription factors are essential in mediating tissue-specific gene expression (Maniatis *et al.*, 1987). In recent years developmental genes coding for potential transcriptional regulatory proteins have been identified from *Drosophila* to man (Gehring, 1987; Bopp *et al.*, 1986; He *et al.*, 1989; Schöler *et al.*, 1990; Weigel and Jäckle, 1990; Garrell and Campuzano, 1991; Chowdhury *et al.*, 1987). The zinc finger domain first characterized in *Xenopus* transcription factor IIIA (TFIIIA) (Ginsberg *et al.*, 1984; Miller *et al.*, 1985) and in *Drosophila* gap genes Krüppel (Rosenberg *et al.*, 1986) and hunchback (Tautz *et al.*, 1987) has been demonstrated to present a gene family of several hundred in the mammalian genome (Chowdbury *et al.*, 1987; Bellefroid *et al.*, 1989; Thiesen, 1990a; Bray *et al.*, 1991).

Zinc Finger Proteins in Neurobiology

The function of most individual zinc finger proteins awaits to be determined. Initial data demonstrate that the zinc finger protein Krox20 (Wilkenson *et al.*, 1989a) and homeobox protein H2B (Wilkenson *et al.*, 1989b) are involved in specifying developmental pathways of murine hindbrain development (Sham *et al.*, 1993). A targeted mutation of Krox20 led to a loss of rhombomeres 3 and 5 resulting in a disorganization of trigeminal, facial, and vestibular ganglia (Swiatek and Gridley, 1993; Schneider-Maunoury *et al.*, 1993). Furthermore, zinc finger proteins Krox20 (Chavrier *et al.*, 1988) and Zif268 (Christy and Nathans, 1989) are rapidly and transiently activated by electroconvulsive shock treatment (ECT), dopamine receptor activation, and opiate withdrawal (Bhat *et al.*, 1992). Zif268 mRNA levels and long-term potentia-

Methods in Neurosciences, Volume 26

tion (LTP) seem to be regulated by similar synaptic mechanisms (Cole *et al.*, 1989). Blockade of afferent visual activity with intraocular injections of tetrodotoxin results in rapid, dramatic reduction of Zif268 mRNA levels (Worley *et al.*, 1991). Zinc finger protein NGFI-C expression is restricted in the rat to the brain and other neural tissues (Crosby *et al.*, 1992). The murine zinc finger-containing gene mKR2 is expressed in the central and peripheral nervous system of adult animals (Chowdhury *et al.*, 1988). The zinc finger protein NTfin 12 encoding 19 zinc finger tandem repeats has been shown to be highly expressed in the neuroectoderm overlaying the mesoderm at the neurulation stage (Noce *et al.*, 1992). Several zinc finger genes have been reported to be expressed in oligodendrocytes (Pott *et al.*, 1993). The zinc finger protein NK10 cloned from mouse cerebellum has been shown to be differentially expressed during murine cerebellum development (Lange *et al.*, 1994). Most likely, zinc finger proteins are implicated in regulating developmental and differentiation processes of mammalian organs, evidenced by the genomic analysis of mutations in the Wilms' tumor suppressor gene (Call *et al.*, 1990; Gessler *et al.*, 1990; Pelletier *et al.*, 1991) and of the GLI-3 gene (Kinzler *et al.*, 1988; Vortkamp *et al.*, 1991).

Principle of DNA–Protein Interactions

In general transcription factors bind specific DNA target sites in a sequence-specific manner (Pabo and Sauer, 1992). Numerous transcription factors increase their DNA binding specificities by forming homo- or heterodimers (Landschulz *et al.*, 1988). Transcription factors that bind DNA as a dimer utilize larger DNA target sites. The dimeric form of yeast DNA binding protein GAL4 recognizes a DNA sequence of 17 nucleotides (Johnston, 1987). The recognition of functional DNA target sites by transcription factors *in vivo* is partly dependent on their binding to specific DNA target sites and is partly supported by their assembly in multimeric DNA protein complexes. Most likely, proteins that directly interact with transcription factors establish multimeric protein complexes that enhance specific DNA protein interactions in the nucleus. Opposed to multimeric protein complexes that might interact at more than one specific contact site with genomic DNA, the availability of putative DNA target sites *in vivo* is considerably influenced by nucleosomal packaging of DNA into chromatin (Kornberg and Lorch, 1992).

To characterize the DNA binding specificities of individual DNA binding proteins, elegant methods for determining DNA target sites *in vitro* have been developed by making use of randomized oligonucleotides (Oliphant *et al.*, 1989; Thiesen, 1990b; Thiesen *et al.*, 1990). A technique using PCR for reamplification of selected oligonucleotides was initially described as target detection assay (TDA) (Thiesen and Bach, 1990; Thiesen, 1990c) and modified by Pollock and Treisman (1990). Herein, a PCR-based procedure is described for making use of genomic DNA fragments for identifying putative DNA target sites. The principle of this method has originally been developed by Kinzler and Vogelstein (1989).

Principles and Objectives

DNA Recognition of the Zinc Finger Domain

In general, DNA binding proteins consist of distinct protein domains with diverse functions. Zinc finger proteins contain at least two functional domains, the nucleic acid (DNA and/or RNA) binding domain exemplified by the zinc finger domain and an effector domain that determines the function of the transcription factor. One effector domain, the highly conserved Krüppel-Associated Box (KRAB), has been identified as displaying a strong transcriptional repressor and silencing activity (Margolin et al,. 1994; Meyer et al., 1994).

Initially, the zinc finger domain is characterized by tandemly repeated motifs having the consensus $TGEKPYXCX_{2-4}CX_3FX_5LX_2HX_{3-4}H$ in common (Ashworth and Denny, 1991). The contiguous stretch of nucleotides corresponding to the H/C linker region—this region connects individual zinc finger with each other—consists of seven highly conserved amino acids (HTGEKPY) (Berg, 1990). The conserved cysteines and histidines of one zinc finger repeat chelate one zinc atom (Diakun et al., 1986) which stabilizes the characteristic zinc finger structure represented by a β-sheet structure followed by an α-helix (Pavletich and Pabo, 1991). Zinc finger structures of this kind were originally predicted by Miller et al. in 1985 and confirmed by the analysis of DNA protein crystals derived from zinc finger proteins Zif268 (Pavletich and Pabo, 1991) and for GLI-1 (Pavletich and Pabo, 1993). In these analysis individual amino acid residues within the α-helical zinc finger region of Zif268 and GLI-1 have been identified to interact with two to four nucleotides of their DNA target sites. In transcription factor SP1 (Kadonaga et al., 1986) mutations of these amino acid residues lead to new DNA binding specificities (Thiesen and Bach, 1991a).

Though not all fingers might be employed in directly binding DNA in a sequence-specific manner (Clemens et al., 1993), Krüppel-type zinc finger domains are thought to be capable of utilizing large stretches of DNA for recognition. For example, the 19 fingers of NTfin12 (Noce et al., 1992) might be assumed to span a DNA binding region of 57 nucleotides under the assumption that each finger spans 3 nucleotides (3 nt t × 19 fingers). Thus, in theory, zinc finger proteins with multiple consecutive zinc fingers have the property of recognizing *in vivo* only a few functional target sites per genome. This characteristic might enable the cloning of functional DNA target genes merely based on *in vitro* genomic target site selection methods.

General Strategy of Selecting Genomic Target Sites

The method being described in detail herein is based on techniques developed by Kinzler and Vogelstein (1989, 1990) and has been modified by using recombinant fusion proteins between glutathione S-transferase (GST) and zinc finger domains. Glutathione-Sepharose affinity chromatography (Smith and Johnson, 1988) is used for purifying the fusion protein and for separating DNA protein complexes from unbound DNA (Fainsod *et al.*, 1991; Costa-Giomi *et al.*, 1992). The principle of identifying genomic DNA target sites is that a purified DNA binding protein selects high-affinity DNA binding sites from a pool of genomic DNA sequences. Genomic DNA fragments that bind with various affinities are selected by glutathione-Sepharose beads that have been loaded with GST-fusion protein. The DNA fragments bound best by the DNA protein complexes are deliberated, amplified by the polymerase chain reaction (PCR), and subjected to further rounds of selection. The stringency of selection determines with what efficiency high-affinity binding sites can be identified. The polymerase chain reaction can be employed after the ends of genomic DNA fragments have been tagged with catch linkers (Kinzler and Vogelstein, 1989). In general, the selection procedure follows the same principles that have been described for the TDA (Thiesen, 1990c; Thiesen and Bach, 1990).

Experimental Procedures

Materials and Stock Solutions

All basic techniques for molecular biology have been exclusively described by Sambrook *et al.* (1989), including materials and working solutions. Enzymes and buffers have been used as recommended by commercial suppliers. Additional equipment, stock solutions, and culture media are listed below.

Equipment

Hybaid Intelligent Heating Block
Biometra, Göttingen, Germany

Sonicator, Labsonic U
Nadelsonde T 40
Braun Diessel Biotech, Melsungen, Germany

UV Stratalinker 1800 autocrosslink
Stratagene, Heidelberg, Germany

Slotblot Kammer
BIO-DOT SF
Bio-Rad, München, Germany

Buffers

$1 \times$ DNA–protein binding buffer
  50 mM HEPES, pH 7.5
  50 mM KCl
  5 mM MgCl$_2$
  10 μM ZnSO$_4$
  1 mM dithiothreitol (DTT)
  20% glycerine

$1 \times$ DNA–protein wash buffer
  50 mM HEPES, pH 7.5
  150 mM KCl
  5 mM MgCl$_2$
  10 μM ZnSO$_4$
  1% Triton X-100
  0.05% sodium dodecyl sulfate (SDS)

$1 \times$ DNA–protein disassociation buffer
  500 mM Tris–HCl, pH 9.0
  20 mM EDTA
  10 mM NaCl
  0.2% SDS

Bacterial Culture Media

YT-medium
  0.8% tryptone
  0.5% yeast extract

> 85m*M* NaCl
> pH 7.4

> YT-agar plates
> 0.8% tryptone
> 0.5% yeast extract
> 85 m*M* NaCl
> 1.5% agar
> pH 7.4

Glutathione S-Transferase-Fusion Proteins: Generation and Purification

Recombinant DNA binding proteins for DNA target site selections can be generated using prokaryotic or eukaryotic expression systems. By making use of the pGEX expression vectors (Pharmacia, Uppsala), GST fusion proteins can be generated harboring the DNA binding domain of interest and GST as fusion partner that enables the purification of the GST-fusion protein by a glutathione-Sepharose column (Pharmacia, Uppsala).

Preparation of Genomic DNA for PCR Amplification

1. Cut 10 μg of genomic DNA with frequently cutting restriction enzymes [RSA I (GT/AC), *Hae*III (GG/CC), and *Alu*I (AG/CT)] and 1 U/μg DNA in 400 μl of appropriate restriction buffer at 37°C overnight.

2. Determine average length of genomic DNA fragments on a 2% agarose gel. The average size should be around 300 nt.

3. Do standard phenol/chloroform extraction of the DNA digest, precipitate and wash genomic DNA fragments with ethanol, dry and resuspend DNA pellet in 18.5 μl H$_2$O.

4. Order or synthesize two oligonucleotides (catch linker A 5' GAGTA-GAATTC TAATATCTC 3' and catch linker B 3' CTCATCTTAAGATTA-TAGAG 5', Kinzler and Vogelstein, 1989).

5. Phosphorylate both catch linkers (32 μg of each linker is kinased by 40 U/μl polynucleotide kinase (Boehringer-Mannheim, Mannheim, Germany) in 100 μl kinase buffer [(50 m*M* Tris–HCl, pH 7.5, 10 m*M* MgCl$_2$, 5 m*M* DTT, 100 μ*M* spermidine, and 1 m*M* adenosine triphosphate (ATP)].

6. Do phenol/chloroform extraction, precipitate [10 μl 3*M* sodium acetate, pH 5.2, and 250 μl ethanol (100%)], wash oligonucleotides with 70% ethanol, dry pellet, and resuspend oligonucleotides in 75 μl H$_2$O.

7. Anneal kinased oligonucleotides A and B (3 min, 95°C) and cool down to room temperature.

8. Ligate 10 μg of cut blunt-ended genomic DNA with 30 μg of double-stranded catch linkers with 1 U/μl T4 DNA ligase (New England Biolabs, Schwalbach, FRG) in 100 μl ligase buffer (50 mM Tris–HCl, pH 7.8, 10 mM MgCl2, 10 mM DTT, 1 mM ATP, 25 μg/ml BSA) at 14°C overnight.

9. Digest ligation mix with restriction enzyme *Xho*I (1 U/μl) (Boehringer-Mannheim) in 1.2 ml of reaction buffer (5 mM Tris–HCl, pH 7.5, 1 mM MgCl$_2$, 10 mM NaCl, 0.1 mM DTE) for 2 hr at 37°C.

10. Do phenol/chloroform extraction, precipitate with 120 μl 3M sodium acetate, pH 5.2, and 3 ml ethanol (100%), wash with 70% ethanol, dry at room temperature, and resuspend pellet in 10 μl H$_2$O.

Selection and Amplification of Genomic DNA Target Sites

1. Incubate 500 ng of genomic catch linker DNA with 400 ng GST-fusion protein bound to 1 μl glutathione-Sepharose (Pharmacia, Uppsala) in the presence of 5.4 μg poly [(dI-dC)] in 20 μl binding buffer (50 mM HEPES, pH 7.5, 50 mM KCl, 5 mM MgCl$_2$, 10 μM ZnCl$_2$, 1 mM DTT, 20% glycerol) for 30 min at room temperature.

2. Wash glutathione-Sepharose beads 2× with 1.5 ml wash buffer (50 mM HEPES, 150 mM KCl, 5 mM MgCl$_2$, 10 μM ZnSO4, 1% Triton X-100, 0.5% SDS) at room temperature.

3. Elute bound DNA fragments with 100 μl dissociation buffer (500 mM Tris–HCl, pH 9.0, 20 mM EDTA, 10 mM NaCl, 0.2% SDS) for 50 min at 50°C.

4. Do phenol/chloroform extraction and ethanol precipitation by adding 10 μl 3 M NaAc, pH 5.2, 500 ng glycogen, and 250 μl 100% ethanol; wash DNA pellet with 70% ethanol; air-dry; and resuspend in 20 μl H$_2$O.

5. Do PCR on 1/10 of selected DNA using 300 ng catch linker A and B, 2.5 U *Taq* polymerase (GIBCO-BRL Gaithersburg, MD), 0.5 μl detergent W1 (GIBCO-BRL) in 50 μl PCR reaction buffer (50 mM KCl, 10 mM Tris–HCl, pH 8.4, 2.5. mM MgCl$_2$, 0.1 mM DTT, 1 mM dNTP, 0.04% gelatin) and do 25 cycles, denaturate 1 min/90°C, anneal 2 min/45°C, and extend 2 min/70°C.

6. Do phenol/chloroform of amplified DNA and precipitate as described in step 4.

7. Repeat step 1 to step 6 several times. Depending on the zinc finger region of interest the stringency of selection can be increased by changing the ratio of synthetic DNA and/or the ratio between genomic DNA and GST-fusion protein. By increasing the KCl concentration and/or adding 1,10-*o*-phenanthroline to the elution buffer, DNA fragments bound with different affinities can be eluted stepwise (Thiesen, 1990c).

8. Cut amplified DNA fragments with *Eco*RI and clone them in appropriate cloning vectors that have been cut with *Eco*RI and dephosphorylated prior to ligation.

Characterization of Selected Genomic Target Sites

After genomic DNA fragments selected by DNA binding proteins of interest have been cloned, various techniques can be used for further characterizing their specific DNA target sites. DNA fragments that have been most abundantly selected can be identified by hybridization studies, homologous or consensus sequences can be determined by sequence analysis of randomly chosen fragments, and individual binding sites can be further characterized by electrophoretic mobility shift assays (EMSA) and by DNase I footprinting analysis. Finally, *in vivo* assays can be designed to verify *in vivo* the function of these target sites. In the end, these fragments can be used for searching expressed target genes located in the neighborhood of these DNA target sites. Detailed protocols of standard techniques describing the analysis of DNA protein interactions are described in Ausubel *et al.* (1988).

Application

Zinc Finger Protein NK10 Expressed in Mouse Cerebellum

The principles of using PCR for amplifying genomic DNA fragments have been used to determine genomic target sites for a murine zinc finger protein designated NK10 which has been cloned and characterized by Lange *et al.* (1994). The organization of the zinc finger domains specific to NK10 is outlined in Fig. 1. Regions of zinc finger domains have been designated

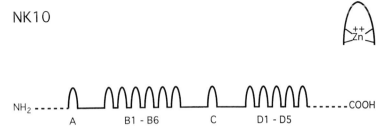

FIG. 1   Structure of zinc finger protein NK10. Regions of zinc finger domains have been designated region A, B, C, and D.

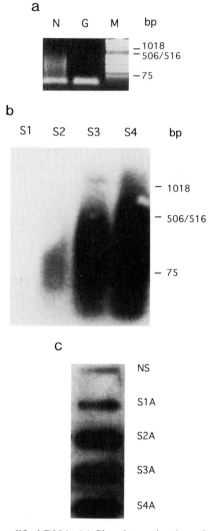

Fig. 2   Selection of amplified DNA. (a) Size determination of selected DNA. Geno-mic DNA were PCR amplified from selections performed with GST-NK10-fusion proteins (lane N) or with GST protein alone (lane G). The average size of amplified genomic DNA is in the range of 300 bp (lane N) compared to the size marker (GIBCO-BRL) in lane M. (b) PCR on selected DNA. Equal amounts of PCR-amplified DNA were labeled with $[\alpha\text{-}^{32}]dCTP$, separated on a agarose gel, transferred to Nytran membrane (NY13N; Schleicher & Schüll, Dassel), and exposed to a Kodak X-ray film. Lane S1 represents the genomic DNA from the first selection, lane S2 to lane S4 the genomic DNA from consecutive rounds of selections. (c) Determination for enrichment of specific sequences. A slot-blot assay was performed to demonstrate

region A, B, C, and D. Region A and C are presented by single finger domains, whereas finger region B encompasses six tandemly repeated zinc fingers and region D five zinc fingers. For determining genomic DNA target sites, the zinc finger regions B–D were cloned into a pGEX expression vector according to the protocol outlined above. The expression of GST-NK10-fusion protein was induced by isopropyl-β-D-thiogalactopyranoside (IPTG) and the GST-NK10-fusion protein purified using glutathione-Sepharose beads.

To determine whether genomic DNA fragments can be selected by GST-NK10-fusion protein, genomic DNA fragments that had been modified with catch linkers were subjected to one round of DNA selection and PCR amplification. DNA fragments of an average size range of 300 bp were exclusively amplified when GST-NK10-fusion protein was employed in the selection procedure (Fig. 2a). After four rounds of selection the proportion of DNA fragments was determined that was specifically bound by NK10 protein and increased from PCR cycle to PCR cycle. Then, 1/20 of the amplified DNA was subjected to five PCR cycles, the DNA was extracted by phenol/chloroform, and a second PCR amplification of three cycles was done in presense of 0.5 μCi [α-^{32}P]dCTP (3000 Ci/mM; Amersham, Braunschweig). Equal amounts of DNA were separated on a 2% agarose gel, transferred to Nytran membrane (NY13N; Schleicher & Schüll, Dassel), and exposed to a Kodak (Rochester, NY) X-ray film (Fig. 2b). Lane S1 represents genomic DNA from the first selection; lane S2 to lane S4 represent genomic DNA from consecutive rounds of selection. This analysis demonstrates that the complexity of amplified DNA fragments has been reduce from one cycle of selection to the next cycle of selection.

In addition, a slot-blot assay (Fig. 2c) was performed to demonstrate that specific DNA sequences have been enriched from one PCR-based selection step to the next. Amplified DNA (100 ng) derived from each selection step was loaded per slot on Nytran membrane NY13N by utilizing a BioRad slot-blot chamber (Bio-Rad, Munich, FRG). Prior to loading, the Nytran membrane soaked in 0.3 M NaOH for 5 min at room temperature. The

---

that specific DNA sequences have been enriched from one PCR-based selection step to the next. A total of 100 ng of PCR-amplified DNA was loaded on Nytran membrane NY13N (lane NS, nonselected DNA; lane S1A, DNA from first round of selection; lane S2A, DNA from second round of selection; lane S3A, DNA from third round of selection; and lane S4A, DNA from fourth round of selection). PCR-amplified DNA derived from the fourth round of PCR selection (S4) were used as specific hybridization probe. Genomic sequences present in slot S4A have been enriched stepwise from the nonselected DNA fraction (NS) to the fourth round of selection, see slot S4A.

transferred DNA was renatured with 100 μl of 0.3 M NaOH for 10 min at room temperature. After the slots were rinsed with 250 μl 0.3 M NaOH, the Nytran membrane was neutralized in 0.5 M Tris–HCl, pH 7.0, 1.5 M NaCl. The DNA was cross-linked to the NY13N membrane by UV Strata-linker 1800 autocross-link (Stratagene, La Jolla, CA). Amplified DNA derived from the fourth round of PCR selection (S4) was used as a specific hybridization probe. Comparing the slots in Fig. 2c, genomic sequences present in slot S4A have been enriched stepwise from the nonselected DNA fraction (NS) to the fourth round of selection in slot S4A by the GST-NK10-fusion protein.

Characterization of Target Sites Specific for Zinc Finger Protein NK10

After genomic DNA fragments derived from four rounds of selection and PCR amplification were selected and cloned a few cloned fragments were subjected to further analysis. In particular, EMSA analysis was utilized to determine the sequence specificity and the affinity of the selected genomic DNA.

Cloned DNA fragment S4A51 was cut with *Eco*RI, purified from a agarose gel, and labeled by a filling-in reaction with 0.2 U/μl Klenow (Boehringer-Mannheim), using 20 μCi [α-^{32}-P]dATP (3000 Ci/mmol; Amersham, Braunschweig) in 20 μl 7 mM Tris–HCl, pH 7.5, 7 mM MgCl$_2$, 50 mM Nacl, 5 mM DTT, 1 mM dCTP, 1 mM dGTP, 1 mM dTTP for 30 min at 37°C. In a standard EMSA reaction micture labeled fragments of 50000 cpm were incubated in presence of 10 ng poly [(dI)-(dC)] with 100 ng GST protein (Fig. 3a, lane N) for 30 min at room temperature in 10.5 μl (100 mM NaCl, 10 mM Tris–HCl, pH 8.0, 1 mM DTT, 10 μM ZnSO$_4$, 10% glycerol). The DNA protein complexes were separated on a 6% polyacrylamide gel (30% acrylamide, 0.8% bisacrylamide) in 0.25× TBE (1× TBE: 0.1 M Tris–HCl, 0.1 M borate, 0.25 mM EDTA, pH 8.3) for 4 hr at 4°C using 10 V/cm. Afterward the gel was transferred to Whatman (Clifton, NJ) 3MM paper, dried, and exposed to Kodak XAR at −80°C for 1–24 hr in the presence of one intensifying screen. A reasonable bandshift becomes visible in presence of 100 ng GST-NK10-fusion protein. The presence of two shifted bands indicates that probably more than one protein can bind to the selected DNA fragment (Fig. 3a).

To assess the affinity of sequence specific DNA recognition, competition experiments were performed using a 42-bp fragment derived from clone S4A51 (Fig. 3b). Experimental procedures were done as described in Fig. 3a. In lane P, no protein was added to the DNA fragment; in lane O, 100 ng GST-NK10-fusion protein were used without any competitor; in lanes of

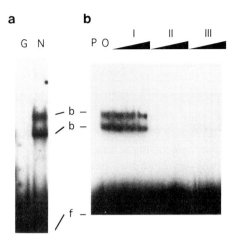

FIG. 3   Characterization of selected genomic DNA fragments. (a) EMSA analysis of PCR-selected DNA fragment. Cloned DNA fragment S4A51 was labeled with 35,000–75,000 cpm, incubated in presence of 10 ng poly[(dI)-(dC)] with GST protein (lane G) or 100 ng of GST-NK10-fusion protein (lane N) and an EMSA was performed. Genomic DNA fragment is bound by GST-NK10-fusion protein. (b) Competition experiments on PCR selected DNA fragment. Competition experiments were performed using the 42-bp insert of S4A51 (50,000 cpm). In lane P, no protein was added to the DNA fragment; in lane O, 100 ng GST-NK10-fusion protein was used without any competitor; in lanes of segment I, increasing amounts (25, 100, and 250 ng) of double-stranded catch linkers (20 bp) were added; in lanes of segment II, the insert itself (25, 100, and 250 ng) was used as competitor DNA; and in lanes of segment III, a 24p-bp oligonucleotide (25, 100, and 250 ng) has been applied that constitutes the consensus sequences of the selected oligonucleotides. The retarded DNA protein complexes are indicated by a b and the free oligonucleotides by f.

segment I, increasing amounts (25, 100, and 250 ng) of double-stranded catch linkers (20 bp) were added; in lanes of segment II, the insert itself (25, 100, 250 ng) was used as competitor DNA; and in lanes of segment III, a 24-bp oligonucleotide (25, 100, 250 ng) has been applied that constitutes the consensus sequences of nine selected genomic fragments. This analysis demonstrates that genomic DNA fragment S4A51 binds sequence specifically to the zinc finger domain of NK10.

Comparison of Genomic Target Site Selection versus Random Oligonucleotide Selection Systems

In general, two PCR-based methods of selecting DNA fragments by DNA binding proteins have been developed, one uses genomic DNA (Kinzler and

Vogelstein, 1989, 1990), the other randomized oligonucleotides (Thiesen, 1990b,c; Thiesen and Bach, 1990). However, the principle of using randomized oligonucleotides is not appropriate for selecting DNA binding sites for more than $N = 23$ random positions, since in these cases not all putative DNA binding sites will be generated in a standard ologonucleotide synthesis (Thiesen, 1990c). In these circumstances the complexity of the genome is by far less than the compexity of randomized ologonucleotides that have to be generated.

The advantage of using genomic DNA for determining DNA target sites of tandemly repeated zinc finger proteins is that DNA fragments derived from the authentic genome are selected by their own zinc finger proteins. If the assumption "DNA binding specificities of zinc finger proteins increase with the number of zinc finger repeats" should turn out to be correct, zinc finger proteins with multiple zinc fingers should even facilitate the direct identification of functional DNA target sites and genes. In this case, selected DNA fragments can be used to identify expressed genes localized in the neighborhood to the genomic target sites.

Critical Appraisal

With the advent of PCR technology the amplification of tiny amounts of DNA has become a routine in molecular biology. However, much care has to be taken to get rid of contaminations (Thiesen et al., 1990). In particular, the quality of selecting DNA fragments that bind with high affinity to the DNA binding protein of choice is depending on the fact that non-DNA sequence-specific interactions that occur during the selection procedures have to be minimized. Since all individual zinc fingers present in one zinc finger domain have the potential of participating in sequence-specific DNA recognition, functional DNA target sites might only be successfully identified once it is guaranteed that the DNA binding domain under study has reached its protein conformation found in vivo. The most important step in optimizing the selection procedure is based on the nature of the DNA binding protein used. Recombinant zinc finger proteins should be properly folded in the presence of zinc since metal reconstitution experiments of Sp1 have shown that variations of zinc concentrations modulate DNA–protein interactions of SP1 with its DNA cognate binding site (Thiesen and Bach, 1991b).

Glutathione S-transferase-fusion proteins facilitate the generation and purification of soluble recombinant DNA binding domains. However, two major concerns have to be excluded. First, the GST domain should not alter the DNA binding properties of the protein under study and, second, the GST protein portion itself should not take part in the selection procedure. Furthermore, zinc finger domains tend to form insoluble inclusion bodies that have to be solubilized for obtaining proper selection (Kinzler and Vogelstein, 1989). In this respect it is worth mentioning that Wolfram Meyer at the Basel Institute for Immunology developed an efficient method for purifying and renaturating zinc finger proteins from inclusion bodies (personal communication). Nevertheless, one of the major setbacks using the techniques described above is that naked DNA is being used. Any chromatin-associated specifications of functional DNA binding sites are not taken into considerations. However, it would be fascinating if immunoprecipitation methods used for determining chromatin-associated DNA target sites (Gould *et al.*, 1990) could be combined with the elegance of PCR-based selection methods.

Summary

Randomized oligonucleotide approaches as well as genomic DNA fragments have been used in conjunction with the polymerase chain reaction to identify DNA target sites and potential DNA target genes. All techniques currently used incorporate principles developed and discussed in manuscripts by Oliphant *et al.* (1989), by Kinzler and Vogelstein (1989), and by Thiesen and Bach (1990). Besides others, DNA binding sites have been identified specific for GLI-1 protein (Kinzler and Vogelstein, 1990), specific for retinoic acid receptors (Costa-Giomi *et al.*, 1992), specific for EVI 1 (Delwel *et al.*, 1993; Matsugi *et al.*, 1993), and specific for the chicken CdxA homeobox gene (Margalit *et al.*, 1993).

However, the determination of functional target genes for DNA binding proteins remains one of the challenges in the near future in order to decipher the function of hundreds of zinc finger genes present in the mammalian genome.

Acknowledgments

This manuscript is dedicated to the memory of Prof. Dr. W. Wille (1947–1992) who initiated the research project described above. He was Professor for Neurosciences at the Genetic Institute at the University of Cologne. His scientific interests were focused on studies concerning molecular aspects of mammalian neuronal development.

The experimental work was financed by the Deutsche Forschungsgemeinschaft (SFB 243) and through Galvachem GmbH, D-50259 Pulheim, Germany. We thank Peter Lane for critical reading of the manuscript. The Basel Institute for Immunology was founded and is supported by F. Hoffmann-LaRoche & Co. Ltd., CH-4005 Basel, Switzerland.

References

Ashworth, A., and Denny, P. (1991). *Mamm. Genome* **1,** 196.

Ausubel, F. M., Brent, R., Kingston, R. E., Moore, D. D., Seidman, J. M., Smith, J. A., and Struhl, K. (1988). "Current Protocols in Molecular Biology." Greene and Wiley (Interscience), New York.

Bellefroid, E. J., Lecocq, P. J., Benhida, A., Poncelet, D. A., Belayew, A., and Martial, J. A. (1989). *DNA* **8,** 377.

Berg, J. M. (1990). *Annu. Rev. Biophys. Biophys. Chem.* **19,** 405.

Bhat, R. V., Worley, P. F., Cole, A. J., and Baraban, J. M. (1992). *Mol. Brain Res.* **13,** 263.

Bopp, D., Burri, M., Baumgartner, S., Frigerio, G., and Noll, M. (1986). *Cell (Cambridge, Mass.)* **47,** 1033.

Bray, P., Lichter, P., Thiesen, H. J., Ward, D. C., and Dawid, I. B. (1991). *Proc. Natl. Acad. Sci. U.S.A.* **88,** 9563.

Call, K. M., Glaser, T., Ito, C. Y., Buckley, A. J., Pelletier, J., Haber, D. A., Rose, E. A., Kral, A., Yeger, H., Lewis, W. H., Jones, C., and Housman, P. E. (1990). *Cell (Cambridge, Mass.)* **60,** 509.

Chaudhari, N., and Hahn, W. E. (1983). *Science* **220,** 924.

Chavrier, P., Zerial, M., Lemaire, P., Almendrahl, J., Bravo, R., and Charnay, P. (1988). *EMBO J.* **7,** 29.

Chowdhury, K., Deutsch, U., and Gruss, P. (1987). *Cell (Cambridge, Mass.)* **48,** 771.

Chowdhury, K., Dressler, G., Breier, G., Deutsch, U., and Gruss, P. (1988). *EMBO J.* **7,** 1345.

Christy, B., and Nathans, D. (1989). *Proc. Natl. Acad. Sci. U.S.A.* **86,** 8737.

Clemens, K. R., Wolf, V., McBryant, S. J., Zhang, P., Liao, X., Wright, P. E., and Gottesfeld, J. M. (1993). *Science* **260,** 530.

Cole, A. J., Saffen, D. W., Baraban, J. M., and Worley, P. F. (1989). *Nature (London)* **340,** 474.

Costa-Giomi, M. P., Gaub, M.-P., Chambon, P., and Abarzúa, P. (1992). *Nucleic Acids Res.* **12,** 3223.

Crosby, S. D., Veile, R. A., Donis-Keller, H., Baraban, J. M., Bhat, R. V., Simburger, K. S., and Milbrandt, J. (1992). *Proc. Natl. Acad. Sci. U.S.A.* **89,** 4739.

Delwel, R., Funabiki, T., Kreider, B. L., Morishita, K., and Ihle, J. N. (1993). *Mol. Cell. Biol.* **13,** 4291.

Diakun, G. P., Fairall, L., and Klug, A. (1986). *Nature (London)* **324,** 689.

Fainsod, A., Margalit, Y., Haffner, R., and Gruenbaum, Y. (1991). *Nucleic Acids Res.* **19,** 4005.

Fraser, S., Keynes, R., and Lumsden, A. (1990) *Nature (London)* **344,** 431.

Garrell, J., and Campuzano, S. (1991.) *BioEssays* **13,** 493.

Gehring, W. J. (1987). *Science* **236,** 1245.

Gessler, M., Poustka, A., Gavenee, W., Neve, R. L., Orkin, S. H., and Bruns, G. A. P. (1990). *Nature (London)* **343,** 774.

Ginsberg, A. M., King, B. O., and Roeder, R. G. (1984). *Cell (Cambridge, Mass.)* **39,** 479.

Gould, A. P., Brookman, J. J., Strutt, D. I., and White, R. A. H. (1990). *Nature (London)* **348**, 308.

He, X., Freacy, M. N., Simmons, D. M., Ingraham, H. A., Swanson, L. W., and Rosenfeld, M. G. (1989). *Nature (London)* **340**, 35.

Johnston, M. (1987). *Microbiol. Rev.* **51**, 458.

Kadonaga, J. T., Jones, K. A., and Tjian, R. (1986). *Trends Biochem. Sci.* **11**, 20.

Kinzler, K. W., and Vogelstein, B. (1989). *Nucleic Acids Res.* **17**, 3645.

Kinzler, K. W., and Vogelstein, B. (1990). *Mol. Cell. Biol.* **10**, 634.

Kinzler, K. W., Ruppert, J. M., Bigner, S. H., Trent, J. M., Law, M. L., O'Brian, S. J., Wong, A. J., and Vogelstein, B. (1988). *Nature (London)* **332**, 371.

Kornberg, R. D., and Lorch, Y. (1992). *Annu. Rev. Cell Biol.* **8**, 563.

Landschulz, W. H., Johnson, P. F., and McKnight, S. L. (1988). *Science* **240**, 1759.

Lange, R. *et al.* (1994). Submitted.

Maniatis, T., Goodburn, S., and Fischer, J. A. (1987). *Science* **236**, 1237.

Margalit, Y., Yarus, S., Shapira, E., Gruenbaum, Y., and Fainsod, A. (1993). *Nucleic Acids Res.* **21**, 4915.

Margolin, J. F., Friedman, J. R., Meyer, W. K. H., Vissing, H., Thiesen, H. J., and Rauscher, F. J. (1994). *Proc. Natl. Acad. Sci. U.S.A.* **91**, 4509–4513.

Matsugi, T., Kreider, B. L., Delwel, R., Cleveland, J. L., Askew, D. S., and Ihle, J. N. (1993). *Mol. Cell. Biol.* (in press).

Meyer, W. K.-H., Georgiev, O., Gerber, H.-P., Margolin, J. F., Friedman J. R., Rauscher, F. J., III, and Thiesen, H.-J. (1994). Submitted for publication.

Miller, J., McLachlan, A. D., and Klug, A. (1985). *EMBO J.* **4**, 1609.

Noce, T., Fujiwara, Y., Ito, M., Takeushi, T., Hashimoto, N., Yamanouchi, M., Higashinakagawa, T., and Fujimoto, H. (1992). *Dev. Biol.* **155**, 409.

Oliphant, A. R., Brandl, C. J., and Struhl, K. (1989). *Mol. Cell. Biol.* **9**, 2944.

Pabo, C. O., and Sauer, R. T. (1992). *Annu. Rev. Biochem.* **61**, 1053.

Pavletich, N. P., and Pabo, C. O. (1991). *Science* **252**, 809.

Pavletich, N. P., and Pabo, C. O. (1993). *Science* **261**, 1701.

Pelletier, J., Bruening, W., Kashtan, C. E., Mauer, S. M., Manivel, J. C., Striegel, J. E., Houghton, D. C., Junien, C., Habib, R., Fouser, L., Fine, R. N., Silverman, B. L., Haber, D. A., and Housman, D. (1991). *Cell (Cambridge, Mass.)* **67**, 437.

Pollock, R., and Treisman, R. (1990). *Nucleic Acids Res.* **18**, 6197.

Pott, U., Holz, A., and Schwab, M. E. (1993). *Experientia* **49**, A66.

Rosenberg, U. B., Schroeder, C., Priess, A., Kienlin, A., Cote, S., Riede, I., and Jaeckle, H. (1986). *Nature (London)* **319**, 336.

Sambrook, J., Fritsch, E. F., and Maniatis, T. (1989). "Molecular Cloning: A Laboratory Manual," 2nd ed. Cold Spring Harbor Lab., Cold Spring Harbor, NY.

Schneider-Maunoury, S., Topilko, P., Seitanidou, T., Levi, G., Cohen-Tannoudji, M., Pournin, S., Babinet, C., and Charnay, P. (1993). *Cell (Cambridge, Mass.)* **75**, 1199.

Schöler, H. R., Ruppert, S., Suzuki, N., Chowdhury, K., and Gruss, P. (1990). *Nature (London)* **344**, 435.

Sham, M. H., Vesque, C., Nonchev, S., Marshall, H., Frain, M., Das Gupta, R.,

Whiting, J., Wilkinson, D., Charnay, P., and Krumlauf, R. (1993). *Cell (Cambridge, Mass.)* **72,** 183.

Smith, D. B., and Johnson, K. S. (1988). *Gene.* **67,** 31.

Sutcliffe, J. G. (1988). *Annu. Rev. Neurosci.* **11,** 157.

Swiatek, P. J., and Gridley, T. (1993). *Genes Dev.* **7,** 2071.

Tautz, D., Lehmann, R., Schnürch, H., Schuh, R., Seifert, E., Kienlin, A., Jones, K., and Jäckle, H. (1987). *Nature (London)* **327,** 383.

Thiesen, H. J. (1990a). *New Biol.* **2,** 363.

Thiesen, H. J. (1990b). *DNA Protein Eng. Tech.* **2,** 93.

Thiesen, H. J. (1990c). ''Immunological Methods,'' Vol. 4, p. 61. Academic Press, Orlando, FL.

Thiesen, H. J., and Bach, C. (1990). *Nucleic Acids Res.* **18,** 3203.

Thiesen, H. J., and Bach, C. (1991a). *FEBS Lett.* **283,** 23.

Thiesen, H. J., and Bach, C. (1991b). *Biochem. Biophys. Res. Commun.* **176,** 551.

Thiesen, H. J., Casorati, G., Lauster, R., and Wiles, M. V. (1990). ''Immunological Methods,'' Vol. 4, p. 35. Academic Press, Orlando, FL.

Vortkamp, A., Gessler, M., and Grzeschik, K. H. (1991). *Nature (London)* **352,** 539.

Weigel, D., and Jäckle, H. (1990) *Cell (Cambridge, Mass.)* **63,** 455.

Wilkenson, D. G., Bhatt, S., Chavrier, P., Bravo, R., and Charnay, P. (1989a). *Nature (London)* **337,** 461.

Wilkenson, D. G., Bhatt, S., Cook, M., Boncinelli, E., and Krumlauf, R. (1989b). *Nature (London)* **341,** 405.

Worley, P. F., Christy, B. A., Nakabeppu, Y., Bhat, R. V., Cole, A. J., and Baraban, J. M. (1991). *Proc. Natl. Acad. Sci. U.S.A.* **88,** 5106.

[28] DNA Extraction from Archived Specimens by Sonication

Robert A. Robinson and Michael J. Heller

Introduction

The analysis of DNA from archived tissues is an important clinical research and diagnostic tool. The analyses of these preserved tissues, which are most commonly formalin-fixed and paraffin-embedded, allow for the retrospective study of a variety of genetic changes or even the presence of infectious agents. Prior to polymerase chain reaction (PCR), genetic analysis of fixed tissue was carried out using *in situ* hybridization, dot-blot hybridization, or Southern blotting (1–5). These methodologies have traditionally provided some degree of success but are sometimes limited in sensitivity, involve complex procedures, or cannot detect degraded DNA which is found in old fixed tissue. PCR analysis provides a simple and sensitive method for analysis of DNA from fixed tissue (6, 7). A number of methods exist for isolating DNA from formalin-fixed, paraffin-embedded tissues, but the best procedures in terms of reliably releasing DNA involve a large number of solvent extractions, centrifugations, and long digestion periods with enzyme buffers (8–12). Quicker procedures often do not extract sufficient DNA for analysis or manipulation (13). We have developed a method by which DNA is quickly and efficiently extracted from paraffin-embedded tissue (14, 15). This method utilizes a sonicating water bath to disrupt the tissue samples, and such samples can be prepared in less than 30 min with only solvent extraction in a minimum of steps.

Materials and Methods

Fixation and Embedding

DNA from essentially all formalin-fixed, paraffin-embedded tissues can be extracted with the sonication technique. Since most tissues are routinely formalin-fixed and paraffin-embedded, our methodology has not been applied to the extraction of tissues fixed in other reagents, such as Bouin's solution. Tissues normally remain exposed to formalin for a period of 12–24 hr before paraffin embedding. However fixation of up to 72 hr or even longer is used in some instances. The longer fixation time usually results in less DNA being extracted. This decreased ability to extract DNA is also observed in fixed tissues stored for excessively long periods (>5years). This time-dependent loss is likely due to incomplete formalin extraction in processing of the paraffin blocks, allowing for continued cross-linking or degradation of DNA. Nevertheless, our sonication technique still allows for extraction of DNA in tissues that have been fixed for long periods. We have utilized specimens for PCR analysis successfully that have been embedded in paraffin for over 20 years.

Tissue Sectioning

For most purposes, tissue should be cut at 5–6 μm thickness and one tissue section per 500-μl sterile tube is used per assay depending on the size of the tissue in the paraffin block. However smaller fragments of tissues may require several sections of tissue whereas larger fragments of tissue require only one section. Although precise and uniformly thin (5 μm) sections are preferred, tissue cut without the use of a microtome can be utilized. We have found using a new, clean single-edge razor blade to slice tissue from the block with subsequent mincing to give adequate results. This is a particularly useful technique if selected areas from a tissue block are to be enriched. It is very important not to contaminate the paraffin sections with stray fragments of paraffin-embedded tissue. For this reason, we recommend using disposable microtome blades when using a microtome. By carefully moving the blade after each specimen, up to three different cases may be cut using a single blade. In addition we recommend that tissue sections be cut in an area away from the routine histology laboratory so as to help avoid contamination.

Sample Preparation (Sonication Method)

The main reagents for sonication sample preparation method include a sample preparation buffer with or without micro-sized glass beads. The sample preparation buffer is 50 mM KCl, 10 mM Tris (pH 8.3), 1.5 mM MgCl$_2$, 0.01% gelatin, 0.5% Tween 20, and 0.5 mg/ml proteinase K. The proteinase K is added to the sample preparation buffer just prior to use. Our initial description utilized micro-sized glass beads to help disrupt the tissue. Subsequent studies have shown that it is not always necessary to use these glass beads although they can aid in tissue disruption of tougher tissues. If the beads are to be used the following source of supply and the method needed to clean the beads are as follows: The micro-sized glass beads (DG-500-200 glycerol glass controlled pore, 120–200 mesh, Sigma Chemical Co. St. Louis, MO) are cleaned by the following procedure before use in sample preparation. About 5 g of the glass beads are placed in a 50-ml capped plastic test tube and washed and decanted three times with 50 ml of sterile deionized, distilled water. The glass beads are then washed three times with 50 ml of sterile sample preparation buffer (without proteinase K). After the final wash, the beads are filtered (coarse sintered glass filter or small column with a glass wool plug) to remove the buffer. The glass beads are placed in a petri dish, covered, and dried in an oven at 90°C for 12 hr. The dried beads should be stored in sterile capped Eppendorf tubes or glass vials. All the above procedures are carried out as carefully as possible so as not to contaminate the beads. The 5 ml of cleaned beads will provide enough material for hundreds of sample preparations. Sonication of samples is carried out in a Branson Model 2200 (Branson Ultrasonics, Danbury, CT) sonicating water bath with temperature control. Human placental DNA obtained from the Sigma Chemical Company (D-7011) is used as a standard or reference DNA in the PCR experiments. Stock solutions at 100 ng/μl are made up in 1× PCR buffer and checked by OD at 260 nm. Subsequent dilutions, in 1× PCR buffer, are prepared at 10, 1, and 0.1 ng/μl levels.

Sample preparation by the sonication method is carried out as follows:

1. Single paraffin section (5 μm thickness) samples are carefully placed in sterile (500 μl) microfuge tubes.
2. 400 μl of xylene is added to each of the sample tubes to deparaffinize the tissue (octane of Histoclear are also acceptable). The tubes are given some slight agitation, shaking, or vortexing and allowed to extract for about 1 min.
3. The tubes are spun for 2 min at high speed in a microcentrifuge.
4. The xylene is removed from the tube with an Eppendorf pippetor. Care must be taken not to lose the delicate tissue section and still remove as much xylene as possible. The tissue section can be gently squeezed against the inside of the tube with the pipette tip to help remove xylene.
5. The samples are usually left to dry by evaporation at room temperature but can be dried by heating in a block or with a blow drier for 1 or 2 min. For large or thick sections, an extra minute or two may be necessary. Again, care has to be taken not to contaminate the samples.
6. If the micro-sized glass beads are used, about 2–5 mg of cleaned glass beads and 100 μl of the sample preparation buffer (with proteinase K at 0.5 mg/ml) are now added to each sample tube. Otherwise only the sample preparation buffer is added. The tubes are tightly capped and placed in a thin Styrofoam raft which floats them in the sonicating water bath, but leaves

the bottom of the tubes immersed in the sonicating water. We normally use a piece of Styrofoam approximately 3 x 4 cm in area and approximately 2–3 mm thick. The tubes are pushed through the foam to the level of the tube cap in order to expose as much of the tube to the sonicating bath as possible.

7. The sample tubes (in the raft) are now placed in the sonicating water bath at approximately 45°C and sonicated for 5 to 10 min, depending on the thickness or amount of intrinsic fibrous tissue. It is advisable to move the raft around in the sonicator bath in order to expose all tubes to the local areas with more intense sonication.

8. After sonication, the samples are boiled for 10 min.

9. After being boiled, the sample tubes are spun 20 sec in a microcentrifuge.

At this point the samples are ready to be used in PCR hybridization reactions. Sample volumes from 1 to 10 μl can be used in PCR reactions. (For the specific experimental results shown, 2 to 5 μl of the original sample, or 5 μl of the subsequent dilutions, are used in the PCR reactions.) In the case of very large tissue sections, it may be necessary to dilute the samples 5- or 10-fold before using them in PCR reactions. If the samples are not going to be used in the near term, they should be frozen.

For some experimental results shown, DNA is isolated from fixed tissue sections using a simple procedure which primarily involves a deparaffinization step and a boiling step (13).

PCR Primers and Conditions

PCR amplification of human genomic and viral target sequences can be used to analyze the DNA extracted from fixed tissues. For the following experimental illustrations, PCR primers were made on an Applied Biosystems, Inc., PCR Mate Model 291 DNA synthesizer. For human genomic DNA analysis two sets of β-globin primers were used: β-globin 3 and 4, (β-globin 3, 5' GAGCCAGGGCTGGGCATAAAAGTCA 3', and β-globin 4, 5' GGAAAATAGACCAATAGGCAGAGAG 3') and β-globin 7 and 8, (β-globin, 7, 5' CTTCTGACACAACTGTGTTCACTAGC 3', and β-globin 8, 5' TCACCACCAACTTCATCCACGTTCAC 3'). Primer pair β-globin 3 and 4 (25-mers) amplify a 309-bp segment of the human β-globin gene, and primer pair β-globin 7 and 8 (26-mers) amplify a 123-bp segment. Viral sequences for cytomegalovirus (CMV) and Epstein-Barr virus (EBV) are detected using CMV 14 and 15 (CMV 14, 5' GTTCGAGTGGACATGCTGCGGCATAG 3', and CMV 15, 5' CATCTCCTCGAAAGGCTCATGAACCT 3') and EBV 1 and 2 (EBV 1, 5' TGTCTGACGAGGGGCCAGGTACAGGAC 3', and EBV

2, 5′ GCAGCCAATGCAACTTGGACGTTTTTC 3′). Primer pair CMV 14 and 15 (26-mers) amplify a 159-bp segment from the CMV/immediate early (exon 4) gene. Primer pair EBV 1 and 2 (27-mers) amplify a 245-bp segment from the EBV IR3 repeat sequence.

Primer pairs β-globin 7 and 8 and CMV 14 and 15, which produce short segments of DNA (<200bp), are specially designed for amplifying DNA isolated from fixed tissue which potentially can be highly degraded. For formalin-fixed, paraffin-embedded tissues, we prefer to design primers that produce short segments since this tissue can be degraded. In addition we have found it important to extend most primers lengths from 18- or 20-mers to 25- to 26-mers when using formalin-fixed, paraffin-embedded tissue.

PCR reagents including Taq polymerase (recombinant), dNTP's, and 1ϕX PCR reaction buffer are obtained from Perkin–Elmer Cetus (Norwalk CT). In some cases 1ϕX PCR reaction buffer (100 mM KCl, 100 mM Tris, pH 8.3, 15 mM MgCl$_2$, 0.1% gelatin) prepared in-house is used in the PCR reactions. PCR reaction mixes are made as shown below.

Component	Volume(μl)	Final concentration
(1) Sterile distilled deionized H$_2$O	x	—
(2) 1ϕX PCR reaction buffer	12	1.2X
(3) dNTP mix	16	200 μM each dNTP
(4) Primers 1 and 2	2	200 μM each primer
(5) Target DNA	2-5	10–10^6 copies
(6) Taq polymerase	0.6	3 units
Final volume (μl)	100	

A volume of 100 μl of mineral oil is placed over the PCR reaction mix. Thermocycling of the samples is carried out on a MJ Research programmable thermal controller using a special 45-cycle program designed for amplifying DNA from fixed tissue sections: (i) Initial denaturation, 94°C for 1.5 min, (ii) annealing, 60°c for 1 min, (iii) extension, 72°C for 0.5 min, (iv) denaturation, 94°C for 1.5 min, (v) cycle, 9 times to step (ii), (vi) annealing, 60°C for 1 min, (vii) denaturation, 93°C for 1 min, (viii) cycle, 34 times to step (vi), and (ix) 4°C for 16 hr (for overnight runs or when samples are not immediately removed after run is complete). It should be pointed out that thermocycling of the samples is always carried out immediately after addition of the Taq polymerase.

Analysis of the PCR reactions is carried out by gel electrophoresis, using 3% agarose gels (18 X 18 cm), run in 1/2X TBE (Tris-borate, EDTA) buffer. Ethidium bromide, for fluorescent visualization of DNA bands, is present in both the gel and running buffer at a concentration of 500 ng/ml. Approximately 16 μl of each PCR reaction, mixed with 8 μl of a 60% glycerol/40%

1X PCR loading buffer, is applied to each well. A φX174 *Hae*III marker, which produces a 1353-, 1078-, 872-, 603-, 310-, (281-, 271-), 234-, 194-, 118-, 72-bp DNA size reference ladder, is also run on each gel. After completion of electrophoresis, the gels are photographed using a Fotodyne UV 300 DNA Transilluminator system.

Results

As with any new technique, it is important to compare the new method against the "gold standard." Fig. 1 shows the PCR detection level for a dilution series of purified DNA against DNA extracted from paraffin-embedded tissue using the sonication extraction method. Human placental DNA was used at known concentrations and amplified with β-globin 3 and 4 primers which produce a 309-bp fragment. Lanes 1–3 are human placental DNA at concentrations of 20, 2, and 0.2 ng, respectively. The β-globin sequence is easily detectable at the 2-ng level, which represents approximately 600 copies of the gene; some banding is still visible at the 0.2-ng or 60-copy level. Lanes 4–6 are human placental DNA, at concentrations of 20, 2, and 0.2 ng, respectively, amplified with β-globin 7 and 8 primers which produce a 123-bp fragment. Again, the β-globin sequence is easily detectable at the 2-ng or 600-copy level, and a light band is still visible at the 0.2-ng or

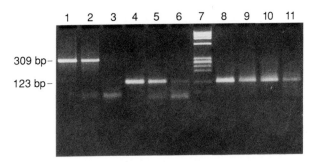

FIG. 1   An ethidium bromide-stained gel comparing dilution series of human placental DNA PCR amplification at known concentrations, with diluted samples of DNA from a normal specimen of fixed lung tissue prepared by the sonication method. Lanes 1–3 are 20, 2, and 0.2 ng, respectively, of human placental DNA amplified using β-globin primers 3 and 4 which produce a 309-bp fragment. Lanes 4–6 are 20, 2, 0.2 ng, respectively, of human placental DNA amplified using β-globin primers 7 and 8 which produce a 123-bp fragment. Lane 7 is a φX174 *Hae*III ladder with bands from 72 to 1353 bp. Lanes 8–11 are 5 μl of the original 100-μl sample, 1/10 dilution, 1/100 dilution, and 1/1000 dilution, respectively, of a sonicated lung tissue section with β-globin primers 7 and 8 (123 bp fragment)

60-copy level. (A no target DNA control, run for this experiment is shown in Fig. 2, lane 5.) Lane 7 shows the ϕX174 *Hae*III reference ladder, which corroborates the 309- and 123-bp bands produced in the PCR reactions. The next set of results shown in Fig. 1 are the PCR detection levels for a dilution series of DNA isolated from a normal specimen of fixed lung tissue prepared by the sonication method. Lanes 8–11 represent 5μl of the original 100-μl sample preparation, 1/10 dilution, 1/100 dilution, and 1/1000 dilution, respectively, amplified in PCR reactions with β-globin 7 and 8 primers. The 123-bp band is easily detectable at the 1/100 dilution, and a light band is still visible at the 1/1000 dilution level.

Because our method takes the same comparatively short amount of time to perform as does a simple deparaffinization/boiling extraction, we thought it appropriate to compare this methodology with the sonication extraction technique. In Fig. 2, lanes 1–4 on the gel represent 5μl of the original 100μl sample preparation (Sonication Methods), 1/10 dilution, 1/100 dilution, and 1/1000 dilution, respectively, amplified in PCR reactions with β-globin primers 3 and 4. The 309-bp band is clearly detectable down to the 1/1000 dilution for DNA prepared by the sonication method. Lane 5 represents 5 μl of a no

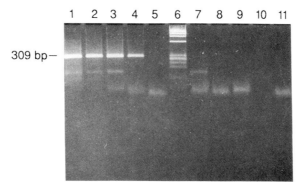

FIG. 2   An ethidium bromide-stained gel comparing the sonication method with the deparaffinization/boiling method. Lanes 1–4 are 5 μl of the original 100-μl sample, a 1/10 dilution, a 1/100 dilution, and a 1/1000 dilution, respectively of a long tissue section prepared by the sonication method and amplified with β-globin primers 3 and 4 (309-bp fragment). Lane 5 is a no target DNA control containing primers 3 and 4. Lane 6 is a ϕX 174 *Hae*III ladder. Lanes 7–10 are 5 μl of the original 100-μl sample, 1/10 dilution, 1/100 dilution, and 1/1000 dilution, respectively, of a lung tissue section prepared by the deparaffinization/boiling method and amplified with β-globin primers 3 and 4. Lane 11 is another no target DNA control sample. There is an artifactual band seen at approximately 650 base pairs in lane 9. From Heller *et al.* (14), used with permission. © 1991 Eaton Publishing.

target DNA control sample that was carried through the complete sonication method procedure and amplified with β-globin 3 and 4 primers. Lanes 7–10 represent 5μl of the original sample preparation (simple deparaffinization/ boiling method), 1/10 dilution, 1/100 dilution, and 1/1000 dilution, respectively, amplified with β-globin 3 and 4 primers. A very faint 309-bp band is present only in lane 7, which represents the highest DNA concentration. Lane 11 represents another no target DNA control sample, amplified with β-globin 3 and 4, showing no detectable band present.

The sonication sample preparation method was tested on a wide variety of different tissue types (all formalin-fixed, paraffin-embedded), including a 10-year-old specimen. Each of the samples was amplified using β-globin primers 7 and 8, which produce a 123-bp fragment. Two microliters of the original sample preparation (100 μl) was used in the PCR reactions. In Fig. 3 lane 1 is breast tissue; lane 2 is testes; land 3 is adrenal cortex; lane 4 is lymph node; lane 5 is salivary gland; lane 6 is the φX174 HaeIII ladder; lane 7 is thyroid gland; lane 8 is liver (10-year-old sample); lane 9 is skin; lane 10 is heart; lane 11 is a no target control sample. The 123-bp band is clearly visible for all the different tissue samples; the no target controls shows no band.

To demonstrate the viability of the sonication method for extragenomic DNA detection, Fig. 4 shows lung tissues which were known to have been infected with either CMV or EBV. Normal (uninfected) lung tissue sections were prepared as the negative controls. Lane 1 is DNA from the CMV-

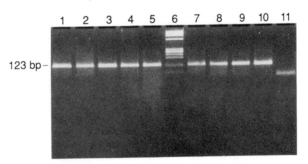

FIG. 3   An ethidium bromide-stained gel showing amplified DNA from a number of different formalin-fixed, paraffin-embedded tissues prepared by the sonication method. Each of the samples was amplified using β-globin primers 7 and 8, which produce a 123-bp fragment. Lane 1 is breast tissue; lane 2 is testis; lane 3 is adrenal cortex; lane 4 is lymph node; lane 5 is salivary gland; lane 6 is φX 174 HaeIII ladder; lane 7 is thyroid gland; lane 8 is liver (from a 10-year-old autopsy); lane 9 is skin; lane 10 is heart; and lane 11 is a no target control sample. From Heller et al. (14), used with permission. © 1991 Eaton Publishing.

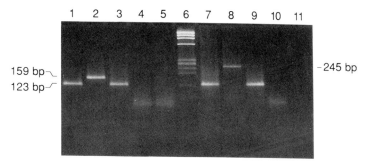

FIG. 4   An ethidium bromide-stained gel showing the detection of cytomegalovirus (CMV) and Epstein–Barr virus (EBV) in lung tissue sections. Lane 1 is DNA from a CMV-positive lung section amplified with β-globin primers 7 and 8; lane 2 is DNA from the same section amplified with CMV primers 14 and 15, which produce a 159-bp fragment. Lane 3 is DNA from a CMV-negative (normal) lung section amplified with β-globin primers 7 and 8, and lane 4 is the same section amplified with CMV primers 14 and 15. Lane 5 is a no target control with CMV primers 14 and 15. Lane 6 is the φX174 *Hae*III ladder. Lane 7 is DNA from an EBV-positive lung section amplified with β-globin primers 7 and 8, and lane 8 is the same section amplified with EBV primers 1 and 2, which produce a 245-bp fragment. Lane 9 is DNA from an EBV-negative (normal) lung section amplified with β-globin primers 7 and 8, and lane 10 is the same section amplified with EBV primers 1 and 2. Lane 11 is a no target control amplified with EBV primers 1 and 2. From Heller *et al.* (14), used with permission. © 1991 Eaton Publishing.

positive lung section amplified with β-globin primers 7 and 8; lane 2 is DNA from the same sample amplified with CMV primers 14 and 15 which produce a 159-bp CMV-specific fragment. The β-globin 123-bp band is present in lane 1 and the CMV-specific 159-bp band is present in Lane 2. Lane 3 is DNA from a CMV-negative (normal) lung section amplified with β-globin primers 7 and 8 and lane 4 is the same sample amplified with CMV primers 14 and 15. The β-globin band is visible in lane 3, however no CMV band is present in Lane 4. Lane 5 is a no target DNA control sample with CMV primers 14 and 15, which shows no band present. Lane 6 is the φX174 *Hae*III reference ladder. Lane 7 is DNA from an EBV-positive lung section amplified with β-globin primers 7 and 8 and lane 8 is the same sample amplified with EBV primers 1 and 2, which produce an EBV-specific 245-bp fragment. The β-globin band is present in lane 7 and the EBV-specific 245-bp band is present in lane 8. Lane 9 is DNA from an EBV-negative (normal) lung section amplified with β-globin primers 7 and 8 and lane 10 is the same sample amplified with EBV primers 1 and 2. The β-globin is present in lane 9;

however, no EBV-specific band is present in lane 10. Lane 11 is a no target control amplified with EBV primers 1 and 2, which shows no band.

After our initial report on sonication, which utilized micro-sized glass beads, we began experimenting with sonication extraction without the use of the beads (15). Figure 5 illustrates a comparison of extraction using beads and extraction without the use of beads. In addition we assessed the utility of the sonication extraction with fresh and fresh-frozen tissue. This experiment compared the same tissues extracted fresh (no fixative), after freezing (again, no fixation), and after fixation in formalin and subsequent paraffin embedding. In this experiment β-globin primers 7 and 8, which amplify a 123-bp fragment were used. Lanes 1–3 represent normal adult kidney that was sonicated fresh (lane 1), frozen (lane 2), or after formalin fixation and paraffin embedding (lane 3). Lanes 4–6 represent fresh, frozen, or paraffin-embedded normal lung tissue, respectively. Tissue obtained at autopsy shows liver (lanes 7 to 9) that was fresh, frozen, or paraffin-embedded, respectively. Lanes 10–18 show the same tissues extracted as described for lanes 1–9 except that no glass beads were added to the sample preparation buffer. Although we believe that the beads can be of use in some tissues that are tougher or fibrous, most of our applications now do not require the beads.

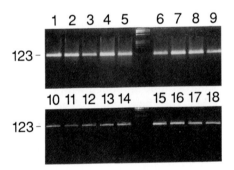

FIG. 5 Comparison of extraction with and without the use of micro-sized glass beads. Lanes 1 to 9 represent extractions using glass beads. Lanes 1 to 3 represent a comparison of identical fresh, frozen, or paraffin-embedded tissue (normal kidney). Lanes 4 to 6 represent similar extractions of normal adult lung that are fresh, frozen, or paraffin-embedded, respectively. Lanes 7 to 9 are from liver tissue also fresh, frozen, or paraffin-embedded. Lanes 10–18 show a similar experiment with same samples extracted without the use of glass beads. Lanes 10–12 correspond to lanes 1–3, respectively; 13–15, to 4–6, respectively; 16–18 to 7–9 respectively. The primers used were β-globin primers 7 and 8. From Heller *et al.* (15), used with permission. © U. S. and Canadian Academy of Pathology.

Discussion and Conclusions

In our initial work on using PCR to amplify human genomic and viral sequences from formalin-fixed, paraffin-embedded tissues, a great deal of effort was expended on examining various sample preparation methods. While there was very little question that the longer, more involved procedures (8–12) gave relatively reliable results, our experience with shorter simplified procedures, such as the deparaffinization/boiling method (13), frequently gave variable results. Thus, a dilemma was always present regarding the choice of sample preparation method. This became an incentive to explore new procedures for sample preparation.

In order to assess the effectiveness of the sonication method for releasing DNA from the sample, it was necessary to make some assumptions about the number of cells (genomic copy number) in a fixed tissue section. Because of the variations in size, shape, and thickness of any given fixed tissue section, one can only make a qualitative estimate of the number of cells in the section without actually counting cells via microscopic examination. Assuming an individual cell diameter of 10 μm, we estimate that a 1 $\times$ 1-cm, 5-μm-thick tissue section is roughly of the order of 10^6 cells. In our 45-cycle PCR reactions, with either primer pairs β-globin 3 and 4 or 7 and 8, it was possible to consistently detect the 0.2-ng (60-copy) level of the human placental DNA standard on ethidium bromide-stained agarose gels (Fig. 1). In our dilution experiments, with DNA extracted from fixed human lung tissue by the sonication method, we were able to still detect both the β-globin 7 and 8, 123-bp band (Fig. 1) and the β-globin 3 and 4, 309-bp band (Fig. 2) at the 1/1000 dilution level. Thus, the 1/1000 dilution appears to be roughly equivalent to 0.2 ng DNA or 60 genomic copy level. Assuming 60 copies for the 1/1000 dilution, extrapolation backward (1/100 dilution = 600 copies, 1/10 dilution = 6000 copies, the 5-μl aliquot of original sample = 60,000 copies) indicates that approximately 10^6 copies of human genomic DNA were in the original 100-μl sample. The dilution experiments suggests (at least qualitatively) that we are extracting most of the DNA from the fixed tissue section.

The experiments comparing the sonication method with the deparaffinization/boiling method (Fig. 2) clearly show the improved efficiency of the sonication method. While DNA from the lung tissue prepared by the sonication method is detectable to the 1/1000 dilution (Fig. 2, lane 4); only the 5-μl aliquot (highest concentration) of original sample prepared by the deparaffinization/boiling method is barely detectable (Fig. 2, lane 7). None of the dilutions from the deparaffinization/boiling method (Fig. 2, lanes 8–10) show the β-globin 3 and 4, 309-bp band.

The sonication method is not limited to any one particular type of tissue.

The range of tissues (formalin-fixed, paraffin-embedded) examined included breast, testes, adrenal cortex, lymph node, salivary gland, thyroid gland, liver, skin, heart, and brain. The experimental results (Fig. 3) indicate DNA was efficiently extracted from all the different tissue, including a 10-year-old liver autopsy specimen (lane 8).

We have also demonstrated that viral target sequences, as well as the human genomic sequences, could be detected in DNA extracted from infected fixed tissue sections by the sonication method. In the viral detection experiments shown in Fig. 4, CMV and EBV sequences (using CMV primers 14 and 15 and EBV primers 1 and 2) were detected in only the lung tissue sections known to be positive. The uninfected lung tissue sections were negative for the CMV and EBV sequences. The human genomic β-globin 7 and 8 sequence was detected in both the infected and uninfected lung tissue sections.

The decision to use microsized glass beads in the sonication extraction is best left to the discretion of the user. We believe that for most applications, the beads should not be utilized since they are expensive, initially time-consuming to prepare, and an additional potential source of contamination. Nevertheless, certain applications, e.g., extracting dense fibrous tissue or bone, might benefit from the addition of the glass beads.

There are several general points concerning sonication extraction we believe should be pointed out. First, it should be noted that the problem of false-negatives due to inhibition of the PCR reaction does occur if too much of the original sample is used in the reactions. Generally, we use 5 μl or less of the original 100 μl sample volume in PCR reactions. In other experiments, we have used up to 10 μl of the original sample. However, if the tissue specimens were larger or thicker than normal and a large sample aliquot was used (10 μl), inhibition of PCR reactions would sometimes occur. We usually try diluting samples that did not amplify in a reaction as a first step in investigating a failed amplification. In addition, examining diluted DNA samples eliminates the possibility that some contaminants carried over from the extracted tissue have inhibited the PCR reactions. Thus, we believe that the potential for false-negatives is eliminated in these experiments when comparing diluted DNA samples These experiments also corroborate why there was so much variability in our earlier results when using the simple deparaffinization/boiling method to prepare tissue for PCR reactions.

Although it was not the primary objective of this work, we would like to strongly emphasize the importance of including proper controls to eliminate false-positive results in PCR reactions. Even when diligent efforts are made to eliminate potential contamination in PCR reactions (particularly from previously amplified samples), it is still possible to get insidious false-positives. Therefore, appropriate controls must be present in PCR experiments. We usually include a control PCR reaction which contains all reagents, including primers, but has no target present.

Thus, in conclusion we believe that the sonication method represents a relatively fast and simple procedure for efficiently extracting DNA from any type of formalin-fixed, paraffin-embedded tissue for subsequent use in PCR reactions. The method can also be used for extracting DNA from frozen tissue sections, tissue cultured cells, or blood and bone marrow smears.

References

1. E. R. Unger, L. R. Budgeon, D. Myerson, and D. J. Brigati, *Am. J. Surg. Pathol.* **10,** (1986)

2. J. Burns, D. R. M. Red Fern, M. M. Esiri, and J. D. McGee, *J. Clin. Pathol.* **39,** 1066 (1986).

3. J. Meinkoth and G. Wahl, *Anal. Biochem.* **138,** 267 (1984).

4. L. Dubeau, L. A. Chandler, J. R. Gralow, P. W. Nichols, and P. A. Jones, *Cancer Res.* **46,** 2964 (1986).

5. S. E. Goelz, S. R. Hamilton, and B. Vogelstein, *Biochem. Biophys. Res. Commun.* **130,** 118 (1985).

6. C. C. Impraim, R. K. Saiki, H. A. Erlich and R. L. Teplitz, *Biochem. Biophys. Res. Commun.* **142,** 710 (1987).

7. D. Shibata, W. J. Martin, and N. Arnheim, *Cancer Res.* **48,** 4564 (1988).

8. M. M. Manos, Y. Ting, D. K. Wright, A. J. Lewis, T R. Broker, and S. M. Wolinksky, *Cancer Cells* **7,** 209 (1989).

9. D. Shibata and E. C. Klatt, *Arch. Pathol. Lab. Med.* **113,** 1239 (1989).

10. D. Shibata, R. K. Brynes, B. Nathwoni, S. Kwok, J. Sninsky, and N. Arnheim, *Am. J. Pathol.* **135,** 697 (1989).

11. B. B. Rogers, L. C. Alpert, E. A. S. Hine, and G. J. Buffone, *Am. J. Pathol.* **136,** 541 (1990).

12. D. K. Wright and M. M. Manos, *in* "PCR Protocols: A Guide to Methods and Applications" (M. A. Innes, D. H. Gelfand, J. J. Sninsky, and T. J. White, eds.), p. 153. Academic Press, San Diego, 1989.

13. D. K. Shibata, N. Arnheim, and W. J. Martin, *J. Exp. Med.* **167,** 225 (1988).

14. M. J. Heller, L. J. Burgart, C. J. TenEyck, M. E. Anderson, T. C. Greiner, and R. A. Robinson, *BioTechniques* **11,** 372 (1991).

15. M. J. Heller, R. A. Robinson, L. J. Burgart, C. TenEyck, and W. W. Wilke, *Mod. Pathol.* **5,** 203 (1992).

Index